Understanding Muscular Dystrophy

Understanding Muscular Dystrophy

Edited by **Carsten Cooper**

FOSTER
ACADEMICS

New Jersey

Published by Foster Academics,
61 Van Reypen Street,
Jersey City, NJ 07306, USA
www.fosteracademics.com

Understanding Muscular Dystrophy
Edited by Carsten Cooper

International Standard Book Number: 978-1-63242-418-1 (Hardback)

Printed in the United States of America.

Contents

Permissions

List of Contributors

Preface

This book was inspired by the evolution of our times; to answer the curiosity of inquisitive minds. Many developments have occurred across the globe in the recent past which has transformed the progress in the field.

Muscular dystrophy is an extremely heterogeneous group of inherited neuromuscular disorders with over 30 distinct types as well as subtypes known and several more to be recognized and sorted. The book presents an elaborative analysis of the different types of muscular dystrophies, genes related to each subtype, disease diagnosis, management as well as available treatment options. Although every distinct type and subtype of muscular dystrophy is related to a distinct causative gene, most of them have overlapping clinical presentations, making molecular diagnosis certain for both patient management as well as disease diagnosis. Discussions regarding the presently available diagnostic approaches that have revolutionized clinical research are presented in this profound book along with reports regarding the ongoing analyses that display a promise for future therapeutic techniques.

This book was developed from a mere concept to drafts to chapters and finally compiled together as a complete text to benefit the readers across all nations. To ensure the quality of the content we instilled two significant steps in our procedure. The first was to appoint an editorial team that would verify the data and statistics provided in the book and also select the most appropriate and valuable contributions from the plentiful contributions we received from authors worldwide. The next step was to appoint an expert of the topic as the Editor-in-Chief, who would head the project and finally make the necessary amendments and modifications to make the text reader-friendly. I was then commissioned to examine all the material to present the topics in the most comprehensible and productive format.

I would like to take this opportunity to thank all the contributing authors who were supportive enough to contribute their time and knowledge to this project. I also wish to convey my regards to my family who have been extremely supportive during the entire project.

Editor

Section 1

Therapy

Muscle Satellite Cells and Duchenne Muscular Dystrophy

Yuko Miyagoe-Suzuki[1], So-ichiro Fukada[2] and Shin'ichi Takeda[1]
*[1]Department of Molecular Therapy, National Institute of Neuroscience,
National Center of Neurology and Psychiatry,
[2]Department of Immunology, Graduate School of Pharmaceutical Sciences,
Osaka University,
Japan*

1. Introduction

Muscle satellite cells are tissue-specific stem cells in skeletal muscle that play central roles in postnatal muscle growth and regeneration, and therefore are a potential source for cell therapy for Duchenne muscular dystrophy (DMD). However, to date, transplantation of satellite cells-derived myoblasts in human has not been successful. To overcome the limitations of transplantation of myoblasts, we need to better understand the molecular and cellular regulation of satellite cells. In this chapter, we summarize recent advances in satellite cell biology and its role in muscular dystrophies. Then we discuss the roles of the muscle tissue microenvironments in muscle regeneration and muscular dystrophies. Recent results emphasize that mutual interactions among myogenic cells, inflammatory cells, and interstitial mesenchymal cells are important for successful muscle regeneration. The latter two are versatile regulators of muscle regeneration. They promote muscle regeneration in healthy muscle, but when muscle fibers fail to regenerate, they promote fibrosis and fatty degeneration to ensure the continuity of the tissue. In the last part of this chapter, we discuss strategies to generate new muscle stem cells from fibroblasts by transcription factor-mediated reprogramming.

2. Muscle satellite cells

Satellite cells are skeletal muscle-specific stem cells located between the muscle basal lamina and myofibers in a quiescent and undifferentiated state (G0). Satellite cells were first identified by electron microscopy by Mauro in 1961 (Mauro 1961). Ultrastructural data suggests that 2-6% of all nuclei in humans are satellite cells (Schmalbruch & Hellhammer 1976). Satellite cells originate from somites or cranial mesoderm and differentiate into Pax3+Pax7+ muscle progenitor cells, and then take the position of satellite cells (Gros et al 2005; Kassar-Duchossoy et al 2005; Relaix et al 2005). A recent paper, however, demonstrated that all satellite cells (MyoD-negative) originate from MyoD-positive progenitors (Kanisicak et al 2009), suggesting that satellite cells are derived from committed myogenic progenitor cells.

During postnatal development, satellite cells divide to provide new myonuclei to growing muscle fibers (Moss & Leblond 1971), and then enter to an undifferentiated quiescent state in adult skeletal muscle (Schultz et al 1978). In mice, vigorous muscle growth due to satellite cell division is observed until three weeks after birth (White et al 2010). During this period, the number of satellite cells decreases, and then it becomes constant for a long time to maintain skeletal muscle homeostasis.

Skeletal muscle regeneration also depends absolutely on satellite cells. When muscle is injured, satellite cells are activated, proliferate, and differentiate into myofibers, and a minor subset self-renew (**Figure 1**). Their dysfunction is responsible for the loss of muscle mass in muscular dystrophies or during aging. Although many studies indicate that stem cells, which are distinct from satellite cells, contribute to the production of myofibers (Ferrari et al 1998; Fukada et al 2002; Gussoni et al 1999; LaBarge & Blau 2002), there is no doubt that satellite cells are the physiological stem cells for skeletal muscle regeneration.

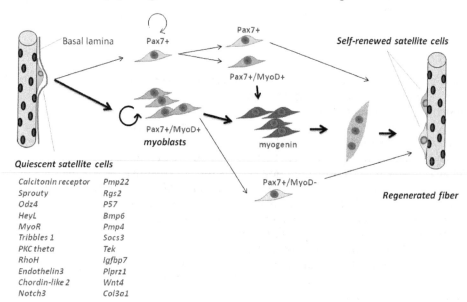

Satellite cells are in a quiescent state in uninjured adult muscle. On injury, satellite cells are activated by mitotic stimuli, vigorously proliferate to reach sufficient cell numbers, and differentiate into myofibers or fuse with pre-existing injured myofibers. A sub-set of cycling satellite cells remains uncommitted by asymmetric division and return to quiescence (Kuang et al 2007). Or a subfraction of MyoD-positive cycling satellite cells withdraw from the cell cycle and returns to the satellite cell niche (Kanisicak et al 2009). Genes up-regulated in quiescent satellite cells are shown as possible regulators of quiescence (Fukada et al 2007).

Fig. 1. Activation, proliferation, differentiation, and self-renewal of satellite cells

2.1 Research tools

Markers: Satellite cells were originally identified by electronic microscopy as mononuclear cells attached to myofibers, but the discovery of M-cadherin expression on satellite cells has made it easier to identify them by light microscopy (Irintchev et al 1994). Pax7 is a marker of satellite cells and is also critical for satellite cell biogenesis, survival and potentially self-renewal (Seale et al 2000). Thanks to an anti-Pax7 monoclonal antibody, which identifies avian, rodent, and human satellite cells (Kawakami et al 1997), Pax7 has become the most widely used marker of satellite cells. Other markers (including c-met, syndecan 3 and 4, SM/C-2.6, integrin-α7, calcitonin receptor, CD34, and CXCR4) have also been established to identify satellite cells by microscopy and flow cytometry (summarized in (Boldrin et al 2010)).

Isolation: Flow cytometric and cell sorting techniques have greatly advanced stem cell studies. Fukada et al. first reported the direct isolation of satellite cells from mouse muscle using their newly developed rat monoclonal antibody, named SM/C-2.6 (Fukada et al 2004). Since then, several groups have reported the purification of satellite cells using CD34, syndecan 4, integrin-α7 or CXCR4 (Boldrin et al 2010; Conboy et al 2010; Fukada et al 2004; Fukada et al 2007; Montarras et al 2005; Sherwood et al 2004; Tanaka et al 2009). A single-fiber culture technique is also widely used for analysis of satellite cells (Rosenblatt et al 1995). In mouse extensor digitorum longus (EDL) muscle, approximately five satellite cells attach to one myofiber, and on isolation of fibers, they are spontaneously activated and migrate from their own myofiber. It is considered that single-fiber culture maintains the satellite cell 'niche' in *in vitro* condition (Collins et al 2005).

Genetic manipulation: Cre-loxP-mediated conditional inactivation of the genes makes it easy to determine the roles of regulatory molecules in a cell of a specific lineage at a specific developmental stage. The Cre-loxP-mediated lineage-tracing system is a powerful method to determine the origins and fates of muscle progenitor cells. These newly established research tools have accelerated research in satellite cell biology. In contrast to the mouse, however, a limited number of markers are available for *in situ* detection of satellite cells in human muscle, and human satellite cells are still isolated by the classical technique.

2.2 Activation, proliferation, differentiation, and self-renewal of satellite cells

Molecular regulators of the activation, proliferation, differentiation, and self-renewal of muscle satellite cells, including paired-box transcription factor Pax7, MyoD families, Six families, epigenetic regulators, or microRNAs, and numerous extracellular components are currently being elucidated (Abou-Khalil et al 2009; Buckingham & Relaix 2007; Chen et al 2010; Crist et al 2009; Dey et al 2011; Dhawan & Rando 2005; Juan et al 2011; Kuang et al 2008; Kuang & Rudnicki 2008; Palacios et al 2010; Yajima et al 2010). Although these molecules are studied mainly on mouse models, similar molecules are believed to regulate human satellite cells.

Self-renewal of satellite cells with stem cell properties is an important process to maintain the stem cell pool throughout life and is one of the main subjects of recent muscle biology research, but it is largely unknown when and how satellite cells self-renew during the regeneration process. Asymmetrical division is proposed to be among the mechanisms by which satellite cells give rise to both stem cells and precursor cells (Conboy & Rando 2002; Conboy et al 2007; Kuang et al 2008; Kuang et al 2007; Shinin et al 2006). It is also possible that some of the activated/proliferating MyoD-positive satellite cells return to the 'niche' of the satellite cells in a stochastic manner. Using MyoD^{iCre} knockin mice and R26R-EYFP or R26R-βgal reporter mice, Kanisicak et al. reported that 99% of satellite cells in limb and body wall muscles originate from MyoD+ progenitors. Their findings suggest that committed MyoD+ myoblasts can return to a dormant state by suppressing MyoD and up-regulating Pax7 (Kanisicak et al 2009). This finding supports the stochastic model and explains well the heterogeneity in myogenic potential within a satellite cell population. Satellite cell activity is impaired in DMD, and how dystrophic environments perturb self-renewal of satellite cells remains to be determined.

Satellite cell behavior is thought to be mainly regulated by the environment. Satellite cells/myoblasts stop dividing just after the size of the regenerated fibers becomes comparable to that of the uninjured muscle and differentiate into myofibers or begin to return to quiescence (Fukada et al 2007; Shea et al 2010). The molecules that signal between the microenvironment and satellite cells are currently being elucidated. Interestingly, Ang1/Tie-2 signaling is such a candidate to regulate self-renewal of satellite cells by controlling the return to quiescence of a subset of them (Abou-Khalil et al 2009).

2.3 Quiescence of satellite cells

Satellite cells are quiescent in uninjured adult muscle. Maintenance of quiescence is important because disruption of cellular quiescence of stem cells leads to a loss of the stem cell pool and impairs tissue repair, but the molecular regulations of satellite cell dormancy are just beginning to be elucidated.

Pax7: Pax7 is highly expressed in quiescent satellite cells and over-expressed Pax7 promote a return to quiescence through repression of MyoD and myogenin (Olguin & Olwin 2004; Olguin et al 2007). Therefore, Pax7 is thought to be central to the maintenance of quiescence. A recent study using a conditional gene inactivation system in mice showed that when Pax7 is inactivated in adult mice, mutant satellite cells can proliferate and reoccupy the sublaminal niche (Lepper et al 2009). Lepper et al. further showed that Pax7 is required in juveniles up to the point when progenitor cells make the transition to quiescence (Lepper et al 2009).

Calcitonin/calcitonin receptor: Fukada et al. performed genome-wide gene expression analysis of quiescent satellite cells freshly isolated from mouse muscle, and reported the molecular signature of quiescent satellite cells (Fukada et al 2007). The authors newly identified genes that are expressed specifically in quiescent satellite cells but down-regulated on activation (including *calcitonin receptor(CTR), Odz4, HeyL/Hesr3, MyoR, tribbles1, PKC theta, Rho H, endothelin 3*)(**Figure 1**), and demonstrated that calcitonin/calcitonin receptor signaling is involved in the maintenance of quiescence of satellite cells (Fukada et al 2007).

Notch: Notch signaling plays a critical role in maintenance of quiescent satellite cells. The *hesr (hes-related,* also known as *hey/herp/hrt/gridlock/chf)* families of bHLH transcriptional repressor genes are the primary target of Notch signaling. Fukada at al. demonstrated that genetic ablation of both *Hesr1* and *Hesr3* genes results in a loss of the satellite cell pool and impairs muscle regeneration (Fukada et al., 2011). Intriguingly, satellite cells lacking both *Hesr1* and *Hesr3* expression ectopically express a proliferation marker, MyoD, and a differentiation marker, myogenin.

Sprouty1 (Spry1): Sprouty1 (Spry1) is a candidate molecule involved in the maintenance of satellite cells. In contrast to Pax7 and Hesr1/Hesr3, however, Sprouty1 is not required for maintenance of the satellite cell pool in uninjured muscle, but it is indispensable for the return to quiescence of the self-renewing satellite cells during repair (Abou-Khalil & Brack 2010; Shea et al 2010). Sprouty1 is a negative regulator of receptor tyrosine kinase (RTK) signaling, which suggests that Sprouty1 plays a role in sensing growth factors within the muscle and regulating satellite cell quiescence during muscle regeneration.

Signals from myofibers seem most important to induce cycling satellite cells to return to the quiescent state and maintain them in the niche, because CTR-positive or Sprouty1-positive satellite cells reappear only at a late stage of regeneration (Fukada et al 2007; Shea et al 2010). Interaction between myofibers and satellite cells through cadherins would be required for the maintenance of the quiescent state of satellite cells. Although M-cadherin-null mice did not show any abnormality in skeletal growth and regeneration, the other cadherin families are thought to compensate for the lack of M-cadherin-deficiency (Hollnagel et al 2002).

2.4 Regulation of satellite cells by non-myogenic cells

Mesenchymal cells in skeletal muscle regulate muscle satellite cells. We previously reported a novel side population subset: CD31(-)CD45(-) SP cells (Uezumi et al 2006). They are resident in skeletal muscle and are activated and vigorously proliferate during muscle regeneration. RT-PCR analysis suggested that CD31(-)CD45(-) SP cells are of mesenchymal lineage, and differentiate into adipocytes, osteogenic cells, and muscle cells after specific induction *in vitro* (Uezumi et al 2006). Motohashi et al. further showed by co-transplantation experiments that CD31(-)CD45(-) SP cells promote proliferation and migration of grafted myoblasts (Motohashi et al 2008). They also showed that CD31(-)CD45(-) SP cells produce a variety of cytokines, cytokine receptors, extra-cellular matrix proteins, matrix met al oproteinase families, and other wound healing-related molecules (Motohashi et al 2008). More recently, Joe et al. identified bipotent fibro/adipogenic progenitor cells (FAPs) in muscle. FAPs are CD31(-)CD45(-)α7integrin(-) CD34(-)Sca1(+), and promote differentiation of satellite cells (Joe et al 2010). Although we speculate that CD31(-)CD45(-) SP cells overlap with FAPs, the relationship between them remains to be determined. Interestingly, these studies suggest that mesenchymal progenitor cells themselves are also regulated by the muscle environment.

Macrophages are also versatile regulators of muscle regeneration, exhibiting opposing activities (pro- and anti-inflammatory effects) (Arnold et al 2007; Mann et al 2011; Segawa et al 2008; Tidball & Villalta 2010; Vidal et al 2008; Villalta et al 2009). Possible interaction among macrophages, mesenchymal progenitor cells, and myogenic cells are summarized in **Figure 2.**

3. Satellite cells and Duchenne muscular dystrophy

Duchenne muscular dystrophy is caused by the absence of dystrophin and characterized by progressive muscle weakness and chronic cycles of degeneration and regeneration of skeletal muscle. Satellite cells and their progeny, myoblasts are thought to gradually lose their proliferative and differentiative capacity, and be eventually exhausted in Duchenne muscular dystrophy, due to repeated activation and proliferation and limited self-renewal capacity (Blau et al 1983; Blau et al 1985; Heslop et al 2000). As a result, muscle regeneration

A. Acute injury

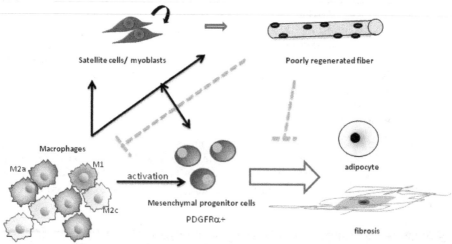

B. Muscular dystrophy

A. In acute muscle injury, resident and infiltrating macrophages first secret pro-inflammatory cytokines, express iNOS, and clear dead fibers by phagocytosis (M1), then release anti-inflammatory cytokines and stimulate myogenesis and fiber growth (M2c: anti-inflammatory macrophages) (Mann et al 2011; Tidball & Villalta 2010). Mesenchymal progenitor cells are rapidly activated, extensively proliferate, and promote proliferation, migration, and differentiation of satellite cells, but almost completely vanish at the completion of myofiber regeneration. M2 macrophages produce pro-fibrotic molecules such as TGF-β and stimulate mesenchymal cells to produce ECM components and ECM-remodeling factors. Successfully regenerated muscle fibers, in turn, seem to calm activated macrophages and mesenchymal cells down.

B. In dystrophic muscle, macrophages continue to release pro-inflammatory cytokines. M2a (alternatively activated) macrophages, which are usually associated with tissue repair, wound-healing and fibrosis, are reported to be abundant in fibrotic muscle of mdx mice, and proposed to be involved in fibrosis development (Vidal et al 2008; Villalta et al 2009). In prolonged inflammation, mesenchymal progenitors differentiate into adipocytes and fibroblastic cells, and promote fatty infiltration and fibrosis. A recent study suggests that regenerated muscle fibers directly inhibit this phenotypic conversion.

Fig. 2. Mutual regulations among macrophages, mesenchymal progenitor cells, and satellite cells in muscle regeneration (model)

is impaired in the advanced state of the disease, and muscle tissue is gradually replaced by adipose and fibrotic tissues. At this stage, gene therapy, exon-skipping therapy, and pharmacological therapy are not effective. Importantly, recent studies show that poor or aberrant muscular regeneration of the diseased muscle cannot be simply ascribed to the exhaustion of satellite cells. Berg et al. recently reported that satellite cells from 10-month-old golden retriever muscular dystrophy dogs, which show severe phenotypes at this age, show proliferation and differentiation potentials equivalent to those of wild-type littermates *in vitro* (Berg et al 2011). The authors suggest that pathological changes in the muscle environment rather than cell-intrinsic defects may be largely implicated in the eventual failure of satellite cell efficacy *in vivo*. For example, prolonged inflammation in dystrophic muscle exposes satellite cells to pro-fibrotic, pro-adipogenic cytokines, and suppresses the myogenic function of satellite cells (reviewed in (Mann et al 2011; Tidball & Villalta 2010). In the next session, we focus on satellite cells in dystrophic conditions, and review the cellular origin of adipogenesis and fibrosis in disease environments. For direct effects of the gene mutations on satellite cells in other muscular dystrophies, please refer to a recent review by Morgan & Zammit (Morgan & Zammit 2010).

3.1 Fibrosis and adipocyte infiltration in DMD muscle

DMD muscle is characterized by chronic inflammation, endomysial fibrosis and adipocyte infiltration (fatty degeneration). It is widely accepted that fibrosis and adipocyte infiltration inhibit not only skeletal muscle function, but also myogenic activities of satellite cells, thereby diminish the amount of target tissue available for therapeutic intervention. Therefore, inhibition of fibrosis and adipogenesis is expected to attenuate DMD progression and increase the success of new cell and gene-based therapies (Mann et al 2011). In fact, many papers show that pharmacological inhibition of fibrosis in *mdx* mice ameliorates the pathology in dystrophin-deficient cardiac and skeletal muscle (Bish et al 2011; Cohn et al 2007; Rafael-Fortney et al 2011; Taniguti et al 2011).

The cellular origin of fatty infiltration has been controversial. Previous studies suggested that satellite cells transdifferentiate into adipocytes and/or fibroblastic cells in pathological conditions. Li et al. reported that TGF-β, a profibrotic cytokine, in skeletal muscle induces the differentiation of C2C12 cells, a myogenic cell line, into fibrotic cells (Li et al 2004). Alexakis et al. also indicated that collagen types I and III were expressed in primary myoblasts derived from mouse satellite cells (Alexakis et al 2007). In contrast, Uezumi et al. (Uezumi et al 2010) and Joe et al.(Joe et al 2010) demonstrated that platelet-derived growth factor receptor alpha (PDGFRα)-positive mesenchymal progenitors or muscle-resident fibro/adipogenic progenitor cells (FAPs) are distinct from satellite cells, and show a strong predisposition towards the generation of adipocytes, and readily differentiate into adipocyte under pathological environments.

Uezumi et al. further provide evidence suggesting that PDGFRα+ mesenchymal progenitors also contribute to fibrosis. The authors demonstrated that PDGFRα+ cells, but not PDGFRα- cells produce fibrosis-related molecules *in vivo* after transplantation, and transforming growth factor (TGF)-βs, known as potent profibrotic cytokines, induce the expression of fibrosis-related genes in PDGFRα+ mesenchymal progenitors, but not in myogenic cells (Uezumi et al 2011). Importantly, imatinib, an inhibitor of several tyrosine kinases including c-abl, c-kit, and PDGFRs, was demonstrated to ameliorate dystrophic phenotypes in *mdx* mice by suppressing the phosphorylation of PDGFRα (Huang et al 2009). In addition, constitutively active PDGFRα-receptor knock-in mice exhibited systemic fibrosis including skeletal muscle tissue (Olson & Soriano 2009). Because PDGFRα is exclusively expressed in mesenchymal progenitors in skeletal muscle, these results strongly suggest that PDGFRα+ mesenchymal progenitors but not satellite cells contribute to connective tissue accumulation in dystrophic muscle.

Mesenchymal progenitor cells never differentiate into adipocytes or produce fibrosis-related molecules in healthy muscle. Why do they preferentially differentiate into collagen-producing fibroblasts or adipocyte in DMD muscle? One plausible explanation is prolonged inflammation due to continuous degeneration/regeneration cycles of muscle and the phenotypic change of macrophages (Mann et al 2011; Tidball & Villalta 2010). Although macrophages promote muscle regeneration (Segawa et al 2008; Tidball & Villalta 2010), macrophages in the advanced stage of mdx are reported to contribute to the development of fibrosis and fatty degeneration by secreting pro-fibrotic and pro-adipogenic cytokines (Mann et al 2011; Tidball & Villalta 2010).

3.2 Limited regenerative potential of human satellite cells

In Duchenne muscular dystrophy, dystrophin deficiency leads to progressive lethal skeletal muscle degeneration. But, dystrophin deficiency does not recapitulate DMD in mice (mdx), which show active regeneration of damaged muscle throughout life, a much milder phenotype than DMD patients, and an almost normal life span.

Sacco et al. demonstrated that mdx mice lacking telomerase activity show shortened telomeres in muscle cells and a severe dystrophic phenotype (Sacco et al 2010). Together with a previous report of a 14-fold greater shortening of telomeres in DMD patients relative to healthy individuals (Decary et al 2000), these studies suggest that a difference in the length of telomeres between humans (5-15 kbs) and mice (>40 kbs) greatly explains the difference in proliferative potential of muscle satellite cells between DMD patients and mdx mice.

On the other hand, Fukada et al. showed that the phenotype of mdx became much more severe when mdx was crossed to with the DBA/2 strain (Fukada et al 2010). The *mdx* mouse (C57BL/10-*Dmd^{mdx}*), first described in 1984, arose in an inbred colony of C57BL/10 mice. Importantly, the proliferation of DBA/2 satellite cells was inferior to that of C57BL/6 (a widely used strain akin to C57BL/10) satellite cells, indicating that the properties of satellite cells and mdx phenotypes greatly depend on the genetic background of the mice.

4. Cell therapy for DMD

In 1989, Partridge et al. demonstrated that transplantation of normal myoblasts restores dystrophin in dystrophin-deficient mdx mice (Partridge et al 1989). In spite of this success, the subsequent myoblast transplantation performed on DMD boys was unsuccessful (Law et al 1992; Mendell et al 1995; Tremblay et al 1993). In this section, we discuss the problems of myoblast-transplantation and other cell sources for cell therapy of DMD.

4.1 Myoblasts transplantation therapy (MTT)

Myoblasts transplantation therapy (MTT) for DMD was tried in the early 90's, but the results were disappointing (Law et al 1992; Mendell et al 1995; Tremblay et al 1993). Although the high-density myoblast transplantation recently performed by Tremblay's team in Canada is promising in some aspects, the effects are still local due to the limited migration and poor survival of grafted cells (Mouly et al 2005; Skuk & Tremblay 2011). In addition, expansion *in vitro* is shown to gradually reduce the regenerative activity of satellite cells (Ikemoto et al 2007; Montarras et al 2005). This is probably because satellite cells have limited proliferative capacities, which are exhausted by expansion in culture. However, currently used culture conditions might simply be inappropriate for the expansion of satellite cells because satellite cells in their niche robustly regenerate injured muscle (Collins et al 2005). Recently, Gilbert et al. pointed out the importance of substrate elasticity in culture (Gilbert et al 2010). When satellite cells were cultured on soft hydrogel substrates that mimic the elasticity of *in vivo* muscle, the cultured cells contributed more extensively to muscle regeneration, indicating that the culture system has much room for improvement. Myoblast transfer therapy is expected to restore muscle function in relatively localized muscle diseases such as oculo-pharyngeal muscular dystrophy (OPMD), by using autologous myoblasts from relatively spared patient muscles (Mouly et al 2005).

4.2 Making satellite cells from non-myogenic cells by reprogramming

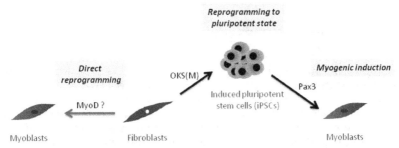

If myogenic cells can be efficiently induced from patient-derived pluripotent stem cells (iPS cells), these cells are candidate sources for cell therapy of muscular dystrophies. On the other hand, direct reprogramming using transcription factors has been reported to successfully convert fibroblasts into clinically relevant cells (neurons, cardiocytes, hepatocytes, chondrocytes, etc). MyoD is a master regulator of myogenesis, but not sufficient to generate myogenic stem cells with high proliferative potential. OKSM: Oct4, Klf4, Sox2 and c-Myc.

Fig. 3. New cell sources for cell therapy of muscular dystrophies

4.3 New cell source for cell therapy of DMD

It is difficult to prepare a large quantity of satellite cells from a donor. In addition, expansion of satellite cells *in vitro* reduces the regenerative activity (Ikemoto et al 2007; Montarras et al 2005). Mesoangioblasts or muscle-derived stem cells (MDSC) are multi-potent stem cells distinct from satellite cells that have been demonstrated to be highly proliferative and able to be delivered to the musculature of the whole body. However, the number of cells, as starting materials, required to restore dystrophin expression in cardiac and respiratory muscle and improve performance of DMD patients remains to be determined in clinical trials. On the other hand, transcription factor-mediated reprogramming of somatic cells into myogenic cells is now being vigorously investigated, and is expected to be a feasible technique in the near future. Two different strategies are proposed to generate myogenic cells from somatic cells **(Figure 3)**. One is to reprogram somatic cells of patients into pluripotent stem cells (iPS cells) using Yamanaka factors, and then induce them to differentiate into transplantable myogenic cells. The other strategy is to directly induce fibroblasts to differentiate into myogenic cells without first passing the cells through a pluripotent state.

4.3.1 Induced pluripotent stem cells (iPS cells)

In 2006, Takahashi and Yamanaka reported that only four factors (Oct4, Klf4, Sox2, and c-Myc, are sufficient to reprogram somatic cells into embryoni stem (ES) cell-like pluripotent stem cells (Takahashi & Yamanaka 2006). The induced cells are called induced pluripotent cells (iPS cells). The next year, the same group and Thompson's group reported the establishment of human iPS cells from skin fibroblasts using slightly different sets of reprogramming factors (Takahashi et al 2007; Yu et al 2007). This technique is groundbreaking, because it enables us to obtain patient-specific iPS cells with pluripotency. Muscular dystrophy patient-specific iPS cells were first reported by Park et al. (Park et al 2008). iPS cells derived from the patients showed human ES-like properties, and therefore may be a promising cell source for cell therapy. If myogenic stem cells can be constantly induced from iPS cells, there will be no limitation in the number of the cells for transplantation. In addition, although a controversial report of immunogenicity appeared recently (Zhao et al 2011), autologous iPS cells are expected to produce tissue-specific stem / progenitor cells that evoke no immune reaction in the host.

4.3.2 Muscle differentiation of ES/iPS cells

The success of iPS cell-based therapy for DMD depends on the efficiency of induction of myogenic progenitor cells from iPS cells. Pax3 and Pax7 have been shown to be a powerful way to derive transplantable myogenic cells from mouse ES cells (Darabi et al 2008; Darabi et al 2011). However, for a clinical trial, integration of viral vectors into the host genome is not desirable. One possibility to avoid the use of viral vectors is to replace Pax3 or Pax7 activity with small bioactive molecules. Purification of myogenic cells from differentiating iPS culture is also important for safe cell transplantation because a culture contains both differentiated and undifferentiated cells. Contamination with undifferentiated cells can cause tumor formation in the host. A research group at Kyoto University described a strategy to sort myogenic cells from differentiating mouse ES cells (Chang et al 2009) or mouse iPS cells (Mizuno et al 2010). The authors cultured embryoid bodies in muscle differentiation medium (10% fetal bovine serum and 5% horse serum in DMEM) for six days and then plated them on Matrigel, and sorted SM/C-2.6-positive cells by FACS before cell transplantation. SM/C-2.6 is a rat monoclonal antibody useful to isolate satellite cells from mouse muscle (Fukada et al 2004). Not all SM/C-2.6-positive cells are myogenic, but the fraction is enriched in myogenic stem cells. Both strategies are promising, but human ES/iPS cells respond to the differentiation signal differently from their mouse equivalents. In addition, human ES/iPS cells differentiate more slowly than their mouse counterparts. In fact, the myogenic differentiation protocol described by Chang et al. for mouse ES/iPS cells was not efficient for human iPS cells (data not shown), and the condition need to be further explored.

4.3.3 Direct reprogramming of fibroblasts by myogenic transcription factors

iPS technology stimulated researchers to seek an appropriate combination of transcriptional factors to reprogram somatic cells into therapeutically relevant cell types *in vitro* and *in vivo* (Hiramatsu et al 2011; Ieda et al 2010; Sekiya & Suzuki 2011; Szabo et al 2010; Vierbuchen et al 2010). However, we already know how to induce myogenic cells from fibroblasts. In 1989, Weintraub and colleagues demonstrated that MyoD is sufficient to convert fibroblasts and numerous other cell types into skeletal muscle (Weintraub et al 1989). This was the first example of transcription factor-based reprogramming of the cell, but this technology has not been successfully applied to regenerative medicine. Recently, Kimura et al. reported that MyoD mediated conversion of fibroblasts *in situ* (Kimura et al 2008). The authors first introduced a tamoxifen-inducible MyoD expression cassette together with a muscle promoter-derived dystrophin expression cassette into mdx-derived fibroblasts, and then transplanted them into mdx muscle. Injection of tamoxifen into the mdx mice resulted in the appearance of dystrophin-positive myofibers in transplanted muscle, but many of them were small and clustered in the interstitial space. Pax3, Pax7 and their co-factors are also candidate transcription factors to reprogram fibroblasts into highly proliferative, systemically transplantable stem cells.

5. Conclusion

Satellite cells are skeletal muscle-specific stem cells involved in muscle growth and regeneration. Their dysfunctions are reported in several pathological conditions. Recent studies emphasize that, in addition to exhaustion of satellite cells, the microenvironment greatly influences satellite cell behaviors. Therefore both satellite cells and their microenvironment are targets of regenerative medicine. Satellite cells are also expected to be a source for cell transplantation therapy, but preparation of viable satellite cells from donors in a large quantity is not realistic. To overcome this limitation, the transcription factor-mediated reprogramming technique is now in the spotlight. MyoD was the first direct reprogramming factor discovered. However, it is not sufficient to generate high-quality myogenic cells from fibroblasts. To overcome this problem, we must fully understand the molecular and cellular regulation of satellite cells. Fortunately, we are now starting to do this.

6. Acknowledgment

We thank all members of Department of Molecular Therapy for valuable discussion.

7. References

Abou-Khalil R, Brack AS. 2010. Muscle stem cells and reversible quiescence: the role of sprouty. *Cell Cycle* 9:2575-80

Abou-Khalil R, Le Grand F, Pallafacchina G, Valable S, Authier FJ, et al. 2009. Autocrine and paracrine angiopoietin 1/Tie-2 signaling promotes muscle satellite cell self-renewal. *Cell Stem Cell* 5:298-309

Alexakis C, Partridge T, Bou-Gharios G. 2007. Implication of the satellite cell in dystrophic muscle fibrosis: a self-perpetuating mechanism of collagen overproduction. *Am J Physiol Cell Physiol* 293:C661-9

Arnold L, Henry A, Poron F, Baba-Amer Y, van Rooijen N, et al. 2007. Inflammatory monocytes recruited after skeletal muscle injury switch into antiinflammatory macrophages to support myogenesis. *J Exp Med* 204:1057-69

Berg Z, Beffa LR, Cook DP, Cornelison DD. 2011. Muscle satellite cells from GRMD dystrophic dogs are not phenotypically distinguishable from wild type satellite cells in ex vivo culture. *Neuromuscul Disord* 21:282-90

Bish LT, Yarchoan M, Sleeper MM, Gazzara JA, Morine KJ, et al. 2011. Chronic losartan administration reduces mortality and preserves cardiac but not skeletal muscle function in dystrophic mice. *PLoS One* 6:e20856

Blau HM, Webster C, Pavlath GK. 1983. Defective myoblasts identified in Duchenne muscular dystrophy. *Proc Natl Acad Sci U S A* 80:4856-60

Blau HM, Webster C, Pavlath GK, Chiu CP. 1985. Evidence for defective myoblasts in Duchenne muscular dystrophy. *Adv Exp Med Biol* 182:85-110

Boldrin L, Muntoni F, Morgan JE. 2010. Are human and mouse satellite cells really the same? *J Histochem Cytochem* 58:941-55

Buckingham M, Relaix F. 2007. The role of Pax genes in the development of tissues and organs: Pax3 and Pax7 regulate muscle progenitor cell functions. *Annu Rev Cell Dev Biol* 23:645-73

Chang H, Yoshimoto M, Umeda K, Iwasa T, Mizuno Y, et al. 2009. Generation of transplantable, functional satellite-like cells from mouse embryonic stem cells. *FASEB J* 23:1907-19

Chen JF, Tao Y, Li J, Deng Z, Yan Z, et al. 2010. microRNA-1 and microRNA-206 regulate skeletal muscle satellite cell proliferation and differentiation by repressing Pax7. *J Cell Biol* 190:867-79

Cohn RD, van Erp C, Habashi JP, Soleimani AA, Klein EC, et al. 2007. Angiotensin II type 1 receptor blockade attenuates TGF-beta-induced failure of muscle regeneration in multiple myopathic states. *Nat Med* 13:204-10

Collins CA, Olsen I, Zammit PS, Heslop L, Petrie A, et al. 2005. Stem cell function, self-renewal, and behavioral heterogeneity of cells from the adult muscle satellite cell niche. *Cell* 122:289-301

Conboy IM, Rando TA. 2002. The regulation of Notch signaling controls satellite cell activation and cell fate determination in postnatal myogenesis. *Dev Cell* 3:397-409

Conboy MJ, Cerletti M, Wagers AJ, Conboy IM. 2010. Immuno-analysis and FACS sorting of adult muscle fiber-associated stem/precursor cells. *Methods Mol Biol* 621:165-73

Conboy MJ, Karasov AO, Rando TA. 2007. High incidence of non-random template strand segregation and asymmetric fate determination in dividing stem cells and their progeny. *PLoS Biol* 5:e102

Crist CG, Montarras D, Pallafacchina G, Rocancourt D, Cumano A, et al. 2009. Muscle stem cell behavior is modified by microRNA-27 regulation of Pax3 expression. *Proc Natl Acad Sci U S A* 106:13383-7

Darabi R, Gehlbach K, Bachoo RM, Kamath S, Osawa M, et al. 2008. Functional skeletal muscle regeneration from differentiating embryonic stem cells. *Nat Med* 14:134-43

Darabi R, Pan W, Bosnakovski D, Baik J, Kyba M, Perlingeiro RC. 2011. Functional Myogenic Engraftment from Mouse iPS Cells. *Stem Cell Rev*

Decary S, Hamida CB, Mouly V, Barbet JP, Hentati F, Butler-Browne GS. 2000. Shorter telomeres in dystrophic muscle consistent with extensive regeneration in young children. *Neuromuscul Disord* 10:113-20

Dey BK, Gagan J, Dutta A. 2011. miR-206 and -486 induce myoblast differentiation by downregulating Pax7. *Mol Cell Biol* 31:203-14

Dhawan J, Rando TA. 2005. Stem cells in postnatal myogenesis: molecular mechanisms of satellite cell quiescence, activation and replenishment. *Trends Cell Biol* 15:666-73

Ferrari G, Cusella-De Angelis G, Coletta M, Paolucci E, Stornaiuolo A, et al. 1998. Muscle regeneration by bone marrow-derived myogenic progenitors. *Science* 279:1528-30

Fukada S, Higuchi S, Segawa M, Koda K, Yamamoto Y, et al. 2004. Purification and cell-surface marker characterization of quiescent satellite cells from murine skeletal muscle by a novel monoclonal antibody. *Exp Cell Res* 296:245-55

Fukada S, Miyagoe-Suzuki Y, Tsukihara H, Yuasa K, Higuchi S, et al. 2002. Muscle regeneration by reconstitution with bone marrow or fetal liver cells from green fluorescent protein-gene transgenic mice. *J Cell Sci* 115:1285-93

Fukada S, Morikawa D, Yamamoto Y, Yoshida T, Sumie N, et al. 2010. Genetic background affects properties of satellite cells and mdx phenotypes. *Am J Pathol* 176:2414-24

Fukada S, Uezumi A, Ikemoto M, Masuda S, Segawa M, et al. 2007. Molecular signature of quiescent satellite cells in adult skeletal muscle. *Stem Cells* 25:2448-59

Fukada S, Yamaguchi M, Kokubo H, Ogawa R, Uezumi A, et al. 2011. Hesr1 and Hesr3 are essential to generate undifferentiated quiescent satellite cells and to maintain satellite cell numbers. *Development*. 138:4609-19.

Gilbert PM, Havenstrite KL, Magnusson KE, Sacco A, Leonardi NA, et al. 2010. Substrate elasticity regulates skeletal muscle stem cell self-renewal in culture. *Science* 329:1078-81

Gros J, Manceau M, Thome V, Marcelle C. 2005. A common somitic origin for embryonic muscle progenitors and satellite cells. *Nature* 435:954-8

Gussoni E, Soneoka Y, Strickland CD, Buzney EA, Khan MK, et al. 1999. Dystrophin expression in the mdx mouse restored by stem cell transplantation. *Nature* 401:390-4

Heslop L, Morgan JE, Partridge TA. 2000. Evidence for a myogenic stem cell that is exhausted in dystrophic muscle. *J Cell Sci* 113 (Pt 12):2299-308

Hiramatsu K, Sasagawa S, Outani H, Nakagawa K, Yoshikawa H, Tsumaki N. 2011. Generation of hyaline cartilaginous tissue from mouse adult dermal fibroblast culture by defined factors. *J Clin Invest* 121:640-57

Hollnagel A, Grund C, Franke WW, Arnold HH. 2002. The cell adhesion molecule M-cadherin is not essential for muscle development and regeneration. *Mol Cell Biol* 22:4760-70

Huang P, Zhao XS, Fields M, Ransohoff RM, Zhou L. 2009. Imatinib attenuates skeletal muscle dystrophy in mdx mice. *Faseb J* 23:2539-48

Ieda M, Fu JD, Delgado-Olguin P, Vedantham V, Hayashi Y, et al. 2010. Direct reprogramming of fibroblasts into functional cardiomyocytes by defined factors. *Cell* 142:375-86

Ikemoto M, Fukada S, Uezumi A, Masuda S, Miyoshi H, et al. 2007. Autologous transplantation of SM/C-2.6(+) satellite cells transduced with micro-dystrophin CS1 cDNA by lentiviral vector into mdx mice. *Mol Ther* 15:2178-85

Irintchev A, Zeschnigk M, Starzinski-Powitz A, Wernig A. 1994. Expression pattern of M-cadherin in normal, denervated, and regenerating mouse muscles. *Dev Dyn* 199:326-37

Joe AW, Yi L, Natarajan A, Le Grand F, So L, et al. 2010. Muscle injury activates resident fibro/adipogenic progenitors that facilitate myogenesis. *Nat Cell Biol* 12:153-63

Juan AH, Derfoul A, Feng X, Ryall JG, Dell'Orso S, et al. 2011. Polycomb EZH2 controls self-renewal and safeguards the transcriptional identity of skeletal muscle stem cells. *Genes Dev* 25:789-94

Kanisicak O, Mendez JJ, Yamamoto S, Yamamoto M, Goldhamer DJ. 2009. Progenitors of skeletal muscle satellite cells express the muscle determination gene, MyoD. *Dev Biol* 332:131-41

Kassar-Duchossoy L, Giacone E, Gayraud-Morel B, Jory A, Gomes D, Tajbakhsh S. 2005. Pax3/Pax7 mark a novel population of primitive myogenic cells during development. *Genes Dev* 19:1426-31

Kawakami A, Kimura-Kawakami M, Nomura T, Fujisawa H. 1997. Distributions of PAX6 and PAX7 proteins suggest their involvement in both early and late phases of chick brain development. *Mech Dev* 66:119-30

Kimura E, Han JJ, Li S, Fall B, Ra J, et al. 2008. Cell-lineage regulated myogenesis for dystrophin replacement: a novel therapeutic approach for treatment of muscular dystrophy. *Hum Mol Genet* 17:2507-17

Kuang S, Gillespie MA, Rudnicki MA. 2008. Niche regulation of muscle satellite cell self-renewal and differentiation. *Cell Stem Cell* 2:22-31

Kuang S, Kuroda K, Le Grand F, Rudnicki MA. 2007. Asymmetric self-renewal and commitment of satellite stem cells in muscle. *Cell* 129:999-1010

Kuang S, Rudnicki MA. 2008. The emerging biology of satellite cells and their therapeutic potential. *Trends Mol Med* 14:82-91

LaBarge MA, Blau HM. 2002. Biological progression from adult bone marrow to mononucleate muscle stem cell to multinucleate muscle fiber in response to injury. *Cell* 111:589-601

Law PK, Goodwin TG, Fang Q, Duggirala V, Larkin C, et al. 1992. Feasibility, safety, and efficacy of myoblast transfer therapy on Duchenne muscular dystrophy boys. *Cell Transplant* 1:235-44

Lepper C, Conway SJ, Fan CM. 2009. Adult satellite cells and embryonic muscle progenitors have distinct genetic requirements. *Nature* 460:627-31

Li Y, Foster W, Deasy BM, Chan Y, Prisk V, et al. 2004. Transforming growth factor-beta1 induces the differentiation of myogenic cells into fibrotic cells in injured skeletal muscle: a key event in muscle fibrogenesis. *Am J Pathol* 164:1007-19

Mann CJ, Perdiguero E, Kharraz Y, Aguilar S, Pessina P, et al. 2011. Aberrant repair and fibrosis development in skeletal muscle. *Skelet Muscle* 1:21

Mauro A. 1961. Satellite cell of skeletal muscle fibers. *J Biophys Biochem Cytol* 9:493-5

Mendell JR, Kissel JT, Amato AA, King W, Signore L, et al. 1995. Myoblast transfer in the treatment of Duchenne's muscular dystrophy. *N Engl J Med* 333:832-8

Mizuno Y, Chang H, Umeda K, Niwa A, Iwasa T, et al. 2010. Generation of skeletal muscle stem/progenitor cells from murine induced pluripotent stem cells. *FASEB J* 24:2245-53

Montarras D, Morgan J, Collins C, Relaix F, Zaffran S, et al. 2005. Direct isolation of satellite cells for skeletal muscle regeneration. *Science* 309:2064-7

Morgan JE, Zammit PS. 2010. Direct effects of the pathogenic mutation on satellite cell function in muscular dystrophy. *Exp Cell Res* 316:3100-8

Moss FP, Leblond CP. 1971. Satellite cells as the source of nuclei in muscles of growing rats. *Anat Rec* 170:421-35

Motohashi N, Uezumi A, Yada E, Fukada S, Fukushima K, et al. 2008. Muscle CD31(-) CD45(-) side population cells promote muscle regeneration by stimulating proliferation and migration of myoblasts. *Am J Pathol* 173:781-91

Mouly V, Aamiri A, Perie S, Mamchaoui K, Barani A, et al. 2005. Myoblast transfer therapy: is there any light at the end of the tunnel? *Acta Myol* 24:128-33

Olguin HC, Olwin BB. 2004. Pax-7 up-regulation inhibits myogenesis and cell cycle progression in satellite cells: a potential mechanism for self-renewal. *Dev Biol* 275:375-88

Olguin HC, Yang Z, Tapscott SJ, Olwin BB. 2007. Reciprocal inhibition between Pax7 and muscle regulatory factors modulates myogenic cell fate determination. *J Cell Biol* 177:769-79

Olson LE, Soriano P. 2009. Increased PDGFRalpha activation disrupts connective tissue development and drives systemic fibrosis. *Dev Cell* 16:303-13

Palacios D, Mozzetta C, Consalvi S, Caretti G, Saccone V, et al. 2010. TNF/p38alpha/polycomb signaling to Pax7 locus in satellite cells links inflammation to the epigenetic control of muscle regeneration. *Cell Stem Cell* 7:455-69

Park IH, Arora N, Huo H, Maherali N, Ahfeldt T, et al. 2008. Disease-specific induced pluripotent stem cells. *Cell* 134:877-86

Partridge TA, Morgan JE, Coulton GR, Hoffman EP, Kunkel LM. 1989. Conversion of mdx myofibres from dystrophin-negative to -positive by injection of normal myoblasts. *Nature* 337:176-9

Rafael-Fortney JA, Chimanji NS, Schill KE, Martin CD, Murray JD, et al. 2011. Early treatment with lisinopril and spironolactone preserves cardiac and skeletal muscle in duchenne muscular dystrophy mice. *Circulation* 124:582-8

Relaix F, Rocancourt D, Mansouri A, Buckingham M. 2005. A Pax3/Pax7-dependent population of skeletal muscle progenitor cells. *Nature* 435:948-53

Rosenblatt JD, Lunt AI, Parry DJ, Partridge TA. 1995. Culturing satellite cells from living single muscle fiber explants. *In Vitro Cell Dev Biol Anim* 31:773-9

Sacco A, Mourkioti F, Tran R, Choi J, Llewellyn M, et al. 2010. Short telomeres and stem cell exhaustion model Duchenne muscular dystrophy in mdx/mTR mice. *Cell* 143:1059-71

Schmalbruch H, Hellhammer U. 1976. The number of satellite cells in normal human muscle. *Anat Rec* 185:279-87

Schultz E, Gibson MC, Champion T. 1978. Satellite cells are mitotically quiescent in mature mouse muscle: an EM and radioautographic study. *J Exp Zool* 206:451-6

Seale P, Sabourin LA, Girgis-Gabardo A, Mansouri A, Gruss P, Rudnicki MA. 2000. Pax7 is required for the specification of myogenic satellite cells. *Cell* 102:777-86

Segawa M, Fukada S, Yamamoto Y, Yahagi H, Kanematsu M, et al. 2008. Suppression of macrophage functions impairs skeletal muscle regeneration with severe fibrosis. *Exp Cell Res* 314:3232-44

Sekiya S, Suzuki A. 2011. Direct conversion of mouse fibroblasts to hepatocyte-like cells by defined factors. *Nature* 475:390-3

Shea KL, Xiang W, LaPorta VS, Licht JD, Keller C, et al. 2010. Sprouty1 regulates reversible quiescence of a self-renewing adult muscle stem cell pool during regeneration. *Cell Stem Cell* 6:117-29

Sherwood RI, Christensen JL, Conboy IM, Conboy MJ, Rando TA, et al. 2004. Isolation of adult mouse myogenic progenitors: functional heterogeneity of cells within and engrafting skeletal muscle. *Cell* 119:543-54

Shinin V, Gayraud-Morel B, Gomes D, Tajbakhsh S. 2006. Asymmetric division and cosegregation of template DNA strands in adult muscle satellite cells. *Nat Cell Biol* 8:677-87

Skuk D, Tremblay JP. 2011. Intramuscular cell transplantation as a potential treatment of myopathies: clinical and preclinical relevant data. *Expert Opin Biol Ther* 11:359-74

Szabo E, Rampalli S, Risueno RM, Schnerch A, Mitchell R, et al. 2010. Direct conversion of human fibroblasts to multilineage blood progenitors. *Nature* 468:521-6

Takahashi K, Tanabe K, Ohnuki M, Narita M, Ichisaka T, et al. 2007. Induction of pluripotent stem cells from adult human fibroblasts by defined factors. *Cell* 131:861-72

Takahashi K, Yamanaka S. 2006. Induction of pluripotent stem cells from mouse embryonic and adult fibroblast cultures by defined factors. *Cell* 126:663-76

Tanaka KK, Hall JK, Troy AA, Cornelison DD, Majka SM, Olwin BB. 2009. Syndecan-4-expressing muscle progenitor cells in the SP engraft as satellite cells during muscle regeneration. *Cell Stem Cell* 4:217-25

Taniguti AP, Pertille A, Matsumura CY, Santo Neto H, Marques MJ. 2011. Prevention of muscle fibrosis and myonecrosis in mdx mice by suramin, a TGF-beta1 blocker. *Muscle Nerve* 43:82-7

Tidball JG, Villalta SA. 2010. Regulatory interactions between muscle and the immune system during muscle regeneration. *Am J Physiol Regul Integr Comp Physiol* 298:R1173-87

Tremblay JP, Malouin F, Roy R, Huard J, Bouchard JP, et al. 1993. Results of a triple blind clinical study of myoblast transplantations without immunosuppressive treatment in young boys with Duchenne muscular dystrophy. *Cell Transplant* 2:99-112

Uezumi A, Fukada S, Yamamoto N, Takeda S, Tsuchida K. 2010. Mesenchymal progenitors distinct from satellite cells contribute to ectopic fat cell formation in skeletal muscle. *Nat Cell Biol* 12:143-52

Uezumi A, Ito T, Morikawa D, Shimizu N, Yoneda T, et al. 2011.Fibrosis and adipogenesis originate from a common mesenchymal progenitor in skeletal muscle. *J Cell Sci.* 124: 3654-64.

Uezumi A, Ojima K, Fukada S, Ikemoto M, Masuda S, et al. 2006. Functional heterogeneity of side population cells in skeletal muscle. *Biochem Biophys Res Commun* 341:864-73

Vidal B, Serrano AL, Tjwa M, Suelves M, Ardite E, et al. 2008. Fibrinogen drives dystrophic muscle fibrosis via a TGFbeta/alternative macrophage activation pathway. *Genes Dev* 22:1747-52

Vierbuchen T, Ostermeier A, Pang ZP, Kokubu Y, Sudhof TC, Wernig M. 2010. Direct conversion of fibroblasts to functional neurons by defined factors. *Nature* 463:1035-41

Villalta SA, Nguyen HX, Deng B, Gotoh T, Tidball JG. 2009. Shifts in macrophage phenotypes and macrophage competition for arginine metabolism affect the severity of muscle pathology in muscular dystrophy. *Hum Mol Genet* 18:482-96

Weintraub H, Tapscott SJ, Davis RL, Thayer MJ, Adam MA, et al. 1989. Activation of muscle-specific genes in pigment, nerve, fat, liver, and fibroblast cell lines by forced expression of MyoD. *Proc Natl Acad Sci U S A* 86:5434-8

White RB, Bierinx AS, Gnocchi VF, Zammit PS. 2010. Dynamics of muscle fibre growth during postnatal mouse development. *BMC Dev Biol* 10:21

Yajima H, Motohashi N, Ono Y, Sato S, Ikeda K, et al. 2010. Six family genes control the proliferation and differentiation of muscle satellite cells. *Exp Cell Res* 316:2932-44

Yu J, Vodyanik MA, Smuga-Otto K, Antosiewicz-Bourget J, Frane JL, et al. 2007. Induced pluripotent stem cell lines derived from human somatic cells. *Science* 318:1917-20

Zhao T, Zhang ZN, Rong Z, Xu Y. 2011. Immunogenicity of induced pluripotent stem cells. *Nature* 474:212-5

2

Duchenne Muscular Dystrophy: Therapeutic Approaches to Restore Dystrophin

Pietro Spitali and Annemieke Aartsma-Rus

Leiden University Medical Center,
The Netherlands

1. Introduction

Duchenne muscular dystrophy (DMD) is a progressive neuromuscular disorder. The first symptoms involve the lower limbs and appear between the third and fifth year. Due to weakness of the knee and hip extensors, patients rise from a sitting position using the Gower's maneuver. Muscle weakness progresses to the shoulder girdle-, upper arm and trunk-muscles and patients loose ambulation before the age of 12 (Emery, 1993). Histological changes involve variation in fiber size with atrophic and hypertrophic fibers, degeneration and regeneration of the muscle fibers, infiltration of inflammatory cells and fibrosis. The fiber necrosis results in leakage of the enzyme creatine kinase (CK), resulting in very high serum CK levels in DMD patients (20,000 to 50,000 U/L compared to 80 to 250 U/L in unaffected individuals). These levels decline as patients get older and the overall muscle mass decreases progressively. The pathology is caused by mutations in the *DMD* gene, which was known to be on the X chromosome long before the responsible gene was cloned due to an X-linked recessive inheritance pattern. The protein product of the gene is a 427 KDa protein called dystrophin. In the early 80s several groups were collaborating on the regional cloning of the gene responsible for DMD (Burghes et al., 1987; Monaco et al., 1985) which happened to co-localize with the locus for Becker muscular dystrophy (BMD) (Kingston et al., 1984). This is a milder disease, where patients are diagnosed in adolescence or adulthood, remain ambulant longer and survival is generally only slightly decreased (Emery, 2002). After a couple of years Monaco and colleagues confirmed that deletions in the identified locus caused DMD (Monaco et al., 1985) and BMD (Hoffman et al., 1988). In the following years, the coding sequence of the gene was identified, which turned out to occupy a huge genomic region. The complete cDNA and protein product of the *DMD* gene were published in 1987 (Hoffman et al., 1987; Koenig et al., 1987). The cloning of the genomic and coding sequence of the *DMD* gene allowed the development of tools for the molecular diagnosis of DMD. Deletions of one or more exons were found to be most common (65% of patients) and mainly localized in two hotspot regions in the gene (exons 2-20 and 45-53). This led Chamberlain and colleagues to develop a multiplex PCR able to detect the most frequent mutations (Chamberlain et al., 1988). This technique has been used for years, but recently multiple ligation-dependent probe amplification (MLPA) has been developed that allows an exact characterization of exons involved in deletions and duplications (Janssen et al., 2005; Schwartz & Duno, 2004). For small mutations a more labour-intensive method of PCR analysis of each exon, followed by direct sequencing is required (Spitali et al., 2009). The study of mutations and clinical features in DMD and BMD patients led to a deeper understanding of the disease, the gene and disease causing mutations. This made it possible to correlate genotype and phenotype and explain the discrepancy that mutations in one gene could lead to a severe DMD and a milder BMD phenotype. In 1989 two groups postulated that frame disrupting mutations were responsible for DMD while BMD was caused by frame maintaining mutations (Koenig et al., 1989; Monaco, 1989). This has been crucial for the development of certain potential therapies such as exon skipping and microdystrophins.

2. Dystrophin and the associated glycoprotein complex (DGC)

Dystrophin consists of 3685 amino acids and is a 427 kDa protein (Koenig et al., 1988). Dystrophin is composed of 4 domains, the first 240 N-terminal aminoacids define the actin-binding domain, which contains two actin-binding sites (Jarrett & Foster, 1995; Koenig & Kunkel, 1990). This domain is followed by a central rod shaped domain, consisting of 24 spectrin-like repeat units interrupted by 4 proline-rich hinge regions (Koenig & Kunkel, 1990). It has been demonstrated that an extra actin binding domain is present between repeats 11 and 17 (Rybakova et al., 1996) and that repeat 16 and 17 contain an nNOS binding site (Lai et al., 2009). The cysteine-rich domain encompasses aminoacids 3080 to 3360 and includes 15 cysteines, two EF hand motifs and a ZZ domain (Koenig et al., 1988) and binds to β-dystroglycan. Finally the C-terminal domain consists of the last 325 amino acids involved in protein-protein interactions. Dystrophin is part of the dystrophin-associated glycoprotein complex (DGC) (Figure 1). The cysteine-rich and C-terminal domains of dystrophin bind to several parts of the DGC, which can be divided into the dystroglycan complex, the sarcoglycan-sarcospan complex and the cytoplasmatic, dystrophin containing complex (Blake et al., 2002; Yoshida et al., 1994). In skeletal muscle the dystroglycan complex consists of α-dystroglycan and β-dystroglycan, which are both heavily glycosylated (Ibraghimov-Beskrovnaya et al., 1992). Dystrophin binds to β-dystroglycan, a transmembrane protein that binds to the extra-cellular α-dystroglycan; α-dystroglycan on its part binds to the extracellular matrix component laminin-2 (Hohenester et al., 1999; Rentschler et al., 1999; Suzuki et al., 1994). The sarcoglycan-sarcospan complex includes α-, β-, γ- and δ-sarcoglycan and sarcospan (Blake et al., 2002). The cytoplasmatic part of the DGC includes dystrophin itself, syntrophin and α-dystrobrevin, which binds to both dystrophin and syntrophin (Ahn et al., 1996). Alpha-syntrophin also binds to dystrophin and, additionally, it recruits the enzyme nNOS to the sarcolemma (Ahn & Kunkel, 1995; Brenman et al., 1995; Yoshida et al., 1995), although it has been recently demonstrated that the recruitment of nNOS by dystrophin repeats 16 and 17 is more important (Lai et al., 2009). Dystrophin also binds to and influences microtubules organization in the cytoplasm (Prins et al., 2009). In BMD patients, internally deleted dystrophins maintaining the N-terminal and C-terminal domains are able to bind to the DGC complex at the sarcolemma (Matsumura et al., 1994; Matsumura et al., 1993; Mirabella et al., 1998), while in DMD patients the absence of dystrophin results in the complete loss or decrease of other DGC proteins, and in the loss of nNOS at the sarcolemma (Brenman et al., 1995; Ervasti et al., 1990; Ohlendieck & Campbell, 1991). The function of the DGC is still largely unknown. However, since the complex forms a mechanical link between the cytoskeleton and the extracellular matrix, it is assumed that the DGC has a function in maintaining sarcolemma stability during contraction (Matsumura & Campbell, 1994).

3. Pathology

Dystrophin loss leads to a high susceptibility of muscle fibers to injury after repeated eccentric contractions. This results in a chronic inflammation state, which provokes damage and necrosis. Muscle tissue is lost and replaced by fibrosis after exhausted cycles of damage and repair. Recent data suggest that stretched contractions activate reactive oxygen species (ROS) production, which causes opening of stretch-activated channels (SACs) and Ca2+ entry via src kinase activation induced by caveolin-3 (Allen et al., 2010). Oxidative stress may amplify the process inducing activation of the inflammatory transcription factor NF-κB, and thus functional impairment of force-generating capacity (Lawler, 2011).

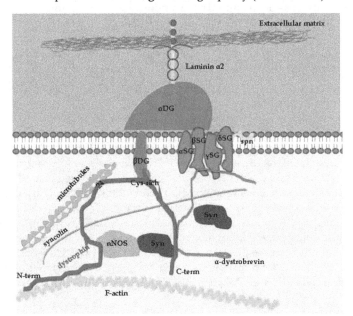

Fig. 1. Schematic representation of the dystrophin associated glycoprotein complex (DGC). αDG: α-dystroglycan; βDG: β-dystroglycan; αSG: α-sarcoglycan; βSG: β-sarcoglycan; γSG: γ-sarcoglycan; δSG: δ-sarcoglycan; spn: sarcospan; N-term: dystrophin aminoterminal domain; Cys-rich: dystrophin cystein rich domain; C-term: dystrophin carboxyterminal domain; nNOS: neuronal nitric oxide synthase; Syn: syntrophin.

4. Current treatment

There is currently no therapy for DMD. Nevertheless the lifespan and quality of life of DMD patients has significantly improved during the last 2 decades due to improved health care, especially assisted ventilation (Eagle et al., 2002). The mean age of death in the 1960s was 14.4 years, whereas for those ventilated since 1990 it was 25.3 years. The chances of survival to 25 years have increased from 0% in the 1960s to 4% in the 1970s and 12% in the 1980s, and that the impact of nocturnal ventilation has further improved this chance to 53% for those ventilated since 1990. Another crucial step has been the use of corticosteroids (mainly prednisone (Moxley, III & Pandya, 2011) and deflazacort (Biggar et al., 2001)), which reduce the inflammatory response in patients' muscle and the accompanied damage and fibrosis, thus longer maintaining muscle quality. The benefit of corticosteroids has been clearly demonstrated for DMD patients in a double-blind randomized controlled trial in more than 100 boys (Mendell et al., 1989). Corticosteroids treatment extends the ambulation of patients for about 2 years and reduces scoliosis (King et al., 2007). The prolonged use of corticosteroids has however known side effects, which include weight gain, hypertension, bone demineralization, vertebral compression fractures and sometimes behavior disorders. Guidelines for DMD patients' management have been published in order to harmonize the standards of clinical practice (Bushby et al., 2010a; Bushby et al., 2010b).

There are numerous therapeutic approaches under development for DMD. Some aim at addressing specific issues of pathology such as Idebenone, or green tea extract to reduce oxidative stress (Dorchies et al., 2009; Nagy & Nagy, 1990), or myostatin inhibition to increase muscle mass (Bish et al., 2011; Dumonceaux et al., 2010), while others directly aim at dystrophin restoration. In this chapter we will focus on the latter.

5. Therapeutic approaches

5.1 Stop codon read-through

This approach has been developed to address nonsense mutations, which are responsible for 14% of DMD cases (Aartsma-Rus et al., 2009). The rationale is to use a compound that interacts with the translation machinery to incorporate an amino acid instead of terminating protein translation at the site of a premature stop codon. This will result in a protein that is – aside from a one amino acid change at the location of the stop mutation – completely normal (Aurino & Nigro, 2006; Kaufman, 1999; Linde & Kerem, 2008; Malik et al., 2010a). This approach can also induce read-through of real stop codons, but this is thought to be less efficient due to differences in sequence context and location of real vs. aberrant stop codons (Manuvakhova et al., 2000). So far, three compounds have been reported induce efficient read-through stop codons in the DMD mRNA.

5.1.1 Gentamicin

Gentamicin is an aminoglycoside antibiotic binding to the 40S ribosomal subunit when this recognizes a stop codon (Palmer et al., 1979; Singh et al., 1979; Yoshizawa et al., 1998). This causes the insertion of an amino acid at the stop codon position. It has first been shown that it can act on each type of stop codon without any preference in vitro (Howard et al., 2004). Gentamicin (and negamycin) can induce the read-through stop codon in the mdx mouse (Arakawa et al., 2003; Barton-Davis et al., 1999), the most used mouse model for DMD which carries a nonsense mutation in exon 23 (Danko et al., 1992). However, in another report gentamicin was unable to restore dystrophin expression in the same mouse model (Dunant et al., 2003). It was later revealed that there are a number of gentamicin isomers, which all have different read-through efficiencies, and that different gentamicin batches consist of different mixes of these isomers, which can explain these controversial results (Aartsma-Rus et al., 2010; Yoshizawa et al., 1998). Three different clinical trials have been undertaken in

DMD patients using gentamicin (Malik et al., 2010b; Politano et al., 2003; Wagner et al., 2001). In the last one Malik and colleagues used the most active gentamicin isomer and treated the patients for 6 months. For 3 out of 12 patients the number of dystrophin positive fibers increased as assessed by immune histochemical analysis, while the effect was less clear by western blot analysis, as dystrophin was already visible before treatment, possibly due to spontaneous read-through or exon skipping (see below). Since chronic gentamicin use, is known to result in reversible kidney toxicity and irreversible ototoxicity, long term treatment with gentamicin – which would be required for DMD patients – is not realistic.

5.1.2 Ataluren

Ataluren, also called PTC124, was identified via in vitro screening in a luciferase assay. It is more selective for premature stop codons than regular ones, and it can be taken orally unlike gentamicin, which is administered intravenously. Studies in the mdx mouse showed that dystrophin expression could be restored after subcutaneous ataluren treatment (Welch et al., 2007). The compound was first tested in healthy volunteers where it was well tolerated (Hirawat et al., 2007). Then different doses were tested in DMD patients and an increase in dystrophin was reported for 18/38 patients (http://www.drugs.com/clinical_trials/ptc-therapeutics-announces-additional-results-phase-2-study-ptc124-duchenne-muscular-dystrophy-2308.html). In a subsequent placebo-controlled phase IIb trial 174 DMD and BMD patients were treated with two doses or placebo for 48 weeks, and then all were treated with the high dose in an open label extension study (Finkel, 2010). Treatment was well tolerated, but the primary outcome – set at 30 meter increase compared to placebo treated patients in the six minute walk test (6MWT) - was not reached, and the extension study was put on hold. From the data released (http://ptct.client.shareholder.com/releasedetail.cfm?ReleaseID=518941) it could be inferred that the low dose worked better than the high dose. It has been postulated that ataluren efficiency works through a bell shaped curve, which could explain this finding. Dystrophin analysis is pending, and different analyses of subgroups of patients is currently ongoing, as well as studies to identify the most optimal dose. Recently (May 2011) Genzyme and PTC Therapeutics announced that they are planning a follow-up clinical study for DMD patients who previously participated in the clinical trials in the UK, Europe, Israel and Australia, starting December 2011. This will provide access to ataluren to patients who have been involved in earlier clinical trials, as the trial in the USA had already been reinititated.

It has been recently published that the results obtained with the in vitro luciferase screening used to identify ataluren may have been biased, as atluren derivatives can stabilize the luciferase enzyme, giving rise to a false positive (Auld et al., 2010; Auld et al., 2009). However, it has been shown that ataluren has at least some read-through potential (Du et al., 2008; Welch et al., 2007), though it is uncertain whether the levels of dystrophin restoration will be sufficient to restore muscle function.

5.1.3 RTC13

RTC13 is a new compound for stop codon read through. Promising preliminary data were presented at the 14th annual meeting of the American Society of Gene and Cell Therapy (http://www.cureduchenne.org/site/PageServer?pagename=research_index). In the mdx mouse model RTC13 was able to restore dystrophin expression as assessed by western blot and immune-fluorescent analyses. Muscle fiber uptake was improved compared to the previous tested compounds. After 6 weeks of treatment mice showed improvement in muscle strength that was dependent on dystrophin recovery. Serum CK levels dropped and no toxicity was detected. Research to assess if RTC13 oral treatment is feasible is ongoing.

5.1.4 Nonsense mediated decay

A modifying factor which can play a role in the stop codon-read through is nonsense-mediated decay (NMD). This mechanism breaks down mRNAs that carry premature stop codons, thus resulting in less target mRNAs for stop codon read through compounds. It is known that NMD efficiency varies among individuals, for different stop codons, location within the mRNA, and sequence context. In a study of cystic fibrosis patient-derived cell cultures carrying premature stop mutations in their *CFTR* gene, it was shown that NMD was more active in patients who did not respond to gentamicin treatment than in patients who did respond to gentamicin patients (Linde et al., 2007). When NMD was blocked in non-responders' cells, they became more responsive to gentamicin treatment (Linde et al., 2007). It is anticipated that NMD influences other stop codon read through approaches.

5.2 Exon skipping

The idea of the exon skipping approach is based on the observation that the milder BMD phenotype is due to mutations in which the mRNA reading frame is maintained, while the more severe DMD phenotype is caused by frame disrupting mutations. The rationale is to restore the open reading frame. Most (~65%) of the DMD causing mutations are deletions (Aartsma-Rus et al., 2009). Scientists have tried to reframe these mutations by inducing the skipping of additional exons adjacent to the out of frame deletions during pre-mRNA splicing (Figure 2). The reframed mRNA will then allow translation into a smaller, partially functional, BMD-like dystrophin protein. Several groups have worked on this approach using antisense oligonucleotides (AONs) or snRNAs to induce the specific exon skipping in patients' cells in vitro and in several animal models.

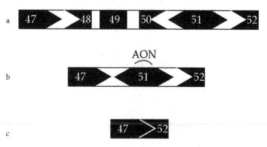

Fig. 2. a. Schematic representation of the DMD genomic region encompassing exons 47 to 52. b. Deletion of exons 48 to 50 leads to an out-of-frame mRNA which can be corrected into an in-frame deletion with the use of antisense oligonucleotides (c).

There are two AON chemistries used in clinical trials for DMD: 2-O-Methyl-Phosphorothioates (2OMePS) and phosphorodiamidate morpholino oligomers (PMOs).

5.2.1 2OMePS studies

2OMePS have a methyl group at the 2'-O position of the ribose, which increases the AON affinity for RNA and avoids RNase H activation of RNA:RNA hybrids (Dominski & Kole, 1993; Sproat et al., 1989). The PS modification is required to further increase the AON nuclease resistance, enhance cellular uptake and increase the serum half-life in vivo.

Proof of principle for the exon skipping approach and dystrophin restoration has been achieved in DMD derived cells and in murine cells (Aartsma-Rus et al., 2003; Errington et al., 2003; Mann et al., 2002; Van Deutekom et al., 2001). To test the feasibility of the approach in vivo the mdx mouse model was mainly used. The premature stop codon in exon 23 leads to a complete absence of dystrophin, and a mild dystrophic phenotype in mice, probably due to a better regenerative capacity. Mouse dystrophin exon 23 is an in frame exon, so it is possible to skip this exon, inducing an exon 22-exon 24 junction which preserves the reading frame. Intramuscular injection of AONs targeting the exon 23 donor splice site resulted in exon 23 skipping and dystrophin synthesis (Lu et al., 2003; Mann et al., 2002). This was accompanied by rescued sarcoglycan expression at the sarcolemma, improved titanic force, while no antibodies against the newly synthesized dystrophin were found in the serum. Gene expression profiling to evaluate AON efficacy and safety was tested in preclinical experiments. AONs were delivered using different carriers (PEI – F127 – Optison) to enhance muscle fibers uptake, or with recombinant adeno-associated virus (rAAV) expressing antisense sequences incorporated in a U7 snRNP gene. Exon skipping induced a shift towards wild type expression levels, which became statistically significant when high exon skipping levels were induced ('t Hoen et al., 2006). Since AON-PEI complexes worsened the muscle inflammation, while F127 and Optison did not enhance AON efficacy in vivo, following experiments were performed using naked AONs. These studies all tested local intramuscular injection, while whole body treatment is required for DMD. It is known that 2OMePS AONs have a favorable serum half-life, as the PS backbones binds to serum proteins with low affinity, which prevents renal filtration and excretion in urine. Normally, 2OMePS AONs are primarily taken up by liver and kidney and the uptake in muscle is poor. However, due to the dystrophic pathology of skeletal muscle in DMD patients, AON uptake is up to 10-fold higher, resulting in sufficient AON levels for exon skipping and dystrophin restoration in skeletal muscles in mdx mice after systemic AON administration (Heemskerk et al., 2009; Lu et al., 2005). In a comparison of intravenous, subcutaneous and intraperitoneal delivery, subcutaneous and intraperitoneal delivery showed the most preferable pharmacokinetic and pharmacodynamic profiles (lower uptake by liver and kidney), while slightly higher exon skipping levels were achieved by intravenous injections (Heemskerk et al., 2010). Based on these results and the relative easy and low invasiveness of subcutenaous injection, this delivery route was selected for systemic clinical trials.

5.2.1.1 Clinical trials with 2OMePS

Since the exon skipping is a mutation specific approach clinical experimentation started with the largest patient cohort that would potentially benefit of skipping a single exon, i.e. exon 51 (13% of all DMD patients (Aartsma-Rus et al., 2009)). Deep phenotypic screening of two BMD patients carrying deletions that could result from exon 51 skipping, showed that these dystrophins can be largely functional (Helderman-van den Enden AT et al., 2010). A first clinical trial was coordinated by Prosensa/GSK in collaboration with the Leiden

University Medical Center, using an AON targeting exon 51 (PRO051, currently called GSK2402968). This trial involved 4 patients who were each injected intramuscularly with 0.8 mg GSK2402968 in their tibialis anterior muscle. This induced specific exon 51 skipping and dystrophin recovery in 64-97% of muscle fibers at levels of 17-35% and 3-12% when quantified by immune-histochemical and western blot analysis, respectively) (Van Deutekom et al., 2007). After these encouraging results, the same AON was used in a subsequent Phase I/IIb clinical trial in which patients were subcutaneously injected and divided into 4 cohorts of 3 patients each based on the dose used (0.5 - 2 - 4 - 6 mg/kg). The AON was well tolerated, and patients showed a dose dependent dystrophin recovery in 60-100% of fibers (Goemans et al., 2011). Dystrophin amounts were quantified via fluorescent signal intensities in immune-histochemical analysis (4 to 11% dystrophin recovery) and via western blot analysis (2 to 20% dystrophin recovery). All patients were included in an open label extension study where they received weekly, subcutaneous treatments of the highest dose (6 mg/kg). The 6-minutes walk test was used as a functional outcome parameter and for most of the patients an improvement in walking distance was found after 3 months (Goemans et al., 2011). This trial did not have a placebo group, so these results, while promising, have to be interpreted with caution. A phase III double blind clinical trial in 180 DMD patients is ongoing to determine whether long term treatment with 6 mg/kg/week GSK2402968 is safe and effective ((http://clinicaltrials.gov/ct2/show/NCT01254019?term=duchenne&rank=4). Furthermore, a trial comparing weekly and biweekly dosing at 6 mg/kg is ongoing (http://clinicaltrials.gov/ct2/show/NCT01153932?term=duchenne&rank=11). Finally, a phase I double-blind, escalating dose, randomized, placebo-controlled study assessing pharmacokinetics, safety, and tolerability in non-ambulant DMD patients is ongoing (http://clinicaltrials.gov/ct2/show/NCT01128855?term=GSK2402968&rank=3) in which patients will receive different dosages (3 - 6 - 9 -12 mg/kg).

5.2.2 PMOs

PMOs contain a morpholino moiety instead of the ribose sugar and phosphoroamidate intersubunit linkages instead of phosphodiester bonds (Kurreck, 2003). PMOs have an affinity for RNA that is comparable to DNA oligos, are nuclease resistant and non-toxic (Summerton, 1999). Their backbone is uncharged, which makes them difficult to transfect in vitro, and as they do not bind serum proteins, their serum half-life is limited as they are filtered out by the kidneys. PMOs have been shown to induce exon skipping and dystrophin restoration in the mdx mouse after intramuscular (Gebski et al., 2003) and systemic injections (Alter et al., 2006; Malerba et al., 2011a; Wu et al., 2010). Upon direct comparison with 2OMePS they were shown to be more effective in inducing exon 23 skipping in the mdx mouse (Heemskerk et al., 2009). However, in all studies exon skipping and dystrophin restoration was only observed in skeletal muscle and not in heart, or only at very low levels unless heroic doses (up to 3 g/kg!) or microbubbles to improve uptake in heart were used (Alter et al., 2009; Wu et al., 2010). It has become clear that repeated low dose injections are more effective than single high dosage injections (Malerba et al., 2011b; Malerba et al., 2009), probably because of the fast PMOs clearance from the body by the kidneys (Heemskerk et al., 2010). Survival studies show that high doses of PMOs could correct the pathology and were well tolerated (Wu et al., 2011b). PMOs have also been used to restore dystrophin expression in the canine model of Duchenne, the golden retriever muscular dystrophy model (GRMD). GRMD dogs carry a splice site mutation in intron 6 leading exon 7 skipping. The skipping of exons 6 and 8 produces an in-frame exon-exon junction. Three dogs have been treated with an equimolar mixture of 3 morpholinos (2 targeting exon 6 and 1 targeting exon 8 in a cumulative dose of 120-200 mg/kg). PMOs were injected 5 to 11 times at weekly or biweekly intervals and tissue examination was performed 2 weeks after the last injection. Dystrophin restoration was achieved showing that exon skipping represents a possible choice also for complex mutations for which more than one exon needs to be skipped (Yokota et al., 2009).

5.2.2.1 Clinical trials with PMOs

Before starting clinical studies optimization of PMOs targeting exon 51 was done in cells and in the hDMD mouse (Arechavala-Gomeza et al., 2007). Clinical studies in DMD patients using PMOs targeting exon 51 (AVI-4658) were performed in the UK by the MDEX consortium in collaboration with AVI Biopharma. Local intramuscular injection in the extensor digitorum longus (EDL) muscle induced exon skipping and dystrophin restoration. After baseline correction for the controlateral, saline injected muscle, 44 to 79% of dystrophin positive fibers were observed (Kinali et al., 2009) at 22-32% of wild type levels (controlateral muscle showed dystrophin levels between 4 and 14%). This led to a Phase I/IIb clinical trial in which 19 patients received 12 weekly intravenous doses of PMO. Patients were divided in cohorts based on six different doses (0.5 – 1 – 2 – 4 - 10 - 20 mg/kg). PMOs were not toxic and well tolerated. The 2 high dosage cohorts showed an increase in the fluorescent intensity per fiber and dystrophin was restored in 7/19 patients. Three patients responded very well showing up to 55% of dystrophin positive fibers with an increase above 10% in mean fluorescence intensity per fiber (Cirak et al., 2011). Based on the varying response it was concluded that dosing was not yet optimal. In a subsequent study recently initiated, weekly intravenous doses of 30 mg/kg and 50 mg/kg for 24 weeks are tested (http://clinicaltrials.gov/ct2/show/NCT01396239?term=AVI-4658&rank=1).

It is difficult to compare results for the experiments performed with the PMOs and 2OMePS, as they were performed by different groups and different analyses were used to quantify dystrophin. In a direct comparison using equal molar amounts of PMO and 2OMePS in the mdx mouse, PMOs targeting exon 23 showed higher exon skipping percentages and higher dystrophin rescue. However, experiments performed in the hDMD mouse model, carrying a copy of the complete human *DMD* gene, there was no clear difference between 2OMePS and PMO AONs targeting exon 44, 45, 46 and 51 upon intramuscular injection (Heemskerk et al., 2009). Differences in the systemic trials for GSK2402968 and AVI-4658 are probably also due to the different pharmacokinetic and pharmacodynamic properties of the AONs. PMOs are extremely stable, but due to their uncharged nature they are filtered out by the kidney and their serum half-life is ~1 hour, so the time for tissue uptake is limited. The 2OMePS AONs by contrast bind serum proteins due to the PS backbone. This prevents renal clearance and increases their serum half-life to weeks. This may underlie the different staining patterns observed between PMO trials (patchy) and 2OMePS trials (more homogeneous).

5.2.3 AON chemistry development

While results in clinical trials are encouraging, ways to improve delivery to muscle tissues, allowing lower AON dosages would be preferred. Many approaches have been tested. Cell penetrating peptides (Jearawiriyapaisarn et al., 2008; Jearawiriyapaisarn et al., 2010; Wu et al., 2008; Yin et al., 2008), muscle targeting peptides connected to cell penetrating peptides (Yin et al., 2009) and guanidine analogs (Hu et al., 2010; Wu et al., 2009) showed the most promising results in the mdx mouse and in the hDMD mouse model (Wu et al., 2011a). Notably, pPMOs (containing arginine-rich peptides covalently bound to the morpholino AONs) have shown great potential in the mdx mouse, inducing high levels of exon skipping in skeletal muscles and heart and high levels of dystrophin rescue. Promising results using pPMOs have also been achieved in the severe mdx-utrophin$^{-/-}$ mouse model, which is defective for dystrophin and its homologue utrophin gene. Normally these mice do not survive beyond 3 months, but survival was increased to over a year after pPMO treatment (Goyenvalle et al., 2010). Unfortunately, preliminary tests in non-human primates showed mild tubular degeneration in the kidney after 4 weekly injections of 9 mg/kg of pPMOs (Moulton & Moulton, 2010). Additional peptide conjugates will hopefully be less toxic (Yin et al., 2011).

5.2.4 Antisense snRNP mediated exon skipping

Due to AON turnover and clearance, life-long treatment would be required. An alternative approach uses viral vectors expressing antisense sequences incorporated in a small nuclear ribonucleoprotein (snRNP). Adeno-associated viral vectors (AAVs) have been used to deliver the modified snRNPs as they have the best capacity to infect the muscle tissue. Different serotypes have been investigated and two molecular strategies which make use of modified U7 and U1 snRNAs have been developed. These snRNAs ensure an efficiently nuclear localization of the antisense construct, specific exon skipping and sustained dystrophin rescue in the mdx mouse model (Denti et al., 2006a; Denti et al., 2006b; Goyenvalle et al., 2004). Optimization for human exons using splicing enhancers has been also performed (Goyenvalle et al., 2009). Preclinical studies show the long-term benefit of the approach for up to 1 year (Denti et al., 2008). However the clinical translation of this approach is complicated by immune response to the viral vector (see section 5.4). Thus immune-suppression will be required, especially for patients for which multiple injections to treat muscles or muscle groups will be required.

5.3 Gene editing

Gene editing is a process in which the endogenous mutated gene is modified to produce a functional dystrophin, either by correcting the DMD causing mutation or by introducing a second mutation which will rescue the effect of the first mutation. This approach has been developed using chimeric RNA-DNA oligonucleotides (RDOs or "chimeraplasts") which anneal to genomic DNA, inducing homologous recombination between the endogenous gene and the RDO, or activating the mismatch repair system. Proof of principle was demonstrated in the mdx mouse muscle (Rando et al., 2000), in muscle precursor cells in vitro and in vivo (Bertoni & Rando, 2002). It has been demonstrated that correction is more efficient when the RDOs target the coding strand (the non transcribed strand) (Bertoni et al., 2005). Unfortunately, the gene conversion efficiency is as yet too low for clinical application and systemic delivery of RDOs in larger animals needs to be optimized further.

Recently another group has pioneered the use of meganucleases to correct the effect of the genetic mutation. The rationale is to correct the reading frame by introducing a microdeletion or micro-insertion into the *DMD* gene. This is done by specific double strand breaks at the end of an exon which precedes a deletion or at the beginning of an exon following a deletion. Meganucleases can be engineered to specifically cut at a certain genomic position causing non-homologous end joining (NHEJ) or homologous recombination when a donor corrected sequence is present. During this process often small deletions or insertions occur, which can restore the reading frame. Proof of principle for this approach has been recently demonstrated in vitro and after local delivery in vivo, albeit at low levels (Chapdelaine et al., 2010). The challenge of this approach will be the delivery of the meganucleases and the limited recognition of target sequences of meganucleases. The recently developed TALE nuclease system (Miller et al., 2011) allows targeting of almost all human sequences, and may provide a better alternative.

5.4 Gene therapy

Gene therapy approaches focus on providing an exogenous functional copy of the mutated gene. Gene therapy approaches are divided into 2 groups based on the type of delivery method used (viral or non-viral vector mediated). Muscle is a difficult target tissue for viral delivery (see below). Furthermore, the huge size of the *DMD* gene and its 11 Kb long full length cDNA sequence (FLDYS) has been one of the bottlenecks in developing this strategy, until smaller dystrophin versions were developed to make them fit into viral vector capsids. These smaller dystrophin coding sequences, called mini-dystrophins (mDYS) and micro-dystrophins (µDys), were designed based on the observations that BMD patients with minor dystrophic phenotype can carry very large deletions (England et al., 1990).

5.4.1 Viral vector based gene therapy

5.4.1.1 Lentiviral vectors

Lentiviral vectors have been used to treat mdx mice locally restoring dystrophin expression at different efficiencies (Kobinger et al., 2003; Li et al., 2005). Kimura and colleagues showed that a lentivirus encoding µDys intramuscularly injected into 2 weeks old mdx[4cv] mice could restore dystrophin in up to 400-1200 fibers in the tibialis anterior muscle. Mice were sacrificed at 4 different time points (4 weeks – 4 months – 1 year – 2 years) and results were comparable over time. The virus was capable of infecting satellite cells ensuring long-term treatment efficacy (Kimura et al., 2010). However, this may also pose a safety risk, since the transgene expression is ensured by the integration of the viral genome into the host genome. This process can cause neoplastic mutations due to the integration of the viral genome which mainly occurs close to promoter sequences (Maruggi et al., 2009). Systemic delivery of lentiviral vectors to muscle tissue is very challenging, as muscle is post-mitotic and fibers bundles are surrounded by layers of connective tissue that filter out most viruses (>30 nm).

5.4.1.2 Adeno-associated viral vectors

Due to their small size (20 nm) adeno-associated viral vectors (AAVs) are able to efficiently infect muscles. They have been more broadly used for gene therapy for muscle diseases. They do not integrate into the host genome, making them safer than lentiviruses. At least five of the many serotypes known, show a high tropism for muscle tissues (serotypes 1, 2, 6, 8 and 9). Due to the low vector capacity mDYS and µDys have been used and efficiently delivered to skeletal muscle (Gregorevic et al., 2004) and heart. Very promising studies performed in the mdx mouse showed high dystrophin recovery with AAV1 (Wang et al., 2008) and AAV2 (Wang et al., 2000), while studies in the dog model with AAV2, AAV6 (Wang et al., 2007) and AAV8 (Ohshima et al., 2009) raised the issue of cytotoxic immune response against the viral capsid proteins. AAV8 has also been tested in non human primates to delivery human µDys and levels up to 80% were obtained. Unfortunately these levels dropped to 40%when antibodies against the viral vector were present before the injection (Rodino-Klapac et al., 2010).

A clinical study has been also carried out in 6 DMD patients (aged 5-11 years) who received an intramuscular injection into the biceps muscle of a recombinant AAV (rAAV) vector carrying a µDYS gene (Mendell et al., 2010). This µDYS encoded the amino-terminal actin binding domain (ABD), 5 rod repeat domains (R1, R2, R22, R23, and R24), 3 hinge domains (H1, H3 and H4), and the cysteine-rich (CR) domain of the human *DMD* gene. The human cytomegalovirus (CMV) immediate early promoter regulated transgene expression. Vector genomes were packaged in AAV2.5, a serotype 2 capsid variant that contains five AAV1 amino acids (one insertion and four substitutions) in the AAV2 VP1 background. AAV2.5 offers improved muscle transduction properties of AAV1 with minimal recognition by serum neutralizing antibodies. Dystrophin recovery was only very limited (a few fibers for 2 patients). Mendell and colleagues further showed the presence of T-cells recognizing dystrophin epitopes in the circulation of some of the patients. For one patient the recognized epitopes were present in the µDys and deleted in the patient *DMD* gene, so this perhaps was not unexpected. Interestingly, for 2 patients T-cells able to recognize dystrophin expressed in revertant fibers were identified before and after treatment. However, the continuous presence of revertant fibers suggests that the immunity against dystrophin in the blood, did not lead to an auto-immune response in the muscle tissue.

5.5 Cell therapy

Another approach to restore dystrophin expression is based on the use of stem cells with myogenic potential, which can help repair the muscle damage and also delivery a healthy (when donor cells are used) or corrected (when autologous cells are used) *DMD* gene.

Initial efforts focused on the transplantation of adult myoblasts able to fuse with resident damaged muscle fibers creating hybrid muscle fibers (Brussee et al., 1999; Gussoni et al., 1997). However, this approach turned out to be hindered by poor cell survival, inability of the cells to extravagate into the muscle from the circulation, and limited migration of the injected cells within the host muscle (Qu et al., 1998). Results of clinical studies were discouraging (Tremblay et al., 1993). To compensate for the poor migration within muscle, a multiple injection technique has been used (up to 250 injections per square cm) (Skuk et al., 2006), but this is only feasible for small superficial muscles.

Many adult stem cells have been tested for their ability to fuse with muscle fibers in the host dystrophic muscles in murine and canine models. Cells have been grown in vitro and then transplanted in vivo with different efficiencies. Characterization of these cells has been based on their adhesion properties in vitro or on their membrane markers. Muscle side-populations cells, bone-marrow-derived stem cells, muscle-derived stem cells, mesangioblasts, blood and muscle derived CD133+ stem cells and pericytes have been identified (Asakura & Rudnicki, 2002; Benchaouir et al., 2007; Dezawa et al., 2005; Doherty et al., 1998; Gavina et al., 2006; Palumbo et al., 2004; Qu-Petersen et al., 2002). Among all, satellite cells, mesangioblasts and pericytes have shown the most promising characteristics.

Satellite cells are small progenitor cells that lie between the basement membrane and the sarcolemma of the muscle fibers. They are normally in a quiescent state but they can be activated to form new muscle fibers or to fuse with damaged ones upon muscle fiber injury. They are characterized by the expression of *pax3* and *pax7* and they have been shown to restore dystrophin expression after transplantation in dystrophic dog muscle (Montarras et al., 2005). Satellite cells have a great myogenic potential that is unfortunately lost when they are expanded in vitro. Encouraging results obtained in a mouse model led to a phase I clinical trial in DMD patients. Donor satellite cells were isolated from muscle biopsies from first-degree relatives of the affected children and were grown in culture (Daston et al., 1996; Seale et al., 2004). Dystrophin production in muscle fibers was very low (~1%) and no functional or clinical improvement in the children was observed (Peault et al., 2007).

Mesangioblasts express early but not late epithelial markers, they can transmigrate from blood vessels in tissues and they can differentiate in to muscle (Meregalli et al., 2010).

Autologous corrected and donor mesangioblasts have shown to recover dystrophin expression in dystrophic dogs, although some dogs died due to pneumonia which may be caused by accumulation of these cells in the lungs (Sampaolesi et al., 2006). At the moment mesangioblasts are tested in a clinical safety trial in DMD patients.

Pericytes share various markers with mesangioblasts, they can be isolated from skeletal muscle (Dellavalle et al., 2007) and also from non-muscular tissues (Crisan et al., 2008). Dellavalle and coworkers demonstrated that pericytes have high myogenic capacity when injected into SCID/mdx mice. It still needs to be determined whether transplanted pericytes can fully reconstitute the satellite cell niche as real functional stem cells (Morgan & Muntoni, 2007) and whether systemic delivery can be performed.

The main hurdles facing stem cell treatment for DMD are the abundance of muscle (up to 40% of the bodyweight in men), which, combined with the poor efficiency of delivery of cells to muscle tissue (generally (much) below 10%), creates the need for the transplantation of huge numbers of cells in order to generate clinical benefit.

Finally the use of donor stem cells would need constant immune suppression to avoid a specific immune response against the newly formed myofibers. This issue can be solved using autologous stem cells modified ex vivo. However, this process reduces the myogenic properties of cells using current culturing methods, and may impact the behavior of the cells once they are re-injected in the patients.

6. Conclusion

In the last 20-25 years we have seen how basic science findings have been translated into clinical research. Many therapeutic approaches have been developed in vitro, in preclinical animal models and some of them have advanced to the clinical stage. Among all therapeutic approaches the exon skipping is at the moment the most promising for clinical application in the near future.

7. References

't Hoen, P. A., van der Wees, C. G., Aartsma-Rus, A., Turk, R., Goyenvalle, A., Danos, O., Garcia, L., van Ommen, G. J., den Dunnen, J. T., & Van Deutekom, J. C. (April 2006). Gene expression profiling to monitor therapeutic and adverse effects of antisense therapies for Duchenne muscular dystrophy. *Pharmacogenomics.*, Vol.7,No.3, (April 2006), pp. 281-297, ISSN

Aartsma-Rus, A., den Dunnen, J. T., & van Ommen, G. J. (December 2010). New insights in gene-derived therapy: the example of Duchenne muscular dystrophy. *Ann.N.Y.Acad.Sci.*, Vol.1214,No.December 2010), pp. 199-212, ISSN

Aartsma-Rus, A., Fokkema, I., Verschuuren, J., Ginjaar, I., van, D. J., van Ommen, G. J., & den Dunnen, J. T. (March 2009). Theoretic applicability of antisense-mediated exon skipping for Duchenne muscular dystrophy mutations. *Hum.Mutat.*, Vol.30,No.3, (March 2009), pp. 293-299, ISSN

Aartsma-Rus, A., Janson, A. A., Kaman, W. E., Bremmer-Bout, M., den Dunnen, J. T., Baas, F., van Ommen, G. J., & Van Deutekom, J. C. (April 2003). Therapeutic antisense-induced exon skipping in cultured muscle cells from six different DMD patients. *Hum.Mol.Genet.*, Vol.12,No.8, (April 2003), pp. 907-914, ISSN

Ahn, A. H., Freener, C. A., Gussoni, E., Yoshida, M., Ozawa, E., & Kunkel, L. M. (February 1996). The three human syntrophin genes are expressed in diverse tissues, have distinct chromosomal locations, and each bind to dystrophin and its relatives. *J.Biol.Chem.*, Vol.271,No.5, (February 1996), pp. 2724-2730, ISSN

Ahn, A. H. and Kunkel, L. M. (February 1995). Syntrophin binds to an alternatively spliced exon of dystrophin. *J.Cell Biol.*, Vol.128,No.3, (February 1995), pp. 363-371, ISSN

Allen, D. G., Gervasio, O. L., Yeung, E. W., & Whitehead, N. P. (February 2010). Calcium and the damage pathways in muscular dystrophy. *Can.J.Physiol Pharmacol.*, Vol.88,No.2, (February 2010), pp. 83-91, ISSN

Alter, J., Lou, F., Rabinowitz, A., Yin, H., Rosenfeld, J., Wilton, S. D., Partridge, T. A., & Lu, Q. L. (February 2006). Systemic delivery of morpholino oligonucleotide restores dystrophin expression bodywide and improves dystrophic pathology. *Nat.Med.*, Vol.12,No.2, (February 2006), pp. 175-177, ISSN

Alter, J., Sennoga, C. A., Lopes, D. M., Eckersley, R. J., & Wells, D. J. (June 2009). Microbubble stability is a major determinant of the efficiency of ultrasound and microbubble mediated in vivo gene transfer. *Ultrasound Med.Biol.*, Vol.35,No.6, (June 2009), pp. 976-984, ISSN

Arakawa, M., Shiozuka, M., Nakayama, Y., Hara, T., Hamada, M., Kondo, S., Ikeda, D., Takahashi, Y., Sawa, R., Nonomura, Y., Sheykholeslami, K., Kondo, K., Kaga, K., Kitamura, T., Suzuki-Miyagoe, Y., Takeda, S., & Matsuda, R. (November 2003). Negamycin restores dystrophin expression in skeletal and cardiac muscles of mdx mice. *J.Biochem.*, Vol.134,No.5, (November 2003), pp. 751-758, ISSN

Arechavala-Gomeza, V., Graham, I. R., Popplewell, L. J., Adams, A. M., Aartsma-Rus, A., Kinali, M., Morgan, J. E., Van Deutekom, J. C., Wilton, S. D., Dickson, G., & Muntoni, F. (September 2007). Comparative analysis of antisense oligonucleotide sequences for targeted skipping of exon 51 during dystrophin pre-mRNA splicing in human muscle. *Hum.Gene Ther.*, Vol.18,No.9, (September 2007), pp. 798-810, ISSN

Asakura, A. and Rudnicki, M. A. (November 2002). Side population cells from diverse adult tissues are capable of in vitro hematopoietic differentiation. *Exp.Hematol.*, Vol.30,No.11, (November 2002), pp. 1339-1345, ISSN

Auld, D. S., Lovell, S., Thorne, N., Lea, W. A., Maloney, D. J., Shen, M., Rai, G., Battaile, K. P., Thomas, C. J., Simeonov, A., Hanzlik, R. P., & Inglese, J. (March 2010). Molecular basis for the high-affinity binding and stabilization of firefly luciferase by PTC124. *Proc.Natl.Acad.Sci.U.S.A*, Vol.107,No.11, (March 2010), pp. 4878-4883, ISSN

Auld, D. S., Thorne, N., Maguire, W. F., & Inglese, J. (March 2009). Mechanism of PTC124 activity in cell-based luciferase assays of nonsense codon suppression. *Proc.Natl.Acad.Sci.U.S.A*, Vol.106,No.9, (March 2009), pp. 3585-3590, ISSN

Aurino, S. and Nigro, V. (June 2006). Readthrough strategies for stop codons in Duchenne muscular dystrophy. *Acta Myol.*, Vol.25,No.1, (June 2006), pp. 5-12, ISSN

Barton-Davis, E. R., Cordier, L., Shoturma, D. I., Leland, S. E., & Sweeney, H. L. (August 1999). Aminoglycoside antibiotics restore dystrophin function to skeletal muscles of mdx mice. *J.Clin.Invest*, Vol.104,No.4, (August 1999), pp. 375-381, ISSN

Benchaouir, R., Meregalli, M., Farini, A., D'Antona, G., Belicchi, M., Goyenvalle, A., Battistelli, M., Bresolin, N., Bottinelli, R., Garcia, L., & Torrente, Y. (December 2007). Restoration of human dystrophin following transplantation of exon-skipping-engineered DMD patient stem cells into dystrophic mice. *Cell Stem Cell*, Vol.1,No.6, (December 2007), pp. 646-657, ISSN

Bertoni, C., Morris, G. E., & Rando, T. A. (January 2005). Strand bias in oligonucleotide-mediated dystrophin gene editing. *Hum.Mol.Genet.*, Vol.14,No.2, (January 2005), pp. 221-233, ISSN

Bertoni, C. and Rando, T. A. (April 2002). Dystrophin gene repair in mdx muscle precursor cells in vitro and in vivo mediated by RNA-DNA chimeric oligonucleotides. *Hum.Gene Ther.*, Vol.13,No.6, (April 2002), pp. 707-718, ISSN

Biggar, W. D., Gingras, M., Fehlings, D. L., Harris, V. A., & Steele, C. A. (January 2001). Deflazacort treatment of Duchenne muscular dystrophy. *J.Pediatr.*, Vol.138,No.1, (January 2001), pp. 45-50, ISSN

Bish, L. T., Sleeper, M. M., Forbes, S. C., Morine, K., Reynolds, C., Singletary, G. E., Trafny, D., Pham, J., Bogan, J., Kornegay, J. N., Vandenborne, K., Walter, G. A., & Sweeney, H. L. (July 2011). Long-term systemic myostatin inhibition via liver-targeted gene transfer in Golden Retriever Muscular Dystrophy. *Hum.Gene Ther.*, Vol.July 2011), pp.

Blake, D. J., Weir, A., Newey, S. E., & Davies, K. E. (April 2002). Function and genetics of dystrophin and dystrophin-related proteins in muscle. *Physiol Rev.*, Vol.82,No.2, (April 2002), pp. 291-329, ISSN

Brenman, J. E., Chao, D. S., Xia, H., Aldape, K., & Bredt, D. S. (September 1995). Nitric oxide synthase complexed with dystrophin and absent from skeletal muscle sarcolemma in Duchenne muscular dystrophy. *Cell*, Vol.82,No.5, (September 1995), pp. 743-752, ISSN

Brussee, V., Tardif, F., Roy, B., Goulet, M., Sebille, A., & Tremblay, J. P. (June 1999). Successful myoblast transplantation in fibrotic muscles: no increased impairment by the connective tissue. *Transplantation*, Vol.67,No.12, (June 1999), pp. 1618-1622, ISSN

Burghes, A. H., Logan, C., Hu, X., Belfall, B., Worton, R. G., & Ray, P. N. (July 1987). A cDNA clone from the Duchenne/Becker muscular dystrophy gene. *Nature*, Vol.328,No.6129, (July 1987), pp. 434-437, ISSN

Bushby, K., Finkel, R., Birnkrant, D. J., Case, L. E., Clemens, P. R., Cripe, L., Kaul, A., Kinnett, K., McDonald, C., Pandya, S., Poysky, J., Shapiro, F., Tomezsko, J., & Constantin, C. (January 2010a). Diagnosis and management of Duchenne muscular dystrophy, part 1: diagnosis, and pharmacological and psychosocial management. *Lancet Neurol.*, Vol.9,No.1, (January 2010a), pp. 77-93, ISSN

Bushby, K., Finkel, R., Birnkrant, D. J., Case, L. E., Clemens, P. R., Cripe, L., Kaul, A., Kinnett, K., McDonald, C., Pandya, S., Poysky, J., Shapiro, F., Tomezsko, J., & Constantin, C. (February 2010b). Diagnosis and management of Duchenne muscular dystrophy, part 2: implementation of multidisciplinary care. *Lancet Neurol.*, Vol.9,No.2, (February 2010b), pp. 177-189, ISSN

Chamberlain, J. S., Gibbs, R. A., Ranier, J. E., Nguyen, P. N., & Caskey, C. T. (December 1988). Deletion screening of the Duchenne muscular dystrophy locus via multiplex DNA amplification. *Nucleic Acids Res.*, Vol.16,No.23, (December 1988), pp. 11141-11156, ISSN

Chapdelaine, P., Pichavant, C., Rousseau, J., Paques, F., & Tremblay, J. P. (July 2010). Meganucleases can restore the reading frame of a mutated dystrophin. *Gene Ther.*, Vol.17,No.7, (July 2010), pp. 846-858, ISSN

Cirak, S., Arechavala-Gomeza, V., Guglieri, M., Feng, L., Torelli, S., Anthony, K., Abbs, S., Garralda, M. E., Bourke, J., Wells, D. J., Dickson, G., Wood, M. J., Wilton, S. D., Straub, V., Kole, R., Shrewsbury, S. B., Sewry, C., Morgan, J. E., Bushby, K., & Muntoni, F. (August 2011). Exon skipping and dystrophin restoration in patients with Duchenne muscular dystrophy after systemic phosphorodiamidate morpholino oligomer treatment: an open-label, phase 2, dose-escalation study. *Lancet*, Vol.378,No.9791, (August 2011), pp. 595-605, ISSN

Crisan, M., Yap, S., Casteilla, L., Chen, C. W., Corselli, M., Park, T. S., Andriolo, G., Sun, B., Zheng, B., Zhang, L., Norotte, C., Teng, P. N., Traas, J., Schugar, R., Deasy, B. M., Badylak, S., Buhring, H. J., Giacobino, J. P., Lazzari, L., Huard, J., & Peault, B. (September 2008). A perivascular origin for mesenchymal stem cells in multiple human organs. *Cell Stem Cell*, Vol.3,No.3, (September 2008), pp. 301-313, ISSN

Danko, I., Chapman, V., & Wolff, J. A. (July 1992). The frequency of revertants in mdx mouse genetic models for Duchenne muscular dystrophy. *Pediatr.Res.*, Vol.32,No.1, (July 1992), pp. 128-131, ISSN

Daston, G., Lamar, E., Olivier, M., & Goulding, M. (March 1996). Pax-3 is necessary for migration but not differentiation of limb muscle precursors in the mouse. *Development*, Vol.122,No.3, (March 1996), pp. 1017-1027, ISSN

Dellavalle, A., Sampaolesi, M., Tonlorenzi, R., Tagliafico, E., Sacchetti, B., Perani, L., Innocenzi, A., Galvez, B. G., Messina, G., Morosetti, R., Li, S., Belicchi, M., Peretti,

G., Chamberlain, J. S., Wright, W. E., Torrente, Y., Ferrari, S., Bianco, P., & Cossu, G. (March 2007). Pericytes of human skeletal muscle are myogenic precursors distinct from satellite cells. *Nat.Cell Biol.*, Vol.9,No.3, (March 2007), pp. 255-267, ISSN

Denti, M. A., Incitti, T., Sthandier, O., Nicoletti, C., De Angelis, F. G., Rizzuto, E., Auricchio, A., Musaro, A., & Bozzoni, I. (June 2008). Long-term benefit of adeno-associated virus/antisense-mediated exon skipping in dystrophic mice. *Hum.Gene Ther.*, Vol.19,No.6, (June 2008), pp. 601-608, ISSN

Denti, M. A., Rosa, A., D'Antona, G., Sthandier, O., De Angelis, F. G., Nicoletti, C., Allocca, M., Pansarasa, O., Parente, V., Musaro, A., Auricchio, A., Bottinelli, R., & Bozzoni, I. (March 2006a). Body-wide gene therapy of Duchenne muscular dystrophy in the mdx mouse model. *Proc.Natl.Acad.Sci.U.S.A*, Vol.103,No.10, (March 2006a), pp. 3758-3763, ISSN

Denti, M. A., Rosa, A., D'Antona, G., Sthandier, O., De Angelis, F. G., Nicoletti, C., Allocca, M., Pansarasa, O., Parente, V., Musaro, A., Auricchio, A., Bottinelli, R., & Bozzoni, I. (May 2006b). Chimeric adeno-associated virus/antisense U1 small nuclear RNA effectively rescues dystrophin synthesis and muscle function by local treatment of mdx mice. *Hum.Gene Ther.*, Vol.17,No.5, (May 2006b), pp. 565-574, ISSN

Dezawa, M., Ishikawa, H., Itokazu, Y., Yoshihara, T., Hoshino, M., Takeda, S., Ide, C., & Nabeshima, Y. (July 2005). Bone marrow stromal cells generate muscle cells and repair muscle degeneration. *Science*, Vol.309,No.5732, (July 2005), pp. 314-317, ISSN

Doherty, M. J., Ashton, B. A., Walsh, S., Beresford, J. N., Grant, M. E., & Canfield, A. E. (May 1998). Vascular pericytes express osteogenic potential in vitro and in vivo. *J.Bone Miner.Res.*, Vol.13,No.5, (May 1998), pp. 828-838, ISSN

Dominski, Z. and Kole, R. (September 1993). Restoration of correct splicing in thalassemic pre-mRNA by antisense oligonucleotides. *Proc.Natl.Acad.Sci.U.S.A*, Vol.90,No.18, (September 1993), pp. 8673-8677, ISSN

Dorchies, O. M., Wagner, S., Buetler, T. M., & Ruegg, U. T. (May 2009). Protection of dystrophic muscle cells with polyphenols from green tea correlates with improved glutathione balance and increased expression of 67LR, a receptor for (-)-epigallocatechin gallate. *Biofactors*, Vol.35,No.3, (May 2009), pp. 279-294, ISSN

Du, M., Liu, X., Welch, E. M., Hirawat, S., Peltz, S. W., & Bedwell, D. M. (February 2008). PTC124 is an orally bioavailable compound that promotes suppression of the human CFTR-G542X nonsense allele in a CF mouse model. *Proc.Natl.Acad.Sci.U.S.A*, Vol.105,No.6, (February 2008), pp. 2064-2069, ISSN

Dumonceaux, J., Marie, S., Beley, C., Trollet, C., Vignaud, A., Ferry, A., Butler-Browne, G., & Garcia, L. (May 2010). Combination of myostatin pathway interference and dystrophin rescue enhances tetanic and specific force in dystrophic mdx mice. *Mol.Ther.*, Vol.18,No.5, (May 2010), pp. 881-887, ISSN

Dunant, P., Walter, M. C., Karpati, G., & Lochmuller, H. (May 2003). Gentamicin fails to increase dystrophin expression in dystrophin-deficient muscle. *Muscle Nerve*, Vol.27,No.5, (May 2003), pp. 624-627, ISSN

Eagle, M., Baudouin, S. V., Chandler, C., Giddings, D. R., Bullock, R., & Bushby, K. (December 2002). Survival in Duchenne muscular dystrophy: improvements in life expectancy since 1967 and the impact of home nocturnal ventilation. *Neuromuscul.Disord.*, Vol.12,No.10, (December 2002), pp. 926-929, ISSN

Emery, A. E. (July 1993). Duchenne muscular dystrophy--Meryon's disease. *Neuromuscul.Disord.*, Vol.3,No.4, (July 1993), pp. 263-266, ISSN

Emery, A. E. (February 2002). The muscular dystrophies. *Lancet*, Vol.359,No.9307, (February 2002), pp. 687-695, ISSN

England, S. B., Nicholson, L. V., Johnson, M. A., Forrest, S. M., Love, D. R., Zubrzycka-Gaarn, E. E., Bulman, D. E., Harris, J. B., & Davies, K. E. (January 1990). Very mild muscular dystrophy associated with the deletion of 46% of dystrophin. *Nature*, Vol.343,No.6254, (January 1990), pp. 180-182, ISSN

Errington, S. J., Mann, C. J., Fletcher, S., & Wilton, S. D. (June 2003). Target selection for antisense oligonucleotide induced exon skipping in the dystrophin gene. *J.Gene Med.*, Vol.5,No.6, (June 2003), pp. 518-527, ISSN

Ervasti, J. M., Ohlendieck, K., Kahl, S. D., Gaver, M. G., & Campbell, K. P. (May 1990). Deficiency of a glycoprotein component of the dystrophin complex in dystrophic muscle. *Nature*, Vol.345,No.6273, (May 1990), pp. 315-319, ISSN

Finkel, R. S. (September 2010). Read-through strategies for suppression of nonsense mutations in Duchenne/ Becker muscular dystrophy: aminoglycosides and ataluren (PTC124). *J.Child Neurol.*, Vol.25,No.9, (September 2010), pp. 1158-1164, ISSN

Gavina, M., Belicchi, M., Rossi, B., Ottoboni, L., Colombo, F., Meregalli, M., Battistelli, M., Forzenigo, L., Biondetti, P., Pisati, F., Parolini, D., Farini, A., Issekutz, A. C., Bresolin, N., Rustichelli, F., Constantin, G., & Torrente, Y. (October 2006). VCAM-1 expression on dystrophic muscle vessels has a critical role in the recruitment of human blood-derived CD133+ stem cells after intra-arterial transplantation. *Blood*, Vol.108,No.8, (October 2006), pp. 2857-2866, ISSN

Gebski, B. L., Mann, C. J., Fletcher, S., & Wilton, S. D. (August 2003). Morpholino antisense oligonucleotide induced dystrophin exon 23 skipping in mdx mouse muscle. *Hum.Mol.Genet.*, Vol.12,No.15, (August 2003), pp. 1801-1811, ISSN

Goemans, N. M., Tulinius, M., van den Akker, J. T., Burm, B. E., Ekhart, P. F., Heuvelmans, N., Holling, T., Janson, A. A., Platenburg, G. J., Sipkens, J. A., Sitsen, J. M., Aartsma-Rus, A., van Ommen, G. J., Buyse, G., Darin, N., Verschuuren, J. J., Campion, G. V., de Kimpe, S. J., & Van Deutekom, J. C. (April 2011). Systemic administration of PRO051 in Duchenne's muscular dystrophy. *N.Engl.J.Med.*, Vol.364,No.16, (April 2011), pp. 1513-1522, ISSN

Goyenvalle, A., Babbs, A., Powell, D., Kole, R., Fletcher, S., Wilton, S. D., & Davies, K. E. (January 2010). Prevention of dystrophic pathology in severely affected dystrophin/utrophin-deficient mice by morpholino-oligomer-mediated exon-skipping. *Mol.Ther.*, Vol.18,No.1, (January 2010), pp. 198-205, ISSN

Goyenvalle, A., Babbs, A., van Ommen, G. J., Garcia, L., & Davies, K. E. (July 2009). Enhanced exon-skipping induced by U7 snRNA carrying a splicing silencer sequence: Promising tool for DMD therapy. *Mol.Ther.*, Vol.17,No.7, (July 2009), pp. 1234-1240, ISSN

Goyenvalle, A., Vulin, A., Fougerousse, F., Leturcq, F., Kaplan, J. C., Garcia, L., & Danos, O. (December 2004). Rescue of dystrophic muscle through U7 snRNA-mediated exon skipping. *Science*, Vol.306,No.5702, (December 2004), pp. 1796-1799, ISSN

Gregorevic, P., Blankinship, M. J., Allen, J. M., Crawford, R. W., Meuse, L., Miller, D. G., Russell, D. W., & Chamberlain, J. S. (August 2004). Systemic delivery of genes to striated muscles using adeno-associated viral vectors. *Nat.Med.*, Vol.10,No.8, (August 2004), pp. 828-834, ISSN

Gussoni, E., Blau, H. M., & Kunkel, L. M. (September 1997). The fate of individual myoblasts after transplantation into muscles of DMD patients. *Nat.Med.*, Vol.3,No.9, (September 1997), pp. 970-977, ISSN

Heemskerk, H., de, W. C., van, K. P., Heuvelmans, N., Sabatelli, P., Rimessi, P., Braghetta, P., van Ommen, G. J., de, K. S., Ferlini, A., Aartsma-Rus, A., & Van Deutekom, J. C. (June 2010). Preclinical PK and PD studies on 2'-O-methyl-phosphorothioate RNA antisense oligonucleotides in the mdx mouse model. *Mol.Ther.*, Vol.18,No.6, (June 2010), pp. 1210-1217, ISSN

Heemskerk, H. A., de Winter, C. L., de Kimpe, S. J., van Kuik-Romeijn, P., Heuvelmans, N., Platenburg, G. J., van Ommen, G. J., Van Deutekom, J. C., & Aartsma-Rus, A. (March 2009). In vivo comparison of 2'-O-methyl phosphorothioate and morpholino antisense oligonucleotides for Duchenne muscular dystrophy exon skipping. *J.Gene Med.*, Vol.11,No.3, (March 2009), pp. 257-266, ISSN

Helderman-van den Enden AT, Straathof, C. S., Aartsma-Rus, A., den Dunnen, J. T., Verbist, B. M., Bakker, E., Verschuuren, J. J., & Ginjaar, H. B. (April 2010). Becker muscular dystrophy patients with deletions around exon 51; a promising outlook for exon skipping therapy in Duchenne patients. *Neuromuscul.Disord.*, Vol.20,No.4, (April 2010), pp. 251-254, ISSN

Hirawat, S., Welch, E. M., Elfring, G. L., Northcutt, V. J., Paushkin, S., Hwang, S., Leonard, E. M., Almstead, N. G., Ju, W., Peltz, S. W., & Miller, L. L. (April 2007). Safety, tolerability, and pharmacokinetics of PTC124, a nonaminoglycoside nonsense mutation suppressor, following single- and multiple-dose administration to healthy male and female adult volunteers. *J.Clin.Pharmacol.*, Vol.47,No.4, (April 2007), pp. 430-444, ISSN

Hoffman, E. P., Brown, R. H., Jr., & Kunkel, L. M. (December 1987). Dystrophin: the protein product of the Duchenne muscular dystrophy locus. *Cell*, Vol.51,No.6, (December 1987), pp. 919-928, ISSN

Hoffman, E. P., Fischbeck, K. H., Brown, R. H., Johnson, M., Medori, R., Loike, J. D., Harris, J. B., Waterston, R., Brooke, M., Specht, L., & . (May 1988). Characterization of dystrophin in muscle-biopsy specimens from patients with Duchenne's or Becker's muscular dystrophy. *N.Engl.J.Med.*, Vol.318,No.21, (May 1988), pp. 1363-1368, ISSN

Hohenester, E., Tisi, D., Talts, J. F., & Timpl, R. (November 1999). The crystal structure of a laminin G-like module reveals the molecular basis of alpha-dystroglycan binding to laminins, perlecan, and agrin. *Mol.Cell*, Vol.4,No.5, (November 1999), pp. 783-792, ISSN

Howard, M. T., Anderson, C. B., Fass, U., Khatri, S., Gesteland, R. F., Atkins, J. F., & Flanigan, K. M. (March 2004). Readthrough of dystrophin stop codon mutations induced by aminoglycosides. *Ann.Neurol.*, Vol.55,No.3, (March 2004), pp. 422-426, ISSN

Hu, Y., Wu, B., Zillmer, A., Lu, P., Benrashid, E., Wang, M., Doran, T., Shaban, M., Wu, X., & Lu, Q. L. (April 2010). Guanine analogues enhance antisense oligonucleotide-induced exon skipping in dystrophin gene in vitro and in vivo. *Mol.Ther.*, Vol.18,No.4, (April 2010), pp. 812-818, ISSN

Ibraghimov-Beskrovnaya, O., Ervasti, J. M., Leveille, C. J., Slaughter, C. A., Sernett, S. W., & Campbell, K. P. (February 1992). Primary structure of dystrophin-associated glycoproteins linking dystrophin to the extracellular matrix. *Nature*, Vol.355,No.6362, (February 1992), pp. 696-702, ISSN

Janssen, B., Hartmann, C., Scholz, V., Jauch, A., & Zschocke, J. (February 2005). MLPA analysis for the detection of deletions, duplications and complex rearrangements in the dystrophin gene: potential and pitfalls. *Neurogenetics.*, Vol.6,No.1, (February 2005), pp. 29-35, ISSN

Jarrett, H. W. and Foster, J. L. (March 1995). Alternate binding of actin and calmodulin to multiple sites on dystrophin. *J.Biol.Chem.*, Vol.270,No.10, (March 1995), pp. 5578-5586, ISSN

Jearawiriyapaisarn, N., Moulton, H. M., Buckley, B., Roberts, J., Sazani, P., Fucharoen, S., Iversen, P. L., & Kole, R. (September 2008). Sustained dystrophin expression induced by peptide-conjugated morpholino oligomers in the muscles of mdx mice. *Mol.Ther.*, Vol.16,No.9, (September 2008), pp. 1624-1629, ISSN

Jearawiriyapaisarn, N., Moulton, H. M., Sazani, P., Kole, R., & Willis, M. S. (February 2010). Long-term improvement in mdx cardiomyopathy after therapy with peptide-conjugated morpholino oligomers. *Cardiovasc.Res.*, Vol.85,No.3, (February 2010), pp. 444-453, ISSN

Kaufman, R. J. (August 1999). Correction of genetic disease by making sense from nonsense. *J.Clin.Invest*, Vol.104,No.4, (August 1999), pp. 367-368, ISSN

Kimura, E., Li, S., Gregorevic, P., Fall, B. M., & Chamberlain, J. S. (January 2010). Dystrophin delivery to muscles of mdx mice using lentiviral vectors leads to myogenic progenitor targeting and stable gene expression. *Mol.Ther.*, Vol.18,No.1, (January 2010), pp. 206-213, ISSN

Kinali, M., Arechavala-Gomeza, V., Feng, L., Cirak, S., Hunt, D., Adkin, C., Guglieri, M., Ashton, E., Abbs, S., Nihoyannopoulos, P., Garralda, M. E., Rutherford, M., McCulley, C., Popplewell, L., Graham, I. R., Dickson, G., Wood, M. J., Wells, D. J., Wilton, S. D., Kole, R., Straub, V., Bushby, K., Sewry, C., Morgan, J. E., & Muntoni, F. (October 2009). Local restoration of dystrophin expression with the morpholino oligomer AVI-4658 in Duchenne muscular dystrophy: a single-blind, placebo-controlled, dose-escalation, proof-of-concept study. *Lancet Neurol.*, Vol.8,No.10, (October 2009), pp. 918-928, ISSN

King, W. M., Ruttencutter, R., Nagaraja, H. N., Matkovic, V., Landoll, J., Hoyle, C., Mendell, J. R., & Kissel, J. T. (May 2007). Orthopedic outcomes of long-term daily corticosteroid treatment in Duchenne muscular dystrophy. *Neurology*, Vol.68,No.19, (May 2007), pp. 1607-1613, ISSN

Kingston, H. M., Sarfarazi, M., Thomas, N. S., & Harper, P. S. (1984). Localisation of the Becker muscular dystrophy gene on the short arm of the X chromosome by linkage to cloned DNA sequences. *Hum.Genet.*, Vol.67,No.1, (1984), pp. 6-17, ISSN

Kobinger, G. P., Louboutin, J. P., Barton, E. R., Sweeney, H. L., & Wilson, J. M. (October 2003). Correction of the dystrophic phenotype by in vivo targeting of muscle progenitor cells. *Hum.Gene Ther.*, Vol.14,No.15, (October 2003), pp. 1441-1449, ISSN

Koenig, M., Beggs, A. H., Moyer, M., Scherpf, S., Heindrich, K., Bettecken, T., Meng, G., Muller, C. R., Lindlof, M., Kaariainen, H., & . (October 1989). The molecular basis for Duchenne versus Becker muscular dystrophy: correlation of severity with type of deletion. *Am.J.Hum.Genet.*, Vol.45,No.4, (October 1989), pp. 498-506, ISSN

Koenig, M., Hoffman, E. P., Bertelson, C. J., Monaco, A. P., Feener, C., & Kunkel, L. M. (July 1987). Complete cloning of the Duchenne muscular dystrophy (DMD) cDNA and preliminary genomic organization of the DMD gene in normal and affected individuals. *Cell*, Vol.50,No.3, (July 1987), pp. 509-517, ISSN

Koenig, M. and Kunkel, L. M. (March 1990). Detailed analysis of the repeat domain of dystrophin reveals four potential hinge segments that may confer flexibility. *J.Biol.Chem.*, Vol.265,No.8, (March 1990), pp. 4560-4566, ISSN

Koenig, M., Monaco, A. P., & Kunkel, L. M. (April 1988). The complete sequence of dystrophin predicts a rod-shaped cytoskeletal protein. *Cell*, Vol.53,No.2, (April 1988), pp. 219-228, ISSN

Kurreck, J. (April 2003). Antisense technologies. Improvement through novel chemical modifications. *Eur.J.Biochem.*, Vol.270,No.8, (April 2003), pp. 1628-1644, ISSN

Lai, Y., Thomas, G. D., Yue, Y., Yang, H. T., Li, D., Long, C., Judge, L., Bostick, B., Chamberlain, J. S., Terjung, R. L., & Duan, D. (March 2009). Dystrophins carrying spectrin-like repeats 16 and 17 anchor nNOS to the sarcolemma and enhance exercise performance in a mouse model of muscular dystrophy. *J.Clin.Invest*, Vol.119,No.3, (March 2009), pp. 624-635, ISSN

Lawler, J. M. (May 2011). Exacerbation of pathology by oxidative stress in respiratory and locomotor muscles with Duchenne muscular dystrophy. *J.Physiol*, Vol.589,No.Pt 9, (May 2011), pp. 2161-2170, ISSN

Li, S., Kimura, E., Fall, B. M., Reyes, M., Angello, J. C., Welikson, R., Hauschka, S. D., & Chamberlain, J. S. (July 2005). Stable transduction of myogenic cells with lentiviral vectors expressing a minidystrophin. *Gene Ther.*, Vol.12,No.14, (July 2005), pp. 1099-1108, ISSN

Linde, L., Boelz, S., Nissim-Rafinia, M., Oren, Y. S., Wilschanski, M., Yaacov, Y., Virgilis, D., Neu-Yilik, G., Kulozik, A. E., Kerem, E., & Kerem, B. (March 2007). Nonsense-mediated mRNA decay affects nonsense transcript levels and governs response of cystic fibrosis patients to gentamicin. *J.Clin.Invest*, Vol.117,No.3, (March 2007), pp. 683-692, ISSN

Linde, L. and Kerem, B. (November 2008). Introducing sense into nonsense in treatments of human genetic diseases. *Trends Genet.*, Vol.24,No.11, (November 2008), pp. 552-563, ISSN

Lu, Q. L., Mann, C. J., Lou, F., Bou-Gharios, G., Morris, G. E., Xue, S. A., Fletcher, S., Partridge, T. A., & Wilton, S. D. (August 2003). Functional amounts of dystrophin produced by skipping the mutated exon in the mdx dystrophic mouse. *Nat.Med.*, Vol.9,No.8, (August 2003), pp. 1009-1014, ISSN

Lu, Q. L., Rabinowitz, A., Chen, Y. C., Yokota, T., Yin, H., Alter, J., Jadoon, A., Bou-Gharios, G., & Partridge, T. (January 2005). Systemic delivery of antisense oligoribonucleotide restores dystrophin expression in body-wide skeletal muscles. *Proc.Natl.Acad.Sci.U.S.A*, Vol.102,No.1, (January 2005), pp. 198-203, ISSN

Malerba, A., Boldrin, L., & Dickson, G. (August 2011a). Long-term systemic administration of unconjugated morpholino oligomers for therapeutic expression of dystrophin by exon skipping in skeletal muscle: implications for cardiac muscle integrity. *Nucleic Acid Ther.*, Vol.21,No.4, (August 2011a), pp. 293-298, ISSN

Malerba, A., Sharp, P. S., Graham, I. R., Arechavala-Gomeza, V., Foster, K., Muntoni, F., Wells, D. J., & Dickson, G. (February 2011b). Chronic systemic therapy with low-dose morpholino oligomers ameliorates the pathology and normalizes locomotor behavior in mdx mice. *Mol.Ther.*, Vol.19,No.2, (February 2011b), pp. 345-354, ISSN

Malerba, A., Thorogood, F. C., Dickson, G., & Graham, I. R. (September 2009). Dosing regimen has a significant impact on the efficiency of morpholino oligomer-induced exon skipping in mdx mice. *Hum.Gene Ther.*, Vol.20,No.9, (September 2009), pp. 955-965, ISSN

Malik, V., Rodino-Klapac, L. R., Viollet, L., & Mendell, J. R. (November 2010a). Aminoglycoside-induced mutation suppression (stop codon readthrough) as a therapeutic strategy for Duchenne muscular dystrophy. *Ther.Adv.Neurol.Disord.*, Vol.3,No.6, (November 2010a), pp. 379-389, ISSN

Malik, V., Rodino-Klapac, L. R., Viollet, L., Wall, C., King, W., Al-Dahhak, R., Lewis, S., Shilling, C. J., Kota, J., Serrano-Munuera, C., Hayes, J., Mahan, J. D., Campbell, K. J., Banwell, B., Dasouki, M., Watts, V., Sivakumar, K., Bien-Willner, R., Flanigan, K. M., Sahenk, Z., Barohn, R. J., Walker, C. M., & Mendell, J. R. (June 2010b). Gentamicin-induced readthrough of stop codons in Duchenne muscular dystrophy. *Ann.Neurol.*, Vol.67,No.6, (June 2010b), pp. 771-780, ISSN

Mann, C. J., Honeyman, K., McClorey, G., Fletcher, S., & Wilton, S. D. (November 2002). Improved antisense oligonucleotide induced exon skipping in the mdx mouse model of muscular dystrophy. *J.Gene Med.*, Vol.4,No.6, (November 2002), pp. 644-654, ISSN

Manuvakhova, M., Keeling, K., & Bedwell, D. M. (July 2000). Aminoglycoside antibiotics mediate context-dependent suppression of termination codons in a mammalian translation system. *RNA.*, Vol.6,No.7, (July 2000), pp. 1044-1055, ISSN

Maruggi, G., Porcellini, S., Facchini, G., Perna, S. K., Cattoglio, C., Sartori, D., Ambrosi, A., Schambach, A., Baum, C., Bonini, C., Bovolenta, C., Mavilio, F., & Recchia, A. (May 2009). Transcriptional enhancers induce insertional gene deregulation independently from the vector type and design. *Mol.Ther.*, Vol.17,No.5, (May 2009), pp. 851-856, ISSN

Matsumura, K., Burghes, A. H., Mora, M., Tome, F. M., Morandi, L., Cornello, F., Leturcq, F., Jeanpierre, M., Kaplan, J. C., Reinert, P., & . (January 1994). Immunohistochemical analysis of dystrophin-associated proteins in Becker/Duchenne muscular dystrophy with huge in-frame deletions in the NH2-terminal and rod domains of dystrophin. *J.Clin.Invest*, Vol.93,No.1, (January 1994), pp. 99-105, ISSN

Matsumura, K. and Campbell, K. P. (January 1994). Dystrophin-glycoprotein complex: its role in the molecular pathogenesis of muscular dystrophies. *Muscle Nerve*, Vol.17,No.1, (January 1994), pp. 2-15, ISSN

Matsumura, K., Nonaka, I., Tome, F. M., Arahata, K., Collin, H., Leturcq, F., Recan, D., Kaplan, J. C., Fardeau, M., & Campbell, K. P. (August 1993). Mild deficiency of dystrophin-associated proteins in Becker muscular dystrophy patients having in-frame deletions in the rod domain of dystrophin. *Am.J.Hum.Genet.*, Vol.53,No.2, (August 1993), pp. 409-416, ISSN

Mendell, J. R., Campbell, K., Rodino-Klapac, L., Sahenk, Z., Shilling, C., Lewis, S., Bowles, D., Gray, S., Li, C., Galloway, G., Malik, V., Coley, B., Clark, K. R., Li, J., Xiao, X., Samulski, J., McPhee, S. W., Samulski, R. J., & Walker, C. M. (October 2010). Dystrophin immunity in Duchenne's muscular dystrophy. *N.Engl.J.Med.*, Vol.363,No.15, (October 2010), pp. 1429-1437, ISSN

Mendell, J. R., Moxley, R. T., Griggs, R. C., Brooke, M. H., Fenichel, G. M., Miller, J. P., King, W., Signore, L., Pandya, S., Florence, J., & . (June 1989). Randomized, double-blind six-month trial of prednisone in Duchenne's muscular dystrophy. *N.Engl.J.Med.*, Vol.320,No.24, (June 1989), pp. 1592-1597, ISSN

Meregalli, M., Farini, A., Parolini, D., Maciotta, S., & Torrente, Y. (August 2010). Stem cell therapies to treat muscular dystrophy: progress to date. *BioDrugs.*, Vol.24,No.4, (August 2010), pp. 237-247, ISSN

Miller, J. C., Tan, S., Qiao, G., Barlow, K. A., Wang, J., Xia, D. F., Meng, X., Paschon, D. E., Leung, E., Hinkley, S. J., Dulay, G. P., Hua, K. L., Ankoudinova, I., Cost, G. J., Urnov, F. D., Zhang, H. S., Holmes, M. C., Zhang, L., Gregory, P. D., & Rebar, E. J. (February 2011). A TALE nuclease architecture for efficient genome editing. *Nat.Biotechnol.*, Vol.29,No.2, (February 2011), pp. 143-148, ISSN

Mirabella, M., Galluzzi, G., Manfredi, G., Bertini, E., Ricci, E., De, L. R., Tonali, P., & Servidei, S. (August 1998). Giant dystrophin deletion associated with congenital cataract and mild muscular dystrophy. *Neurology*, Vol.51,No.2, (August 1998), pp. 592-595, ISSN

Monaco, A. P. (October 1989). Dystrophin, the protein product of the Duchenne/Becker muscular dystrophy gene. *Trends Biochem.Sci.*, Vol.14,No.10, (October 1989), pp. 412-415, ISSN

Monaco, A. P., Bertelson, C. J., Middlesworth, W., Colletti, C. A., Aldridge, J., Fischbeck, K. H., Bartlett, R., Pericak-Vance, M. A., Roses, A. D., & Kunkel, L. M. (August 1985). Detection of deletions spanning the Duchenne muscular dystrophy locus using a tightly linked DNA segment. *Nature*, Vol.316,No.6031, (August 1985), pp. 842-845, ISSN

Montarras, D., Morgan, J., Collins, C., Relaix, F., Zaffran, S., Cumano, A., Partridge, T., & Buckingham, M. (September 2005). Direct isolation of satellite cells for skeletal muscle regeneration. *Science*, Vol.309,No.5743, (September 2005), pp. 2064-2067, ISSN

Morgan, J. and Muntoni, F. (March 2007). Mural cells paint a new picture of muscle stem cells. *Nat.Cell Biol.*, Vol.9,No.3, (March 2007), pp. 249-251, ISSN

Moulton, H. M. and Moulton, J. D. (December 2010). Morpholinos and their peptide conjugates: therapeutic promise and challenge for Duchenne muscular dystrophy. *Biochim.Biophys.Acta*, Vol.1798,No.12, (December 2010), pp. 2296-2303, ISSN

Moxley, R. T., III and Pandya, S. (August 2011). Weekend high-dosage prednisone: A new option for treatment of Duchenne muscular dystrophy. *Neurology*, Vol.77,No.5, (August 2011), pp. 416-417, ISSN

Nagy, K. and Nagy, I. (November 1990). The effects of idebenone on the superoxide dismutase, catalase and glutathione peroxidase activities in liver and brain homogenates, as well as in brain synaptosomal and mitochondrial fractions. *Arch.Gerontol.Geriatr.*, Vol.11,No.3, (November 1990), pp. 285-291, ISSN

Ohlendieck, K. and Campbell, K. P. (December 1991). Dystrophin-associated proteins are greatly reduced in skeletal muscle from mdx mice. *J.Cell Biol.*, Vol.115,No.6, (December 1991), pp. 1685-1694, ISSN

Ohshima, S., Shin, J. H., Yuasa, K., Nishiyama, A., Kira, J., Okada, T., & Takeda, S. (January 2009). Transduction efficiency and immune response associated with the administration of AAV8 vector into dog skeletal muscle. *Mol.Ther.*, Vol.17,No.1, (January 2009), pp. 73-80, ISSN

Palmer, E., Wilhelm, J. M., & Sherman, F. (January 1979). Phenotypic suppression of nonsense mutants in yeast by aminoglycoside antibiotics. *Nature*, Vol.277,No.5692, (January 1979), pp. 148-150, ISSN

Palumbo, R., Sampaolesi, M., De, M. F., Tonlorenzi, R., Colombetti, S., Mondino, A., Cossu, G., & Bianchi, M. E. (February 2004). Extracellular HMGB1, a signal of tissue damage, induces mesoangioblast migration and proliferation. *J.Cell Biol.*, Vol.164,No.3, (February 2004), pp. 441-449, ISSN

Peault, B., Rudnicki, M., Torrente, Y., Cossu, G., Tremblay, J. P., Partridge, T., Gussoni, E., Kunkel, L. M., & Huard, J. (May 2007). Stem and progenitor cells in skeletal muscle development, maintenance, and therapy. *Mol.Ther.*, Vol.15,No.5, (May 2007), pp. 867-877, ISSN

Politano, L., Nigro, G., Nigro, V., Piluso, G., Papparella, S., Paciello, O., & Comi, L. I. (May 2003). Gentamicin administration in Duchenne patients with premature stop codon. Preliminary results. *Acta Myol.*, Vol.22,No.1, (May 2003), pp. 15-21, ISSN

Prins, K. W., Humston, J. L., Mehta, A., Tate, V., Ralston, E., & Ervasti, J. M. (August 2009). Dystrophin is a microtubule-associated protein. *J.Cell Biol.*, Vol.186,No.3, (August 2009), pp. 363-369, ISSN

Qu, Z., Balkir, L., Van Deutekom, J. C., Robbins, P. D., Pruchnic, R., & Huard, J. (September 1998). Development of approaches to improve cell survival in myoblast transfer therapy. *J.Cell Biol.*, Vol.142,No.5, (September 1998), pp. 1257-1267, ISSN

Qu-Petersen, Z., Deasy, B., Jankowski, R., Ikezawa, M., Cummins, J., Pruchnic, R., Mytinger, J., Cao, B., Gates, C., Wernig, A., & Huard, J. (May 2002). Identification of a novel population of muscle stem cells in mice: potential for muscle regeneration. *J.Cell Biol.*, Vol.157,No.5, (May 2002), pp. 851-864, ISSN

Rando, T. A., Disatnik, M. H., & Zhou, L. Z. (May 2000). Rescue of dystrophin expression in mdx mouse muscle by RNA/DNA oligonucleotides. *Proc.Natl.Acad.Sci.U.S.A*, Vol.97,No.10, (May 2000), pp. 5363-5368, ISSN

Rentschler, S., Linn, H., Deininger, K., Bedford, M. T., Espanel, X., & Sudol, M. (April 1999). The WW domain of dystrophin requires EF-hands region to interact with beta-dystroglycan. *Biol.Chem.*, Vol.380,No.4, (April 1999), pp. 431-442, ISSN

Rodino-Klapac, L. R., Montgomery, C. L., Bremer, W. G., Shontz, K. M., Malik, V., Davis, N., Sprinkle, S., Campbell, K. J., Sahenk, Z., Clark, K. R., Walker, C. M., Mendell, J. R., & Chicoine, L. G. (January 2010). Persistent expression of FLAG-tagged micro dystrophin in nonhuman primates following intramuscular and vascular delivery. *Mol.Ther.*, Vol.18,No.1, (January 2010), pp. 109-117, ISSN

Rybakova, I. N., Amann, K. J., & Ervasti, J. M. (November 1996). A new model for the interaction of dystrophin with F-actin. *J.Cell Biol.*, Vol.135,No.3, (November 1996), pp. 661-672, ISSN

Sampaolesi, M., Blot, S., D'Antona, G., Granger, N., Tonlorenzi, R., Innocenzi, A., Mognol, P., Thibaud, J. L., Galvez, B. G., Barthelemy, I., Perani, L., Mantero, S., Guttinger, M., Pansarasa, O., Rinaldi, C., Cusella De Angelis, M. G., Torrente, Y., Bordignon, C., Bottinelli, R., & Cossu, G. (November 2006). Mesoangioblast stem cells ameliorate muscle function in dystrophic dogs. *Nature*, Vol.444,No.7119, (November 2006), pp. 574-579, ISSN

Schwartz, M. and Duno, M. (2004). Improved molecular diagnosis of dystrophin gene mutations using the multiplex ligation-dependent probe amplification method. *Genet.Test.*, Vol.8,No.4, (2004), pp. 361-367, ISSN

Seale, P., Ishibashi, J., Scime, A., & Rudnicki, M. A. (May 2004). Pax7 is necessary and sufficient for the myogenic specification of CD45+:Sca1+ stem cells from injured muscle. *PLoS.Biol.*, Vol.2,No.5, (May 2004), pp. E130-

Singh, A., Ursic, D., & Davies, J. (January 1979). Phenotypic suppression and misreading Saccharomyces cerevisiae. *Nature*, Vol.277,No.5692, (January 1979), pp. 146-148, ISSN

Skuk, D., Goulet, M., Roy, B., Chapdelaine, P., Bouchard, J. P., Roy, R., Dugre, F. J., Sylvain, M., Lachance, J. G., Deschenes, L., Senay, H., & Tremblay, J. P. (April 2006). Dystrophin expression in muscles of duchenne muscular dystrophy patients after high-density injections of normal myogenic cells. *J.Neuropathol.Exp.Neurol.*, Vol.65,No.4, (April 2006), pp. 371-386, ISSN

Spitali, P., Rimessi, P., Fabris, M., Perrone, D., Falzarano, S., Bovolenta, M., Trabanelli, C., Mari, L., Bassi, E., Tuffery, S., Gualandi, F., Maraldi, N. M., Sabatelli-Giraud, P., Medici, A., Merlini, L., & Ferlini, A. (November 2009). Exon skipping-mediated dystrophin reading frame restoration for small mutations. *Hum.Mutat.*, Vol.30,No.11, (November 2009), pp. 1527-1534, ISSN

Sproat, B. S., Lamond, A. I., Beijer, B., Neuner, P., & Ryder, U. (May 1989). Highly efficient chemical synthesis of 2'-O-methyloligoribonucleotides and tetrabiotinylated derivatives; novel probes that are resistant to degradation by RNA or DNA specific nucleases. *Nucleic Acids Res.*, Vol.17,No.9, (May 1989), pp. 3373-3386, ISSN

Summerton, J. (December 1999). Morpholino antisense oligomers: the case for an RNase H-independent structural type. *Biochim.Biophys.Acta*, Vol.1489,No.1, (December 1999), pp. 141-158, ISSN

Suzuki, A., Yoshida, M., Hayashi, K., Mizuno, Y., Hagiwara, Y., & Ozawa, E. (March 1994). Molecular organization at the glycoprotein-complex-binding site of dystrophin. Three dystrophin-associated proteins bind directly to the carboxy-terminal portion of dystrophin. *Eur.J.Biochem.*, Vol.220,No.2, (March 1994), pp. 283-292, ISSN

Tremblay, J. P., Malouin, F., Roy, R., Huard, J., Bouchard, J. P., Satoh, A., & Richards, C. L. (March 1993). Results of a triple blind clinical study of myoblast transplantations without immunosuppressive treatment in young boys with Duchenne muscular dystrophy. *Cell Transplant.*, Vol.2,No.2, (March 1993), pp. 99-112, ISSN

Van Deutekom, J. C., Bremmer-Bout, M., Janson, A. A., Ginjaar, I. B., Baas, F., den Dunnen, J. T., & van Ommen, G. J. (July 2001). Antisense-induced exon skipping restores dystrophin expression in DMD patient derived muscle cells. *Hum.Mol.Genet.*, Vol.10,No.15, (July 2001), pp. 1547-1554, ISSN

Van Deutekom, J. C., Janson, A. A., Ginjaar, I. B., Frankhuizen, W. S., Aartsma-Rus, A., Bremmer-Bout, M., den Dunnen, J. T., Koop, K., van der Kooi, A. J., Goemans, N. M., de Kimpe, S. J., Ekhart, P. F., Venneker, E. H., Platenburg, G. J., Verschuuren, J. J., & van Ommen, G. J. (December 2007). Local dystrophin restoration with antisense oligonucleotide PRO051. *N.Engl.J.Med.*, Vol.357,No.26, (December 2007), pp. 2677-2686, ISSN

Wagner, K. R., Hamed, S., Hadley, D. W., Gropman, A. L., Burstein, A. H., Escolar, D. M., Hoffman, E. P., & Fischbeck, K. H. (June 2001). Gentamicin treatment of Duchenne and Becker muscular dystrophy due to nonsense mutations. *Ann.Neurol.*, Vol.49,No.6, (June 2001), pp. 706-711, ISSN

Wang, B., Li, J., Qiao, C., Chen, C., Hu, P., Zhu, X., Zhou, L., Bogan, J., Kornegay, J., & Xiao, X. (August 2008). A canine minidystrophin is functional and therapeutic in mdx mice. *Gene Ther.*, Vol.15,No.15, (August 2008), pp. 1099-1106, ISSN

Wang, B., Li, J., & Xiao, X. (December 2000). Adeno-associated virus vector carrying human minidystrophin genes effectively ameliorates muscular dystrophy in mdx mouse model. *Proc.Natl.Acad.Sci.U.S.A*, Vol.97,No.25, (December 2000), pp. 13714-13719, ISSN

Wang, Z., Kuhr, C. S., Allen, J. M., Blankinship, M., Gregorevic, P., Chamberlain, J. S., Tapscott, S. J., & Storb, R. (June 2007). Sustained AAV-mediated dystrophin expression in a canine model of Duchenne muscular dystrophy with a brief course of immunosuppression. *Mol.Ther.*, Vol.15,No.6, (June 2007), pp. 1160-1166, ISSN

Welch, E. M., Barton, E. R., Zhuo, J., Tomizawa, Y., Friesen, W. J., Trifillis, P., Paushkin, S., Patel, M., Trotta, C. R., Hwang, S., Wilde, R. G., Karp, G., Takasugi, J., Chen, G., Jones, S., Ren, H., Moon, Y. C., Corson, D., Turpoff, A. A., Campbell, J. A., Conn, M. M., Khan, A., Almstead, N. G., Hedrick, J., Mollin, A., Risher, N., Weetall, M., Yeh, S., Branstrom, A. A., Colacino, J. M., Babiak, J., Ju, W. D., Hirawat, S., Northcutt, V. J., Miller, L. L., Spatrick, P., He, F., Kawana, M., Feng, H., Jacobson, A., Peltz, S. W., & Sweeney, H. L. (May 2007). PTC124 targets genetic disorders caused by nonsense mutations. *Nature*, Vol.447,No.7140, (May 2007), pp. 87-91, ISSN

Wu, B., Benrashid, E., Lu, P., Cloer, C., Zillmer, A., Shaban, M., & Lu, Q. L. (2011a). Targeted skipping of human dystrophin exons in transgenic mouse model systemically for antisense drug development. *PLoS.One.*, Vol.6,No.5, (2011a), pp. e19906-

Wu, B., Li, Y., Morcos, P. A., Doran, T. J., Lu, P., & Lu, Q. L. (May 2009). Octa-guanidine morpholino restores dystrophin expression in cardiac and skeletal muscles and ameliorates pathology in dystrophic mdx mice. *Mol.Ther.*, Vol.17,No.5, (May 2009), pp. 864-871, ISSN

Wu, B., Lu, P., Benrashid, E., Malik, S., Ashar, J., Doran, T. J., & Lu, Q. L. (January 2010). Dose-dependent restoration of dystrophin expression in cardiac muscle of dystrophic mice by systemically delivered morpholino. *Gene Ther.*, Vol.17,No.1, (January 2010), pp. 132-140, ISSN

Wu, B., Moulton, H. M., Iversen, P. L., Jiang, J., Li, J., Li, J., Spurney, C. F., Sali, A., Guerron, A. D., Nagaraju, K., Doran, T., Lu, P., Xiao, X., & Lu, Q. L. (September 2008). Effective rescue of dystrophin improves cardiac function in dystrophin-deficient mice by a modified morpholino oligomer. *Proc.Natl.Acad.Sci.U.S.A*, Vol.105,No.39, (September 2008), pp. 14814-14819, ISSN

Wu, B., Xiao, B., Cloer, C., Shaban, M., Sali, A., Lu, P., Li, J., Nagaraju, K., Xiao, X., & Lu, Q. L. (March 2011b). One-year treatment of morpholino antisense oligomer improves skeletal and cardiac muscle functions in dystrophic mdx mice. *Mol.Ther.*, Vol.19,No.3, (March 2011b), pp. 576-583, ISSN

Yin, H., Moulton, H. M., Betts, C., Seow, Y., Boutilier, J., Iverson, P. L., & Wood, M. J. (November 2009). A fusion peptide directs enhanced systemic dystrophin exon skipping and functional restoration in dystrophin-deficient mdx mice. *Hum.Mol.Genet.*, Vol.18,No.22, (November 2009), pp. 4405-4414, ISSN

Yin, H., Moulton, H. M., Seow, Y., Boyd, C., Boutilier, J., Iverson, P., & Wood, M. J. (December 2008). Cell-penetrating peptide-conjugated antisense oligonucleotides restore systemic muscle and cardiac dystrophin expression and function. *Hum.Mol.Genet.*, Vol.17,No.24, (December 2008), pp. 3909-3918, ISSN

Yin, H., Saleh, A. F., Betts, C., Camelliti, P., Seow, Y., Ashraf, S., Arzumanov, A., Hammond, S., Merritt, T., Gait, M. J., & Wood, M. J. (July 2011). Pip5 transduction peptides direct high efficiency oligonucleotide-mediated dystrophin exon skipping in heart and phenotypic correction in mdx mice. *Mol.Ther.*, Vol.19,No.7, (July 2011), pp. 1295-1303, ISSN

Yokota, T., Lu, Q. L., Partridge, T., Kobayashi, M., Nakamura, A., Takeda, S., & Hoffman, E. (June 2009). Efficacy of systemic morpholino exon-skipping in Duchenne dystrophy dogs. *Ann.Neurol.*, Vol.65,No.6, (June 2009), pp. 667-676, ISSN

Yoshida, M., Suzuki, A., Yamamoto, H., Noguchi, S., Mizuno, Y., & Ozawa, E. (June 1994). Dissociation of the complex of dystrophin and its associated proteins into several unique groups by n-octyl beta-D-glucoside. *Eur.J.Biochem.*, Vol.222,No.3, (June 1994), pp. 1055-1061, ISSN

Yoshida, M., Yamamoto, H., Noguchi, S., Mizuno, Y., Hagiwara, Y., & Ozawa, E. (July 1995). Dystrophin-associated protein A0 is a homologue of the Torpedo 87K protein. *FEBS Lett.*, Vol.367,No.3, (July 1995), pp. 311-314, ISSN

Yoshizawa, S., Fourmy, D., & Puglisi, J. D. (November 1998). Structural origins of gentamicin antibiotic action. *EMBO J.*, Vol.17,No.22, (November 1998), pp. 6437-6448, ISSN

3

Exon Skipping and Myoblast Transplantation: Single or Combined Potential Options for Treatment of Duchenne Muscular Dystrophy

T. Iannitti[1,*], D. Lodi[2], V. Sblendorio[3], V. Rottigni[4] and B. Palmieri[3]
*[1]Department of Physiology, School of Medicine,
University of Kentucky Medical Center, Lexington,
[2]Department of Nephrology, Dialysis and Transplantation, University of Modena and
Reggio Emilia Medical School, Modena,
[3]Department of General Surgery and Surgical Specialties, University of Modena and
Reggio Emilia Medical School, Surgical Clinic, Modena,
Present address: Unit of Pharmacology, Department of Pharmacobiology,
Faculty of Pharmacy, University of Bari,
[4]Department of General Surgery and Surgical Specialties, University of Modena and
Reggio Emilia Medical School, Surgical Clinic, Modena,
[1]USA
[2,3,4]Italy*

1. Introduction

Edward Meryon, an English doctor, described Duchenne muscular dystrophy (DMD) for the first time, but the symptoms and the histology typical of this condition were firstly described by Duchenne de Boulogne in 1861. The dystrophin gene (dys) was firstly identified by Kunkel and coworkers (Kunkel et al., 1986), while Hoffman and colleagues (Hoffman et al., 1987) identified the gene product dystrophin. This protein is lacking in DMD patients' muscles and, due to its essentiality in membrane stability, its absence induces contraction-related membrane damage and the activation of the inflammatory cascade, leading to muscle failure, necrosis, and fibrosis (Hoffmann and Dressman, 2001; Blake et al., 2002; Palmieri B. and Sblendorio V., 2006). This condition affects primarily human and animal skeletal and cardiac muscle and it is defined as an X-linked recessive disease with the most cases inherited from carrier mothers, and about a third of cases occurring as de novo mutations in the infants. DMD is present at birth, but clinical symptoms are not evident until 3 to 5 years of age (leg weakness, increasing spine kyphosis, and a waddle-like gait) and usually its diagnosis is made on the basis of gait spine abnormalities from 4 to 5 years after birth (Dubowitz et al., 1975; Jennekens et al., 1991). DMD patients display problems in climbing stairs and rising up from the floor; they are unable to run, and in a variable way, most of them lose ambulation by 7 to 12 years (Iannitti et al., 2010). Moreover, other characteristics of this

---

* Corresponding Author

disease are the progressive loss of respiratory function that can lead to respiratory failure, scoliosis, weight loss, cardiomyopathy, and finally death, as a result of respiratory and cardiac complications (Iannitti et al., 2010). The continuous muscle wasting, that characterizes this pathological condition, puts DMD patients, from 8 to 12 years of age, in wheelchairs with scoliosis developing in 90% of boys who use a wheelchair full-time and die in the late teens or early twenties due to respiratory/cardiac failure after a worsening of symptoms (Emery, 1993). In children with DMD, non-progressive abnormalities of the central nervous system have also been observed. In fact, the mean intelligence quotient of these patients is 82 which is 18 points under the mean value of the healthy population, while 30% of the patients have a quotient under 75 (Bresolin et al., 1994).In particular, verbal intelligence is primarily affected and 80% of DMD patients display atypical electroretinography with the most prominent portion of the normal electroretinogram, the wave b, that is absent (Billard et al., 1992; Sigesmund et al., 1994).

Inflammation, mediated by neutrophils, macrophages and cytokines, also seems to be involved in the damage of dystrophic muscles (Whitehead et al., 2006). Gosselin and colleagues (Gosselin et al., 2004) described the important role played by inflammation showing that a persistent inflammatory response has been observed in dystrophic skeletal muscle leading to an alteration in extracellular environment; it includes an increase in inflammatory cells, such as macrophages and elevated levels of various inflammatory cytokines like tumor necrosis factor alpha (TNF-α) that contributes to muscle degeneration, while pro-fibrotic cytokines, such as transforming growth factor beta (TGF-β), can account for a progressive fibrosis. Experimental studies, using the DMD mdx mouse model, support this fact reporting that the depletion of inflammatory cells, such as neutrophils, cromolyn blockade of mast cell degranulation or pharmacological blockade of TNF, reduces necrosis of dystrophic myofibers (DeSilva et al., 1987).

2. Dystrophin

The human dystrophin gene (13.973 nucleotides), dys, maps at the Xp21.1 locus; it is encoded by a 2.25-Mbp gene with 79 exons and 99.4% of its sequence is composed of introns (the fully processed transcript is only 14 Kbp) (Kunkel et al., 1986). The DMD gene can produce different dystrophin isoforms through alternative promoter usage and splicing of pre-mRNA and the predominant isoform is an approximately 427-kDa cytoskeletal protein that consists of 3685 amino acids constituting 5% of sarcolemmal protein and 0.002% of total striated muscle protein (Hoffman et al., 1987; Koenig et al., 1988).

Four domains constitute the structure of full length dystrophin, i.e. an N-terminal "acting binding" domain, a middle "rod" domain consisting of spectrin-like repeats, a cysteine-rich domain encoded by exons 62 to 70 and a C-terminal domain. The last two domains play a key role in the assembly of the dystroglycan complex and in the sarcolemmal function (Petrof, 2002; Palmieri and Sblendorio, 2006). When a mutation and deletion occur in the dystrophin gene, as observed in DMD patients, the protein cannot be produced leading to its complete absence in muscle fibers. Dystrophin belongs to a group of proteins called dystrophin glycoprotein complex (DGC), which also include cytoskeletal actin, the dystroglycan integral membrane proteins, the syntrophins, dystrobrevins and α-catulin (Brown et al., 1997).Dystrophin links the actin intracellular microfilament network to the extracellular matrix and its absence changes the level and localization of DGC, making the sarcolemma fragile and muscle fibers prone to degeneration during repeated cycles of muscle contraction and relaxation. Actin associates with the N-terminal of dystrophin, in a region displaying two calponin homology domains (Corrado et al., 1994; Norwood et al., 2000; Way et al., 1992), while the other proteins bind to the C-terminal region of dystrophin. The association of b-dystroglycan with dystrophin is mediated by a cysteine-rich region of dystrophin that contains a protein module with two highly conserved tryptophans (WW domain) and 2 EF-handlike motifs (Huang et al., 2000; Jung et al., 1995). Furthermore, b-dystroglycan associates with the extracellular protein a-dystroglycan which, in turn, connects to laminin in the extracellular matrix (ECM) (Henry et al., 1998; Henry et al., 1999; Hohenester et al., 1999).Dystrophin, through its association with actin and dystroglycan, represents a key bridge between the ECM and cytoskeleton, playing an important role in the structural integrity of the muscle cell membrane. The absence or disruption of dystrophin, observed in DMD, also exerts some effects on the central nervous system (CNS) function. In fact the dystrophin role in the positioning of receptors and channels is relevant at the synapse level where the neuromuscular junction exerts an important role on the synapse structure and function (Hall et al., 1993; Sanes et al., 1999). Dystrophin is localized in the deep regions of junctional folds at the post-synaptic face (Bewick et al., 1992; Sealock et al., 1991) and, through its association with its complex of proteins (Fig. 1), dystrophin plays both structural and signalling roles.

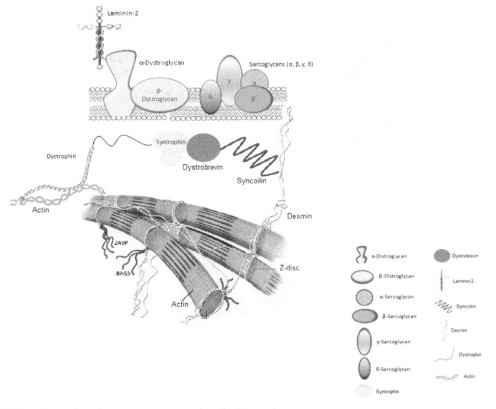

Fig. 1. Complex of proteins associated with dystrophin.

Other clinical aspects of the DMD pathophysiology have been reported. These are cognitive impairment and lower intelligence quotient (IQ) (average = 85) observed in boys with DMD, disordered CNS architecture, abnormalities in dendrites and loss of neurons. Moreover, at the biochemical level, the bioenergetics of the CNS is abnormal, and there is an increase in the concentration of choline-containing compounds, indicative of CNS pathology.

Dystrophin expression is regulated by seven independent promoters, three of which regulate the expression of full-length isoforms, while four intragenic promoters regulate the expression of different short isoforms in various tissues. Two additional isoforms are considered to be full-length and are expressed in the brain. The mutation, that affects dystrophin promoter regions and regulates the expression of brain isoforms, may be the cause of neurological symptoms in some patients with DMD. Each of the additional transcripts results in the expression of multiple dystrophin proteins (Dp) that are indicated according to their molecular weight: Dp427 muscle, Dp427 brain, Dp427 purkinje, Dp260, Dp140, Dp116, and Dp71 (Muntoni et al., 2003).These last four variants contain unique first exons and lack the actin binding domain, suggesting that they may have functions that are different from the ones ascribed to full-length dystrophin. Dp260 in the retina and Dp71 in the brain and other tissues restore the integrity of DGC, but only Dp260, the longest of the short isoforms, restores some functional integrity in the dystrophic muscle. These findings suggest that a better bridge between ECM and actin is more necessary for the improvement of dystrophic muscle function than the one provided by the Dp71 variant.

Alternative splicing of exons 71 to 74 and 78 increases the diversity of transcripts; the first splicing regulates interactions with syntrophins. These exons can be spliced singularly or in a different combination, generating a series of in-frame spliced variants.

The elimination of exons 73 and 74 in any of these transcripts generates a functional protein that lacks the syntrophin binding sites (Yang et al., 1995; Newey et al., 2000). The splicing of exons gives a translational frame shift, producing the substitution of the last 13 amino acids of the predominantly hydrophilic C-terminal region with 31 hydrophobic amino acids. This process is regulated in a developmental and tissue- specific way (Tennyson et al., 1996). The hydrophobic splice variant is abundant in the cerebral cortex and retina and it serves to regulate the binding of dystrophin to α-catulin and its associated proteins (Roberts et al., 1998).

3. Searching criteria and aim

We have been searching Pubmed/Medline, using the key words "Duchenne", "Muscular" and "Dystrophy" combined with "Exon", "Skipping", "Immunosuppressant", "Stem", "Cells", "Myoblast" and "Transplantation", in order to collect and analyze all the recent advances in DMD, focusing on clinical trials performed in humans. This chapter highlights the most promising therapeutic approaches to DMD, i.e. exon skipping and myoblast transplantation with some details about the immunosuppressive therapy.

4. Immunosuppressant drugs

Among the scientific community there is a growing interest in the use of immunosuppressant drugs that may potentially give clinical benefits during the DMD course. The interest is due to the host transplant, potential immunosuppressant schedule that should be suitable to increase myoblast or mesangioblast graft survival supporting, in the meantime, the autologous crippled mass function. Among immunosuppressant drugs, corticosteroids slow DMD progression and, in particular, two corticosteroids, i.e. prednisone and deflazacort have been extensively used because of their ability to improve skeletal muscle function. Research has also focused on the use of suppressing drugs acting against TNF level and suppressing calcineurin signals.

The long-term effects of deflazacort treatment has been investigated according to two treatment protocols from Naples (N) and Toronto (T) in boys, aged between 8 and 15 years, who were affected by DMD and had 4 or more years of deflazacort treatment (Biggar et al., 2001).Thirty seven boys were treated with protocol N, using deflazacort at a dose of 0.6 mg/kg per day for the first 20 days of the month and no deflazacort for the remainder of the month.Vitamin D and calcium were administered daily to boys with osteoporosis. Deflazacort treatment started between 4 and 8 years of age. Thirty two were treated with protocol T, using deflazacort at a dose of 0.9 mg/kg per day, plus vitamin D and calcium daily. Treatment started between 6 and 8 years of age. All boys were monitored every 4 to 6 months and the results were compared with age-matched control subjects in the two groups (19 for protocol N and 30 for protocol T). It was observed that: 1) for the boys treated with protocol N, 97% were ambulatory at 9 years (control, 22%), 35% at 12 years (control, 0%) and 25% at 15 years (control, 0%); 2) for the 32 boys treated with protocol T, 100% were ambulatory at 9 years (control, 48%), 83% at 12 years (control, 0%) and 77% at 15 years (control, 0%); 3) in boys aged 13 and older, scoliosis developed in 30% of boys in protocol N, 16% in protocol T, and 90% of control subjects. 30% of boys, who were treated according to protocol T, had asymptomatic cataracts, but they did not require any treatment. Fractures occurred in 19% of boys in protocol N (controls: 16%) and 16% of boys in protocol T (controls: 20%). Summarizing, long term deflazacort treatment has beneficial effects on both protocols, although protocol T seems to be more effective and it is frequently associated with asymptomatic cataracts.

The same group (Biggar et al., 2006) designed a study involving 54 boys (30 treated with deflazacort), aged between 7 and 15 years, affected by DMD, who were reviewed retrospectively. The boys, untreated with deflazacort, stopped walking at 9.8 ± 1.8 years, while 7 out of 30 treated boys stopped walking at 12.3 ± 2.7 years (P < 0.05). Among the 23 boys who were still walking, 21 were 10 year older; pulmonary function was significantly greater in 15 year old treated boys (88% ± 18%) than in untreated boys (39% ± 20%) (P<0.001). Between 9 and 15 years, the treated boys were shorter and, between 9 and 13 years, the treated boys weighed less. After 13 years, the treated boys maintained their weight, whereas the untreated boys lost weight. Asymptomatic cataracts developed in 10 out of 30 boys who had received deflazacort.

Another clinical study compared the course of 74 boys, aged from 10 to 18 years, and affected by DMD, treated (n = 40) and untreated (n = 34) with deflazacort (Biggar et al., 2006). The treated boys were able to rise from a supine condition to standing, climb stairs, and walk 10 m without aids from 3 to 5 years longer than the untreated boys. After 10 years of age, the treated boys had a significantly better pulmonary function than the untreated boys and, after 15 years of age, 8 out of 17 untreated boys required nocturnal ventilation unlike the 40 treated boys. As for boys older than 15 years of age, 11 out of 17 untreated boys required assistance with feeding unlike the treated boys. Towards 18 years, 30 out of 34 untreated boys had a spinal curve greater than 20° if compared with 4 out of the 40 treated boys. By 18 years of age, 7 out of 34 untreated boys had lost 25% or more of their body weight (treated 0 out of 40) and four of those 7 boys required a gastric feeding tube. By 18 years of age, 20 out of 34 untreated boys had cardiac left ventricular ejection fractions, less than 45% if compared with 4 out of the 40 treated boys and 12 out of 34 died in their second decade (17.6 ± 1.7 years), primarily of cardiorespiratory complications. Two out of 40 boys, treated with deflazacort, died at 13 and 18 years of age from cardiac failure. The treated boys were significantly shorter, did not have excessive weight gain, and 22 out of 40 had asymptomatic cataracts. Long bone fractures occurred in 25% of boys in both the treated and untreated groups. The authors conclude that these long-term observations are the most encouraging. The major benefits of daily deflazacort appear to be the prolonged ambulation, improvement in cardiac and pulmonary functions, delay in the need for spinal instrumentation, and a greater independence for self-feeding. According to the described last two studies, deflazacort has a significant impact on health, quality of life, and healthcare costs for boys with DMD and their families and it is associated with a few side effects.

Houde and coworkers (Houde et al., 2008) collected data over an 8-year period for 79 patients with DMD, 37 of whom were treated with deflazacort. Deflazacort (dose of 0.9 mg/kg adjusted to a maximum of 1 mg/kg according to the side effects) was started when the boys showed a functional decline resulting in ambulating difficulties. The mean length of treatment was 66 months.

The treated boys stopped walking at 11.5 ± 1.9 years, whereas the untreated boys stopped walking at 9.6 ± 1.4 years. The cardiac function, assessed by echocardiography every 6 to 12 months, was better preserved as shown by a normal shortening fraction in treated (30.8% ± 4.5%) versus untreated boys (26.6% ± 5.7%, $P < 0.05$), a higher ejection fraction (52.9% ± 6.3% treated versus 46% ± 10% untreated), and lower frequency of dilated cardiomyopathy (32% treated versus 58% untreated). No change was observed in blood pressure, left ventricle end-diastolic diameter, or cardiac mass. Scoliosis was much less severe in treated (14° ± 22.5°) than in untreated boys (46° ± 224°) and no spinal surgery was necessary in treated boys. Limb fractures occurred in 24% of treated and in 26% of untreated boys, whereas vertebral fractures occurred in the treated group only (7 out of 37 compared with zero in the untreated group). In both groups, weight excess was observed at 8 years of age, and its frequency tripled between the ages of 8 and 12 years. More patients had weight excess in the treated group (13 out of 21 [62%]) than in the untreated group (6 out of 11 [55%]), at 12 years of age. Cataracts developed in 49% of treated patients and, in almost all of these patients, they developed after at least 5 year treatment. This study underlines that deflazacort use in DMD prolongs walking for at least 2 years, slows the decline of vital capacity, and postpones the need for mechanical ventilation. The quality of life seems to improve in terms of prolonged independence in transfers and rolling over in bed, as well as sitting comfortably without having to resort to surgery.

A study determined and compared the long-term effects of prednisone and deflazacort on 49 boys, aged between 12 and 15 years, with DMD over a 7-year follow up period (Balaban et al., 2005). Eighteen boys were treated with prednisone, 12 with deflazacort, and 19 had no drug treatment. Analyzing their lower and upper limb motor functions, pulmonary function, prevalence of surgery for scoliosis and side effects, they reached these results: the boys in the steroid groups were significantly more functional and performed better on all tests than the untreated boys (P < 0.05); there was no significant difference between deflazacort- and prednisone-treated groups (P >0.05); the number of boys having scoliosis surgery among the treated groups was significantly less than the one of untreated boys (P<0.05); the control group's capacity had decreased and was significantly less than the one of both the prednisone and deflazacort treated boys; both deflazacort and prednisone had beneficial effects on the pulmonary function and scoliosis; cataracts, hypertension, behavioural changes, excessive weight gain, and vertebral fracture were noted as serious side effects. The results of this long-term study are very encouraging and both prednisone and deflazacort seem to have a significant beneficial effect on slowing the disease progress. Their use in DMD may prolong ambulation and upper limb function with similar potency. Both steroids are also able to improve pulmonary function, more than delay the need for spinal interventions, with similar therapeutic profiles.

A study was performed in 17 patients affected by DMD, aged between 17 and 22 years, treated with deflazacort (0.9 mg/kg/day) and compared with DMD patients who did not receive any treatment, in order to evaluate the involvement of cardiac and sternocleidomastoid muscles by means of magnetic resonance imaging (MRI) measurement of T2 relaxation time and the left ventricular systolic function (Mavrogeni et al., 2009). This study showed that DMD patients, treated with deflazacort, present a better cardiac and skeletal profile compared to DMD patients without medication (p<0.001).

Dubowitz and colleagues (Dubowitz et al., 2002) reported a 5-year follow up of two 4-year-old boys, with classic DMD with an out-of-frame deletion in the Duchenne gene and absence of dystrophin in their muscle, who had a quite remarkable response to an intermittent, low dosage regime of prednisolone (0.75 mg/kg per day for 10 days each month or alternating 10 days on and 10 days off). In the first case, there was a complete remission of all clinical signs of dystrophy, sustained, almost fully, up to the present time; in the second case, the initial response was almost as marked, sustained for almost 5 years before showing a fairly rapid decline over the ensuing year that resulted in loss of independent ambulation at the age of 10. Both boys remained around the 50th percentile as for height and weight and showed no evidence of demineralization of bone on consecutive dual x-ray absorptiometry scanning of the spine nor any signs of chronic prednisolone toxicity. Although this study involved a limited number of patients, it showed that there might be an optimal window for treatment in the early stages of the disease and further larger-scale controlled studies should be targeted more selectively at this stage of the disease. This report also showed that a regime of low-dosage, intermittent prednisolone, with cycles of 10 day treatment, either per month or alternating with 10 days off treatment, is well tolerated in children affected by DMD.

Markham and colleagues (Markham et al., 2005) studied the effect of steroids in the cardiac function of patients with DMD. They evaluated the left ventricular systolic function and cardiac geometry of those subjects through a transthoracic echocardiogram; 111 patients, aged 21 years or younger, affected by DMD, were selected. They were divided into two groups: untreated (never exposed or treated for less than 6 months) and steroid-treated (steroids were administered longer than 6 months); the subjects did not differ in age, height, weight, body mass index, systolic and diastolic blood pressure, or left ventricular mass. Among the treated patients, 29 received prednisone and 19 received deflazacort. TThis study showed that treatment, either with prednisone or deflazacort, appears to have an impact on the decline in cardiac function seen with DMD. The shortening fraction was significantly lower in the untreated group than in the steroid-treated one. The authors concluded that deflazacort and prednisone were equally effective in preserving the cardiac function. This study shows that the progressive decline in cardiac muscle function can be altered by steroid treatment. In particular steroid treatment brings a clinical improvement in respiratory and cardiac function in DMD patients, during and beyond their treatment period. Moreover, it has the potential to prolong their survival.

A randomized controlled trial of prednisone and azathioprine, involving 99 boys aged between 5 and 15 years and affected by DMD, was conducted with the aim to assess the longer-term effects of prednisone and to determine whether azathioprine, alone or in combination with prednisone, is able to improve strength (Griggs et al., 1993). The patients were divided into 3 groups: placebo; 0.3 mg/kg prednisone per day; 0.75 mg/kg prednisone per day. After 6 months, 2 to 2.5 mg/kg azathioprine per day was added to the first two groups and placebo added to the third group. The study showed that the beneficial effect of prednisone (0.75mg/kg per day) is maintained for at least 18 months and it is associated with a 36% increase in muscle mass. Weight gain, growth retardation, and other side effects were associated with prednisone and azathioprine did not have any beneficial effect. The authors conclude that prednisone beneficial effect is not the result of immunosuppression.

Kirschner et al. (Kirschner et al., 2008) conducted a randomized, multicenter, double-blind placebo-controlled trial. One hundred and fifty three patients were randomized to receive either placebo or 4 mg/kg ciclosporin A (CsA). After 3 months, both groups received additional treatment with intermittent prednisone (0.75 mg/kg, 10 days on/10 days off) for 12 months more. In each group, 73 patients were available for intention to treat analysis. Baseline characteristics were comparable in both groups. There was no significant difference between the two groups concerning primary (manual muscle strength according to the Medical Research Council) and secondary (myometry, loss of ambulation, side effects) outcome measures. Peak CsA values were measured blindly and ranged from 12 to 658 ng/mL (mean, 210 ng/mL) in the verum group. According to this study CsA does not improve muscle strength as a monotherapy and the efficacy of intermittent prednisone in DMD. Calcineurin inhibitors induced chronic nephrotoxicity as reported in a previous study (Naesens et al., 2009).

Sharma and coworkers (Sharma et al., 1993) tested CsA in 15 patients affected by DMD and observed an increase in the muscular force generation, measuring the titanic force and maximum voluntary contraction (MVC) of both anterior tibial muscles. Normally the titanic force and MVC declined during 4 months in patients with DMD. During 8 week CsA treatment (5 mg/kg per day), the titanic force significantly increased (25.8% 6 6.6%) and MVC (13.6% 6 4.0%) occurred in two weeks' time. The CsA side effects, gastrointestinal and flu-like symptoms were transient and self-limiting. Straathof and colleagues (Straathof et al., 2009) retrospectively analyzed 35 DMD patients' data, who were treated with 0.75 mg/kg prednisone per day intermittently, 10 days on/10 days off. Prednisone was started during the ambulant phase at the age 3.5 up to 9.7 years. The median period of treatment was 27 months. The authors reported the following results: the median age at which ambulation was lost was 10.8 years; 9 patients (26%) had excessive weight gain; 8 boys (21%) had a bone fracture that happened when four of those 8 children lost the ability to walk. Treatment was stopped in 2 obese patients, 2 hyperactive boys, and 1 patient after a fracture. Based on the previously described data, the authors conclude that prednisone, 10 days on/10 days off, has relatively few side effects and extends the ambulant phase for 1 year if compared to historical controls.

5. Exon skipping

DMD is caused by mutations in the dystrophin gene (Aartsma-Rus et al., 2006; Muntoni, 2003), leading to disruption of the open reading frame (Fig. 2a). Monaco et al. (Monaco et al., 1988) found that frame shift mutations in the DMD gene will lead to a truncated and non-functional dystrophin. Patients with such mutations present less severe Becker muscular dystrophy. This reading frame rule holds true for ~91% of DMD cases (Aartsma-Rus et al., 2006) and has inspired the development of the exon skipping strategy which employs antisense oligonucleotides (AON). These small synthetic RNA molecules are complimentary to exonic or splice site sequences, thereby, upon hybridization, they are able to modulate exon inclusion by the splicing machinery (Manzur et al., 2009; Trollet et al., 2009; van Ommen et al., 2008). Although the functionality of the resulting protein may vary, this treatment could delay or even stop disease progression and improve function in the remaining muscle (Melis et al., 1998; Helderman-van den Enden et al., 2010). The antisense oligonucleotides are chemically modified to resist nucleases and promote RNA binding and are designed to have high sequence specificity. A lot of studies have provided the proof of principle of the therapeutic feasibility of the AON to reframe dystrophin transcripts and restore dystrophin synthesis, both in vitro (Aartsma-Rus et al., 2002, 2003, 2004) and in vivo using the mdx and DMD mice (Mann et al., 2002; Bremmer-Bout et al., 2004; Heemskerk et al., 2009). In studies in the mdx mouse model, oligonucleotides with chemical properties, similar to the ones of 2'-O-methyl-phosphorothioate (2'OMePS) RNA, were taken up in dystrophin-deficient muscle up to 10 times as much as in healthy muscle tissue, most likely owing to increased permeability of the muscle myofiber membrane. In addition, 4 to 8 weeks' subcutaneous delivery of the oligonucleotides resulted in a steady increase in oligonucleotides levels, exon skipping and dystrophin levels (Heemskerk et al., 2010).

Exon skipping provides a mutation-specific, and so potentially personalized, therapeutic approach for patients with DMD (Fig. 2b). Since mutations cluster around exons 45-55 of DMD, the skipping of one specific exon may be therapeutic for patients with a variety of mutations. The skipping of exon 51 affects the largest subgroup of patients (approximately 13%), including the ones with deletions of exons 45 to 50, 48 to 50, or 52 (Aartsma-Rus et al., 2009). Subsequent clinical trials have shown that two different AON chemistries, either 2'OMePS (van Deutekom et al., 2007) or phosphorodiamidate morpholino oligomer (PMO) (Kinali et al., 2009), targeting DMD exon 51, can restore local dystrophin synthesis in DMD patients with no or minimum side effects. However, some relevant points of pathophysiologic DMD cascade, such as severe muscle wasting, fibrosis and deficient muscle regeneration, may reduce the efficacy of the DMD exon skipping therapy. In addition, as DMD patients suffer from muscle degeneration from their early life, myoblasts undergo extensive division in an attempt to regenerate, eventually leading to exhaustion of the muscle regenerative potential (Yoshida et al., 1998; Hawke et al., 2001; Blau et al., 1985). To overcome these problems, there have been several additional therapies in which myostatin inhibition has received considerable interest (Kemaladewi et al., 2011).

Here we report the three clinical trials based on the exon skipping approach which have been performed to date and we describe the trials that are still ongoing. A study, consisting in the injection of 0.8 mg of PRO051 into the tibialis anterior muscle, was performed by van Deutekom and colleagues (van Deutekom et al., 2007). PRO051 is a 2'OMePS antisense oligoribonucleotide complementary to a 20-nucleotide sequence within exon 51. Four patients with DMD were included in this study and they all had deletions that were correctable by exon-51skipping and had no evidence of dystrophin in the previously made diagnostic muscle biopsy. For every patient mutational status and positive exon-skipping response to PRO051 in vitro were confirmed, and T1-weighted MRI was used to determine the condition of the tibialis anterior muscle. The intramuscular injection of PRO051 induced exon-51 skipping, corrected the reading frame, and thus introduced dystrophin in the muscle in all four patients affected by DMD. PRO051 restored dystrophin to levels between 3-12% or 17- 35%, basing on quantification relative to total protein or myofiber content. The poorest results that were obtained in a patient, who had the most advanced disease, led the authors to underline the importance of using patients at a relatively young age, since in them relatively little muscle tissue has been replaced by fibrotic and adipose tissue. Among the adverse effects, mild local pain at the injection site was reported by a patient. Mild-to-moderate pain, after the muscle biopsy, was also reported. Blistering under the bandages used for wound closure was reported by two patients. In the period of time elapsing between injection and biopsy, flu-like symptoms were observed in two patients and a mild diarrhea in a patient.

A dose escalation intramuscular trial was performed in 7 patients (2 patients received 0 09 mg and 5 patients received 0 9 mg of AVI-4658) who received injections in one extensor digitorum brevis (EDB) muscle, while the contralateral EDB muscle was injected with 900 μL normal saline (Kinali et al., 2009). The 7 patients had deletions in the open reading frame of DMD that are responsive to exon 51 and were selected on the basis of the preservation of EDB muscle, as assessed by MRI, and the response of cultured fi fibroblasts from a skin biopsy to AVI-4658. Muscles were biopsied between 3 and 4 weeks after injection. No adverse events, related to AVI-4658, were reported in this study and they showed an increased dystrophin expression in all treated EDB muscles. Immunostaining of EDB-treated muscle for dystrophin was performed. In the areas of the immunostained sections, that were close to the needle track through which AVI-4658 was given, 44-79% of myofibres had increased expression of dystrophin. In randomly chosen sections of treated EDB muscles, the mean intensity of dystrophin staining ranged from 22% to 32% of the mean intensity of dystrophin in healthy control muscles (mean 26 4%), and the mean intensity was 17% (range 11-21%) greater than the intensity in the contralateral saline-treated muscle. In the dystrophin-positive fibres, the intensity of dystrophin staining was up to 42% of that in healthy muscle. Western blot analysis detected increased expression of dystrophin in the AVI-4658-treated muscle of all patients who received the high dose, and the immunoblot detected expression of dystrophin of the expected molecular weight in all patients. This study has led to a dose-ranging systemic study of AVI-4658 in ambulant patients affected by DMD (ClinicalTrials.gov, number NCT00844597).

A phase 1-2a study has been conducted to assess the safety, pharmacokinetics and molecular and clinical effects of systemically administered PRO051 (Goemans et al., 2011). PRO051 was administered subcutaneously for 15 weeks in 12 patients, with each of four possible doses (0.5, 2.0, 4.0, and 6.0 mg per kilogram of body weight) given to 3 patients. Irritation at the administration site and, during the extension phase, mild and variable

proteinuria and increased urinary α(1)-microglobulin levels were reported. The mean
terminal half-life of PRO051 in the circulation was 29 days. PRO05, at the dose of 2.0 mg per
kilogram or higher, induced specific exon-51 skipping. In 10 patients new dystrophin
expression was observed between approximately 60% and 100% of muscle fibers, as
observed in post-treatment biopsy. New dystrophin expression increased dose-dependently
up to 15.6% of the expression in healthy muscle. After the 12 week extension phase, a
modest improvement was observed in the 6 minute walk test (Netherlands National Trial
Register number, NTR1241).

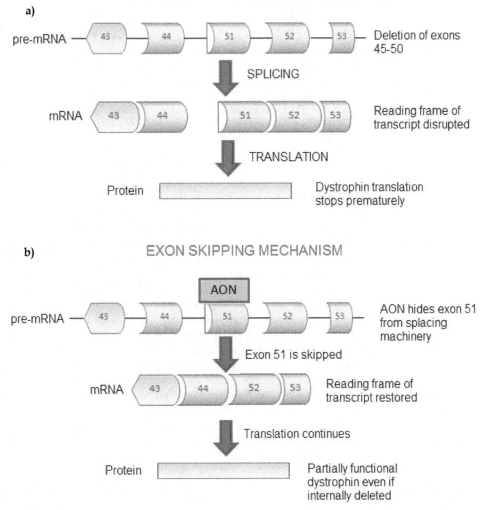

Fig. 2. a) Duchenne muscular dystrophy is caused by mutations in the dystrophin gene,
leading to disruption of the open reading frame; b) Exon skipping mechanism in Duchenne
muscular dystrophy.

6. Ongoing clinical trials

Several clinical trials, involving DMD patients, and based on the exon skipping approach are ongoing. A phase 1 trial is testing a drug (GSK2402968) that has been designed to skip exon 51 of the dystrophin gene, assessing the safety and tolerability of the drug in boys/adolescents who are unable to walk. The absorption and processing of the drug in their bodies will be also studied. This trial is expected to end in September 2011. A Phase 1/2 trial is investigating whether the experimental drug PRO044 is safe and effective as a therapy for people with DMD with a mutation in a specific region of the dystrophin gene, i.e. exon 44. The expecting end date of the trial is December 2011. Another phase 2 trial is investigating GSK2402968 (two different doses), a drug that has been designed to skip exon 51 of the dystrophin gene. The aim of the study is to determine if an intermittent treatment with GSK2402968 will lead to a better long-term safety profile, while maintaining its effectiveness. This trial is expected to end in September 2012. A phase 3 trial is undergoing testing a drug (GSK2402968) that has been designed to skip exon 51 of the dystrophin gene. It will assess the effect of GSK2402968 on the muscle function of boys with DMD and will monitor the safety of the drug. It is expected to end in December 2012 (The information contained in this paragraph has been collected from the website http://www.musculardystrophy.org/research/clinical_trials/0/duchenne+muscular+dyst rophy accessed on 18/05/2011).

7. Cell-based therapy

The cell-based therapy, or cell transplantation, involves different procedures with injected cell pool to correct some functional tissue or organ impairment. Depending on the pathology to be treated, the protocol of cell graft is specific. In genetic disorders, cells are genetically corrected with ex vivo procedure and grafted. In degenerative disorders, cells are amplified and injected. In cancer or infectious pathologies, the cells are selected on the base of immunoreacting or immunomodulating properties, amplified and injected in patients. The cells can derive from other species (xenotransplantation), other subjects (heterologous) or the receiver (autologous). Using cells deriving from other organism, xenotransplantation and heterologous transplantation are associated with the immunosuppressive therapy which reduces host immune-reaction against graft. It is important to decide which cell type to transplant. Based on remaining differentiate ability and plasticity, it is possible to choose the stem cell origin (embryonic, foetal or adult), progenitor cells or terminally committed cells, and collect them from the tissue of interest. Based on remaining differentiated ability and plasticity, it is possible to choose the stem cell origin (embryonic, foetal or adult), progenitor cells or terminally committed cells, from a selected specific tissue and followed by a process and purification before graft. They are frequently amplified and specifically stimulated to increase and improve grafted pool. In autologous transplantation treating genetic disorder, the cells are genetically handled to revert mutation. Depending on localization of the disorder, the cells are locally or systemically injected. The strategies of the cell-based therapy, adopted for DMD, are two: ex vivo genetic correction in autologous cells, followed by graft, or heterologous injection of cells. It allows to evaluate rapidly the improvement or disadvantages of the therapy, avoiding severe complications due to impairment in vital muscles. Heterologous transplantation allows to inject low-handled healthy cells with the certainty of avoiding dys mutations. Unfortunately, the immunosuppressive therapy is necessary to protect graft from host immune system.

8. Cell types

In these last few years, stem cells have received a lot of attention for their potential use in cell-based therapies for various human diseases including DMD (Lodi et al., 2011; Farini et al., 2009). For several years, after they were discovered, the satellite cells were considered as the only cells responsible for the growth and maintenance of the skeletal muscle (Le Grand and Rudnicki, 2007a; Le Grand and Rudnicki, 2007b). With the improvements of cell-isolation technology, a number of markers were described to identify a lot of muscular and nonmuscular subpopulations able to actively participate in myogenesis. Recent works have described the partial identification and characterization of multilineage stem cells derived in culture from numerous adult tissues. In the skeletal muscle itself, rather than satellite cells, alternative adult multi-lineage progenitor cell populations showed to have a myogenic potential: muscle-derived stem cells (MDSCs) (Sarig et al., 2006), muscle side-population (mSP) cells (Wognum et al., 2003) and muscle-derived CD133+ progenitors (Peault et al., 2007). Several works have described how nonmuscular resident stem cells could participate in myogenesis: the bone marrow–derived mesenchymal stem cells (BMMSCs) can differentiate into mesodermal cells, including myoblasts (Pittenger et al., 1999; Prockop, 1997) and adult tissue host cells can also contribute to endodermal and ectodermal cell lineages (Krause et al., 2001; Mezey et al., 2000). A subpopulation of CD133+ cells, that play an important role in myogenic development, has been isolated from blood (Torrente et al., 2004). Furthermore, other stem cells have been identified in the dorsal aorta of avian and mammalian species, the so-called mesoangioblasts (Cossu and Bianco, 2003), while the pericytes were found in the basement membrane of the vessels (Dellavalle et al., 2007).

9. Satellite cells

Satellite cells derive from a progenitor population paired box protein 3 and 7 (Pax3 and Pax7, muscle and neural crest development markers) +/+ localized in the central portion of the dermomyotome, the dorso-lateral part of the somite. During the fetal development, the resident progenitor population generates cells in satellite position around myofibers, which are marked by the expression of Pax7, while the limb muscle satellite cells arise from hypaxial cells expressing Pax3. (Le Grand and Rudnicki, 2007b). The satellite cells are located beneath the basal lamina of mature skeletal muscle fibres, and they are ideally positioned to repair degenerating muscle fibres. These quiescent cells are activated to proliferate upon muscle injury or when heavily used during activities such as weight lifting or running. This proliferation step is necessary to generate sufficient numbers of myoblasts for muscle differentiation and myotube formation. In humans, these mononuclear cells are most plentiful at birth (estimated at 32% of sublaminar nuclei). Their frequency declines postnatally, stabilizing between 1% and 5% of skeletal muscle nuclei in the adult muscle. In humans, the proportion of satellite cells in skeletal muscles also decreases with age, and it could explain the decreased efficiency of muscle regeneration in older subjects. Satellite cells from aged muscle also display reduced proliferative and fusion capacity, as well as a tendency to store fat, thus deteriorating their regeneration potential. Satellite cells present an extended proliferative potential and can repopulate extensively the host's muscle with an efficiency unknown in any other experimental situation (Cooper et al., 2006).

10. Multipotent muscle-derived stem cells

Recent studies have demonstrated the existence of a population of multipotent muscle-derived stem cells (MMDSCs), distinct from satellite cells, with high myogenic potential in vitro, even after being appropriately stimulated to differentiate into other lineages, such as haematopoietic. MMDSCs reside in skeletal muscle sharing the ability to self-renew and differentiate into other mesodermal cell types (Farini et al., 2009). MDSCs were isolated on the base of their adhesion ability. The cells, obtained by enzymatic digestion of muscle tissue, are seeded on a culture dish and, after 1 hour, the medium and non-adherent cells are transferred to another dish (preplating). Then, analogous preplates are repeated at 24 hour intervals until preplate 6 (pp6) is completed. The cells, which rapidly attach to the surface, are mainly fibroblasts (pp1), cells which adhere within 24-48 hours. They are predominantly satellite cells (pp2 – pp4) and the population, which settle at the most slowest speed on a flask, consists of multipotential stem cells (pp-6). The phenotype of fraction pp6 is described as stem cell antigen-1 (sca-1), CD34+ (marker of hematopoietic and satellite cells), CD45-, c-kit- (markers of hematopoietic cells) with the expression of desmin (marker of myogenic cells) on a different level. MDSCs, cultured in vitro, differentiate spontaneously into myotubes, but, when appropriately stimulated, these cells can also give rise either to osteoblasts , chondroblasts , hematopoietic cells or endothelial cells. MDSCs firmly adhere to endothelium in mdx muscles microcirculation and then participate in muscle regeneration, following an intramuscular injection. Interestingly, they have also been found in muscles, after intravenous administration, and their number was higher in muscles, previously injured, than in the control ones. The expression of desmin gradually decreases with subsequent preplates and in pp6 population only about 10-20% of cells are positive for this protein. However, pp6 cells, cultured in standard conditions, spontaneously enter the myogenic pathway that is associated with an increased desmin expression. It has also been demonstrated that the majority of MDSCs is positive as for desmin. The studies, regarding cell viability after transplantation, have shown that more MDSCs survive following intramuscular administration, if compared to more differentiated cells (myoblasts). After the injection of the same number of either MDSCs or early preplate (EP) cells, the contribution to muscle regeneration, 30 and 90 days later, has been even 10 times higher in MDSC group. Marked differences have probably been associated with the distinct immunogenicity between MDSCs and EP cells. The evaluation of major histocompatibility complex (MHC-1) expression in cell membranes of both cell types has revealed that MHC-1 is present in 63% of EP cells, whereas only in 0.5% of MDSCs. However, MDSCs are a much less numerous cell population if compared to "typical" satellite cells which dominate in EP group. Only one clone of MDSCs can be obtained from 10^5 of cells originally isolated from muscle tissue (Lee-Pullen and Grounds, 2005). MMDSCs could also be distinguished by flow cytometry. After staining with Hoechst 33324, it was possible to characterize a cell population, called skeletal muscle side population (SMSP) or simply side population (SP), which is able to extrude dye via ATP-binding cassette G2 (ABCG2) multi-drug resistant pump. SP expresses several surface markers associated with haematopoietic stem cells (HSCs) including CD45, c-kit, Sca-1 and CD34, but no satellite cell markers such as M-cadherin, Pax7 or desmin. SP cells can give rise to all hematopoetic lines, both in vitro and in vivo. The question of myogenic potential is more complex. The SP cells, harvested in vitro, do not differentiate spontaneously into myocytes. However, cell-mediated inductive interactions trigger myogenic potential of SP cells. These cells contain two distinct fractions with myogenic potential, such as CD45+ and CD45-, both exhibiting the potential to constitute myogenic cells after a co-culture with primary myoblasts. In particular, CD45+ SP are able to integrate into regenerating muscle fibres after an intramuscular injection, while the sub-fraction CD45- SP has the potential to give rise to adipocytes and osteocyte. Regardless of hematopoietic and myogenic potential, SP also displays endothelial trait (CD31+). Moreover, it has been shown that SP expresses angiopoietin 2 and the Tie2 receptor, which is bound and activated by angiopoietins. It means, that most of the SP cells share partially signalling pathways with endothelial/hematopoietic precursor cell populations. SP cells demonstrate that lack of Pax7 gene in experimental animals does not influence the number of muscle SP cells. Furthermore, Pax7-/- SP cells can differentiate into myotubes when co-cultured with myoblasts. It indicates that Pax7 gene is not required for myogenic specification of SP cells. Finally, forced expression of MyoD induces myogenic differentiation of Pax7-/- SP cells, but not pax7-/- myoblasts. All these data suggest that SMSP and satellite cells are distinct populations and probably have different origin (Burdzinska et al., 2008).

11. Blood- and muscle-derived CD133+ progenitors

CD133+ cells are considered to be haematopoietic and endothelial stem cells of bone marrow origin that could give rise to both endothelial cells and myoblasts. Circulating human CD133+ cells demonstrate stemness properties and the ability to restore dystrophin expression and eventually regenerate the satellite cells pool in dystrophic scid/mdx mouse after intra-muscular and intra-arterial delivery. Skeletal muscle CD133+ stem cell have the potential to differentiate towards both muscle and endothelium lineages. Dystrophic human CD133+ are able to express an exon-skipped version of human dystrophin, after transduction with a lentivirus, carrying a construct designed to skip exon 51, so their ability to participate in muscle regeneration has been examined after transplantation into scid/mdx mice. The comparison of two distinct CD133+ cell populations, one from blood and one from skeletal muscle, show that the muscle-derived CD133+ stem cells have the potential to differentiate towards both muscle and endothelium lineages. Skipped blood and muscle-derived Δ49–50 stem cells, fused in vivo with regenerative fibres, express a functional human dystrophin and restructure the dystrophin-associated protein complex, as shown by plasmalemmal re-expression of a and b-sarcoglycan proteins. Moreover, being sometimes located beneath the basal lamina, and distributed along freshly isolated fibres, it is interesting to assess whether muscle-derived CD133+ stem cells are able to differentiate into satellite cells. Genetically engineered DMD muscle-derived CD133+ cells show a better muscle regeneration in terms of spreading and number of positive fibres in comparison with the results obtained from blood-derived stem cells. DMD muscle-derived CD133+ cells are more efficient than their blood counterpart in the improvement of morphology and restoration of the normal skeletal muscle function in dystrophic murine muscles. Human CD133+ cells, isolated from muscle or blood, are able to promote muscular- and endothelial-differentiation after intra-arterial and intra-muscular delivery. These cells can be injected safely in DMD patients, not only without side effects, but also promoting an increase in the number of capillaries per muscle fibres. Moreover, DMD CD133+ cells can be genetically modified to re-express a functional dystrophy. Unfortunately, several things need to be ameliorated, such as the potential to enhance proliferation of blood-derived CD133+ cells in culture and storage for repeated treatments, the relative efficiency of blood-derived cells, compared with muscle-derived cells to contribute to muscle nuclei, the strategy to deliver myogenic cells chronically to the various sites of sporadic regeneration that occur in muscular dystrophies (Farini et al., 2009; Peault et al., 2007).

12. Mesenchymal stem cells

Mesenchymal stem cells (MSCs) are conventionally defined as adherent, non-hematopoietic cells expressing markers such as CD90, CD105, and CD73, and being negative for CD14, CD34, and CD45. While originally identified in the bone marrow, MSCs have been extracted from numerous tissues including adipose tissue, heart, Wharton's jelly, dental pulp, peripheral blood, cord blood menstrual blood, and, more recently, Fallopian tube. One of the major properties of MSCs is the ability to differentiate into various tissues. The traditional differentiation properties of MSCs are their ability to become adipocytes, chondrocytes, and osteocytes in vitro, after treatment with induction agents. Non-orthodox differentiation into other tissues, for example, cells resembling neurons, muscles, hepatocytes and pancreatic islets, has also been reported. There is some evidence that MSCs may differentiate selectively into tissues that have been injured. The ease of obtaining bone marrow sample and myogenic potential of MSCs makes this population an attractive candidate for cellular transplantation in cases of diseases associated with muscle dysfunction. However, there are still a lot of controversies around the level of myogenic potential of mesenchymal cells. Numerous studies were focused on the methodology of induction of MSC differentiation into muscle cells. Contrasting results were obtained treating MSCs with DNA methyltransferase inhibitor, such as 5-azacitidine, or galectin-1 as the factor initializing myogenesis of MSCs (Chan et al., 2006; Liu et al., 2003). Regarding BMMSC myogenic potential, interesting results were achieved culturing the cells by a mixture of cytokines and growth factors (fibroblast growth factor beta (βFGF), forskolin, plateled derived growth factor (PDGF), neuregulin and subsequently transfected with gene encoding Notch 1 intracellular domain (NICD). Following this procedure, cells differentiated into muscle cells with the efficacy of 89% (Dezawa et al., 2005). An alternative approach to induce myogenesis in MSCs, is the exposure of these cells to myogenic environment. MSCs, co-cultured with cardiomycytes or satellite cells, differentiated in either cardiac cells or myotubes respectively (Fukuhara et al., 2003; Lee et al., 2005). However, the differentiation rate in these conditions was highly limited. The fate of MSCs, injected into either skeletal or cardiac muscle, was also analyzed (Shi et al., 2004). It has been demonstrated that undifferentiated MSCs can undergo myogenesis after an intramuscular administration, but, similarly to the in vitro studies, the proportion of differentiated cells was barely detectable, only 0,44% of transplanted MSCs fused in myotubes. Gene-corrected DMD MSCs restored dystrophin expression in co-cultured dystrophic myoblasts through spontaneous cell fusion (Goncalves et al., 2006a). Furthermore, a study where dystrophic MSCs transfected by recombinant adenovirus, which contains human microdystrophin cDNA, were injected into mdx mouse, showed that expression of dystrophin was detected in dystrophic tissue (Xiong et al., 2007). A study has also compared MSCs transplantation with and without prior differentiation. Cells were injected around the myocardial infarcted area of a rabbit model. The improvement in left ventricular function, vascular density and reduction of infarcted area did not differ significantly between the two groups. The perspective to transplant undifferentiated mesenchymal stem cells seems to be promising, because it does not require time-consuming and expensive extracorporeal manipulations in cells (Ichim et al., 2010).

13. Mesoangioblasts

Mesoangioblasts are multipotent progenitors of mesodermal tissues, physically associated with the embryonic dorsal aorta in avian and mammalian species. Mesoangioblasts are able to differentiate into various mesodermal phenotypes. Mesoangioblast-like cells have been isolated from vessels of post-natal tissues. Post-natal cells generally express pericytes rather than endothelial cell markers, but they are otherwise similar to their embryonic counterparts in terms of proliferation and differentiation potency. When wild-type or dystrophic, genetically corrected mesoangioblasts are delivered intra-arterially to dystrophic muscle of α-sarcoglycan- null mice (a model for limb girdle muscular dystrophy), they induce a dramatic functional amelioration of the dystrophic phenotype. This is due to the widespread distribution of the donor's cells through the capillary network and to an intrinsic defect of proliferation in the resident satellite cells, a situation that creates a selective advantage for the injected donor cells. To proceed with clinical experimentation, it has been considered to be crucial that the delivery and muscle homing of mesoangioblasts may be optimized to characterize human cells in depth and the protocol needs to be tested in a large animal model. Recently, it has been reported that the enhancing delivery of mesoangioblasts leads to the complete reconstitution of downstream skeletal muscles in α-sarcoglycan-null dystrophic mice. Mesoangioblasts, exposed in vitro to either stromal cell derived factor-1 or TNF-α, have showed enhanced transmigration in vitro and migration into dystrophic muscle in vivo. Transient expression of α-4 integrins or l-selectin have also produced a several-fold increase in migration, both in vitro and in vivo. Mesoangioblasts, transduced with a lentiviral vector expressing human microdystrophin and injected scid/mdx mice and immunosuppressed dystrophic golden retriever muscular dystrophy (GRMD) dogs, have showed a modified mesoangioblasts-induced dystrophin positivity in myofibres. In particular, the results of these injections have been promising in the dystrophic dogs with improvements in their muscle function and mobility together with an increased dystrophin expression. In order to ameliorate the efficiency of the muscle repair by mesoangioblasts, cell migration to skeletal muscle has been improved and unspecific trapping in the capillary filters of the body, such as liver and lung, has been reduced (Farini et al., 2009).

14. Bone marrow stem cells

In the last decade, it has been discovered the contribution of various nonmyogenic cells in the regeneration of skeletal muscle, such as bone marrow-derived cells (BMDCs) and the circulating haematopoietic cells. With the advent of more sensitive markers, it has been demonstrated that BMDCs can enter the sites of muscle regeneration and also contribute to the formation of new muscle fibres. Furthermore, similar cells, resident in skeletal muscle, appeared to reconstitute the bone marrow and via this route, enter again and contribute to the regeneration of skeletal muscle. In this sense, it has been demonstrated that the intravenous injection of either normal HSCs or a novel population of MDSCs into irradiated mdx mice resulted in the reconstitution of the haematopoietic compartment of the transplanted recipients, the incorporation of donor-derived nuclei into muscle, and the partial restoration of dystrophin expression in the affected muscle. Similarly, after the transplantation into immunodeficient mice, BMDCs migrated into areas of induced muscle degeneration, underwent myogenic differentiation, and participated in the regeneration of the damaged fibres. Following the transplantation in irradiated mice ablated of endogenous satellite cells, the transplanted BMDCs were able to occupate the niche of those satellite cells. Furthermore, BMDC satellite cells participated in the regeneration of multinucleated muscle fibres at high frequency, becoming heritably myogenic. As these results were obtained using the whole bone marrow as transplant source, and since it is known to contain haematopoietic and non-haematopoietic progenitors, it is possible to speculate that the bone marrow could contain such progenitors for muscle and blood. On the other hand, a common progenitor with haematopoietic potential could generate myogenic cells due to either physiological stimuli and fusion with a myogenic cell (Farini et al., 2009).

15. Pericytes

Pericytes wrap around the vascular tube and interdigitate with the endothelial cells in the basement membrane of the vessels, playing a fundamental role in the maintenance of microcirculation functionality. Pericytes can be mobilized from the adult bone marrow under ischemic conditions, and utilized for their contractile capabilities and their multiple cytoplasmic processes. It has been demonstrated that pericytes have a high capacity of myogenic differentiation because they give rise to a high number of muscular fibres, when injected into scid/mdx mice. It has been proposed that the pericyte could be released from its position on a vascular tube in the case of a focal injury, functioning as an immunomodulatory and trophic mesenchymal stem cell. The activity of the pericyte ensures that the field of damage remains limited and that tissue-intrinsic progenitors replace the expired cells. As provided by this evidence, these stem cells could represent a good candidate for the muscle therapy because they could be isolated from a muscle biopsy and therefore easily accessible. They can be cultured in vitro without loss of stem-cell properties and are able to regenerate skeletal muscle after muscular and arterial injection. Nevertheless, it would be important to determine whether transplanted pericytes can fully reconstitute the satellite cell niche as a real functional stem cell. More information are needed about the role of pericytes, in both normal and dystrophic skeletal muscle, in order to avoid that the injection of these cells into human dystrophic muscle environment could elicit pericyte-derived tumours.

16. Adipocytes

Adipocytes share the same mesodermal origin with skeletal muscle. An inverse relationship, between skeletal muscle mass and adipose tissue mass, is apparent in murine models of skeletal muscle dystrophic pathology such as mdx where the relative level of fat tissue, within the diseased muscle, has increased. Moreover, in the myostatin-/- mouse, where the skeletal muscle mass has hugely increased, the fat tissue mass is reduced substantially. Moreover, cell culture studies have demonstrated that myogenic cell lines, when made to overexpress adipogenic transcription factors peroxisome proliferator-activated receptor gamma (PPARγ) and CCAAT/enhancer-binding protein alpha (C/EBPα) lose their myogenic marker expression and differentiate into adipocytes, suggesting that the adult myoblasts are capable of being reprogrammed to become adipocytes. Furthermore, the satellite cell population has been shown to be capable of conversion into the adipocyte lineage, given the correct cues. A more recent work has provided good evidence that the adipocyte lineage can also undergo conversion into myoblasts. An adipocyte-specific stem cell population, that expressed high levels of CD13, CD44, CD73 and CD90 and was negative for CD34, CD45, CD56 and CD184, suggesting mesenchymal stem cell-like characteristics, was recently isolated and has shown to display myogenic markers and fuse with maturing myofibres when co-cultured with myoblast cell lines. Furthermore, it has been demonstrated that cells, isolated from the stromal vascular fraction of adipose tissue, which have been shown to differentiate in vitro into adipogenic, chondrogenic, osteogenic and myogenic cells, can spontaneously form myotubes when cultured under standard conditions in vitro. Furthermore, these cells are able to fuse into myotubes following in vitro expansion and following injection into ischaemic murine hind limbs. They also form new myofibres and are capable of restoring dystrophin expression in mdx mice, thus displaying a therapeutic potential. More recently, a more specific CD45- side population of adipocyte progenitor cells, purified from the stromal vascular fraction, has been shown to form myofibres in vivo. An array analysis of murine brown fat precursor cell populations has recently shown that certain myogenic transcription factors, including myogenin, Myf5 and MyoD, are expressed at levels comparable with C2C12 cells within these progenitors. These data are in keeping with the previous lineage-tracing studies that showed a dermomyotomal origin for brown, but not white, fat precursor cells. Moreover, brown fat lineage cells also express the known myogenic microRNAs miR-1 miR-133a and miR-206, suggesting that brown adipocytes share a common ancestor with myogenic cells. Subsequently, it has been demonstrated that the transcription factor PRD1-BF1-RIZ1 homologous domain containing 16 (PRDM16), is sufficient and necessary to drive the conversion of white adipocytes into brown adipocytes, through an up-regulation of uncoupling protein and PPARγ coactivator-1alpha (PGC1-α) expression. It shows to be a key regulator in the formation of the brown fat lineage. PRDM16 drives the brown fat lineage by forming a transcriptional complex with C-terminal binding protein 1 or 2, whereby it acts to repress white fat-specific genes or complexing with PGC1-α, and PPARγ Coactivator 1-beta (PGC1-β) according to which it enhances expression of brown fat genes. Recently, it has been elegantly shown that brown fat cells arise from a Myf5+ common precursor that was previously only thought to form skeletal muscle cells. Furthermore, PRDM16 overexpression causes brown fat cells to undergo a lineage switch, forming skeletal myoblasts through the activation of PPAR-γ, whereas PRDM16- /- brown fat has elevated myogenic gene transcription and reduced uncoupling ability. Subsequently, it has been shown that human skeletal muscle contains a population of brown fat precursor cells that up-regulates uncoupling protein 1 following PPAR-γ agonist treatment. Finally, human adipose tissue-derived mesenchymal stem cells have been shown to differentiate into myofibres spontaneously as well as induce dystrophin expression following co-culture with human DMD myoblasts in vitro through a cell fusion. These data show that adipogenic stem cells may be used for therapeutic applications (Otto et al., 2009).

17. Clinical trials

Myoblast transplantation is a possible treatment for DMD. Promising results in vivo nude/mdx mouse transplantation was obtained and in the 90's a series of clinical trials on DMD patients was conducted. Huard et al. (Huard, et al. 1991; Huard, et al. 1992) transplanted myoblasts from an immunocompatible donor into the limb muscles of 4 DMD patients in the advanced stages of the disease. A different degree of dystrophin was detected by immunostaining in the patients, but this change slowly decayed over time and it was not associated to a strength improvement. Although no immunosuppressive treatment was used, no patient showed any clinical sign of rejection. The effects of myoblast transplantations, without an immunosuppressive treatment on muscle strength and the formation of dystrophin-positive fibers, were studied in five young boys with DMD, using a triple blind design. No increase in the static contraction was detected. The expression of dystrophin in myoblast-injected fibers was generally low and it decreased to control level in 6 months. These results strongly suggest that myoblast transplantations, as well as gene therapy for DMD, cannot be done without immunosuppression (Tremblay et al., 1993). Karpati et al. (Karpati et al., 1993) used cyclophosphamide as an immunosuppressive agent to improve the myoblast transfer; however, subsequent experiments demonstrated that this antitumour drug killed the transplanted myoblasts, as well as any other rapidly proliferating cells. Normal dystrophin was detected, by reverse-transcriptase polymerase chain reaction, in DMD patients after myoblast transplantation, but it was not associated to an increase in the percentage of dystrophin-positive fibers (Gussoni et al., 1992). Immunosuppression of DMD boys by cyclosporine, during myoblast transplantation, improved force generation, but it was not effective in replacing clinically significant amounts of dystrophin in DMD muscle (Miller et al., 1997). Mendell et al. (Mendell et al., 1995) injected myoblast, once a month for six months, in 12 DMD patients, but this treatment failed to improve strength. Law et al. (Law et al., 1992) demonstrated the feasibility and safety of myoblast transplantation, but with a poor clinical improvement. At the end of the 90's, a careful overview of the previous initial trials brought several research teams to identify three problems responsible for the limited results observed: (1) 3 day after the graft, at least 75% of the transplanted myoblasts died (Fan et al., 1996; Guerette et al., 1997; Huard et al., 1994); (2) myoblasts were not able to migrate more than 200 μm away from the intramuscular injection trajectory (Skuk et al., 1999); (3) if immunosuppression was not adequate, the myoblasts were rapidly rejected in less than 2 weeks (Guerette et al., 1994) or were induced to activate apoptosis, such as cyclophosphamide usage (Hardiman et al., 1993; Hong et al., 2002). There are now some solutions to overcome these problems. The rapid death of a large percentage of myoblasts can be compensated by the transplantation of a high number of cells. Indeed the transplantation of 30 million cells per mm^3 has given very good results in monkeys (Skuk et al., 1999). In monkeys, the low migration distance of myoblasts was avoided by a high number of adjacent intramuscular injections, i.e. 100 injections per cm^2 of muscle surface. High density of intramuscular injections of myoblast in 11 DMD patients were also well tolerated. One patient received a total of 4,000 intramuscular injections without any complication. No infection or other complication, related to the procedure, was registered (Skuk et al., 2007). An interesting improvement in myoblast migration injected in muscle was obtained by the modulation of MyoD expression (El Fahime et al., 2000; Smythe and Grounds, 2001). Similarly, it has been observed the restoration of 26–30% dystrophin expression in muscle fibers in the environment of the irradiated muscle, suggesting an improvement in myoblast migration induced by factors released with the irradiated muscle (Cousins et al., 2004; Skuk et al., 2006; Skuk et al., 2007; Skuk et al., 2004). The immunosuppression problem was tackled introducing new drugs. FK506 (Tacrolimus or Prograf®; Astellas Pharma, Deerfield, IL, USA) allowed to obtain very good transplantation results, not only in mice, but also in monkeys (Kinoshita et al., 1996; Kinoshita et al., 1994). Unfortunately, FK506 may induce adverse effects in patients (nephrotoxicity, diabetes, increased risk of cancer) if used on an ongoing, long-term basis (Palmieri et al., 2010). Many therapeutic protocols were developed to induce specific immunological tolerance towards the donor's myoblasts and through the creation of mixed chimerism and central tolerance (Camirand et al., 2004; Stephan et al., 2006). Another support to immunosuppression therapy was the transplantation of genetically modified autologous myoblasts (Floyd et al., 1998; Goncalves et al., 2006b; Quenneville et al., 2007), or avoidance of gradual senescence of differentiated cells, autologous pluripotent stem cells (Di Rocco et al., 2006). Other researchers refocus their efforts to optimise the therapy searching cell populations thought to be more primitive and less immunologic than myoblasts. They include MDSCs (Sarig et al., 2006), mSP cells (Wognum et al., 2003) and muscle-derived CD133+ progenitors (Farini et al., 2009). In a double-blind phase I clinical trial, Torrente et al. (Torrente et al., 2007) transplanted autologous CD133+ cells, extracted from muscle biopsies by intramuscular injection, into eight boys with DMD and sampled after 7 months. The cells were not genetically corrected, their fate was not monitored, and the boys were not immunosuppressed, because the experiment was designed only to test the safety of the implanted cells (grown in culture for only 48 hours). No adverse effects were observed. Afterwards, thanks to these observations, the cell therapy was combined with a genetic approach: ex vivo introduction of corrective genes into dystrophic CD133+ myogenic cells and their subsequent autologous transplantation. The use of exon-skipping for the expression of human dystrophin, within the DMD CD133+ cells, allows the use of the patient's own stem cells, thus minimizing the risk of immunological graft rejection (Riviere et al., 2006). The exon-skipping therapeutic approach is applicable to gene defects up to 70% of DMD patients, and avoids the problems associated with the delivery of the prohibitively large full length dystrophin gene or a (less functional) truncated mini-gene. Blood- and muscle-derived DMD CD133+ cells were isolated and characterized for their ability to express an exon-skipped version of human dystrophin, after infection with a lentivirus carrying a construct designed to skip exon 5 (Denti et al., 2006; Goyenvalle et al., 2004). The skipped blood and muscle-derived Δ49–50 stem cells were able to fuse in vivo with regenerative fibres and expressed, not only a functional human dystrophin, but also the dystrophin-associated proteins a and b-sarcoglycans. However, intramuscular transplantations lead only to local and focused regeneration, whereas DMD pathology affects the whole body musculature and its effective treatment requires some methods to distribute the injected cells to the dispersed sites. In future clinical trials, we speculate that these stem cells, purified from DMD patients, could be ex vivo engineered and reinjected in the initial donor intra-arterially. The intra-arterial injections of the patients'own infected stem cells allow the distribution of the cells to the whole body musculature so that it could be possible to take care of severely affected patients that have a reduced mass body. One of the most important problem to solve, for a future clinical application, is the amelioration in safety procedures of the gene modifications. Ichim et al. (Ichim et al., 2010) reported the case study of a 22 year-old male diagnosed with DMD, treated with a combination of endometrial regenerative cells (ERC) and CD34+ umbilical cord blood. Three months later, the patient received another course of therapy including placental matrix derived mesenchymal stem cells. The improvement in muscular strength, clinical respiratory function and general level of activity are maintained to date. No adverse events have been associated with the stem cell infusion. The innovation introduced by this trial was the usage of "adjuvant" cellular population which provides a more suitable environment for muscle regeneration. The local intramuscular MSCs are able to add chemotactic/ trophic support for the intravenously administered CD34. It has been reported that mesoangioblasts, which reside within the CD34 population, as well as cord blood CD34 cells, have had positive activity on DMD in animal models, although they appear to be short-lived (Jazedje et al., 2009; Nunes et al., 2007; Otto et al., 2009). Mesoangioblasts have been the main contributors to de novo myogenesis and were selectively attracted into the dystrophic tissue. It is known that CD34 cells express very late antigen-4 (VLA-4), which is the ligand for Vascular Cell Adhesion Molecule 1 (VCAM-1), whose expression is elevated in dystrophic muscles (Gavina et al., 2006). Furthermore, CD34 chemokines such as Macrophage inflammatory protein-1 alpha (MIP-1α) and Regulated upon activation normal T-cell expressed and secreted (RANTES) expression have been found in dystrophic muscle (Demoule et al., 2005).

18. Conclusions

According to this review, the attempts to treat DMD with different genetic and cellular approaches open new perspectives in the muscular function restoration, although it is very difficult to predict, at the moment, what strategy will be more successful. From a lifelong perspective, it is reasonable to conceive an integrated schedule of treatment protocols, subdivided by decades of age.On this basis, cell transplantation is supposed to be the final answer to replace the irreversibly impaired muscle mass with healthy myocytes. It is therefore important to choose the best age for the transplant and the best timing schedule is probably before the crash of the muscular framework that will be replaced with fibrous and adipose tissue. Alternatively , in the very early period of life, when the disease is not phenotipically expressed yet, and it is just a genetic biochemical trait, the timing could be perfect for either exon skipping or cell transplant approaches that could be more easily integrated in the muscular structure. Furthermore, in the homologous cell transplantation, a longstanding immunosuppressive phase, which is strongly adversed by the ethical committees, is at the moment mandatory in order to achieve an adequate survival of nonidentical transplanted cells. These cells should be reasonably replaced with a series of transplant sessions in the follow up, as long as their vital cycle will decline to apoptosis. Probably, in the next future,even histocompatible cadaver sources might be helpful in the long run.

As to the cell administration route, the transplant procedure, addressed by Cossu and coworkers (Sampaolesi et al., 2003; Díaz-Manera et al., 2010), through intra-arterial regional perfusion, has to be validated and compared with the more cumbersome repeated intramuscular injections for which automatically injecting devices, a proper anesthesia and, probably, laparoscopic-thoracoscopic schedule will be required, especially for the deep muscles, like diaphragm and heart. In the procedure described by Cossu (Sampaolesi et al., 2006), according to the results obtained in dog models of DMD, the mesangioblasts can easily trespass the endothelial barrier and reach the muscular areas to be restored by new healthy myocytes. On the other hand, in the direct intramuscular injections, the operator chooses the topography of injections, and, on the basis of mathematical and geometrical models, and with the hopeful aid of robotization, a systematic and well arranged replacement of several millions of myocytes can be achieved, during each session, on a very accurately, individually tailored protocol. The exon-skipping approach is very appealing due to the progress observed in the clinical trials, but it is very hard to conceive that this genetic correction of the dystrophin gene will be enough effective to support the muscular strength in the developing child, guaranteeing long lasting surrogate effect if introduced in a lifelong administration schedule. In this scenario, the oral route is certainly preferred to the subcutaneous one, and toxicological studies in mice let us suppose that the compounds are safe, but clinical trials in humans require further commitments, especially regarding the clinical monitoring of the follow up to determine possible side effects.

In conclusion, we think that, at the moment, due to brand new strong technological weapons, we could achieve a normal life span and quality of life for DMD kids and their families. At the same time, we need the collaboration of the centers working on DMD to design new clinical trials in order to reach the best effective therapeutic protocol as soon as possible. In the "Global Village", based on the World Wide Web, it is possible to plan panels of evidence-based medicine clinical studies by a single international World Wide Web based committee, eventually organized by the World Health Organization. This committee will be a powerful instrument to meet the urgent demand of the generation of kids with DMD who claim to achieve the goal of a fully autonomous life.

19. Statement of authorship

The authors hereby certify that all work contained in this review is original work of Tommaso Iannitti, Daniele Lodi, Valeriana Sblendorio, Valentina Rottigni and Beniamino Palmieri. All the information, taken from other articles, including tables and pictures, have been referenced in the "Bibliography" section. The authors claim full responsibility for the contents of the article.

20. Conflict of interest statement

The authors certify that there is no conflict of interest with any financial organization regarding the material discussed in the manuscript.

21. Acknowledgments

The authors contributed equally to this work. This review was not supported by grants.

22. Abbreviations

2'OMePS: 2'-O-methyl-phosphorothioate
ABCG2: ATP Binding Cassette G2
AON: Antisense Oligonucleotide
BMDC: Bone Marrow Derived Cell
BMMSC: Bone Marrow Mesenchymal Stem Cell
βFGF: Fibroblast Growth Factor beta
C/EBPα: CCAAT/Enhancer Binding Protein alpha
CNS: Central Nervous System
CsA: Ciclosporin A
DGC: Dystrophin Glycoprotein Complex
DMD: Duchenne Muscular Dystrophy
Dp: Dystrophin proteins
Dys: Dystrophin

ECM: Extracellular matrix
EDB: Extensor Digitorum Brevis
EP: Early Preplate
ERC: Endometrial Regenerative Cell
GRMD: Golden Retriever Muscular Dystrophy
HSC: Haematopoietic Stem Cell
IQ: Intelligence Quotient
MDSC: Muscle Derived Stem Cell
MHC: Major Histocompatibility Complex
MIP-1α: Macrophage Inflammatory Protein-1 alpha
MMDSC: Multipotent Muscle Derived Stem Cell
MRI: Magnetic Resonance Imaging
MSC: Mesenchymal Stem Cell
mSP: muscle Side Population
MVC: Maximum Voluntary Contraction
N: Naples
NICD: Notch1 Intracellular Domain
NTR: Netherlands National Trial Register
PDGF: Plateled Derived Growth Factor
PGC1-α: PPARγ Coactivator 1-alpha
PGC1-β: PPARγ Coactivator 1-beta
PMO: Phosphorodiamidate Morpholino Oligomer
PPARγ: Peroxisome Proliferator Activated Receptor gamma
pp6: preplate 6
RANTES: Regulated upon Activation, Normal T-cell Expressed and Secreted
SMSP: skeletal muscle side population
SP: Side Population
T: Toronto
TGF-β: Transforming Growth Factor beta
TNF-α: Tumor Necrosis Factor-alpha
VCAM-1: Vascular Cell Adhesion Molecule 1
VLA-4: Very Late Antigen-4

23. References

Aartsma-Rus A, Bremmer-Bout M, Janson AA, den Dunnen JT, van Ommen GJ, van Deutekom JC. Targeted exon skipping as a potential gene correction therapy for Duchenne muscular dystrophy. Neuromuscul Disord 2002;12 Suppl 1:S71-77.

Aartsma-Rus A, Janson AA, Kaman WE, Bremmer-Bout M, den Dunnen JT, Baas F, van Ommen GJ, van Deutekom JC. Therapeutic antisense-induced exon skipping in cultured muscle cells from six different DMD patients. Hum Mol Genet 2003;12:907-14.

Aartsma-Rus A, Janson AA, Kaman WE, Bremmer-Bout M, den Dunnen JT, van Ommen GJ, van Deutekom JC. Antisense-induced multiexon skipping for Duchenne muscular dystrophy makes more sense. Am J hum Genet 2004;74:83-92.

Aartsma-Rus A, Kaman WE, Weij R, den Dunnen JT, van Ommen GJ, van Deutekom JC. Exploring the frontiers of therapeutic exon skipping for Duchenne muscular dystrophy by double targeting within one or multiple exons. Mol Ther 2006;14: 401 - 07.

Aartsma-Rus A, van Deutekom JC, Fokkema IF, van Ommen GJ, den Dunnen JT. Entries in the Leiden Duchenne muscular dystrophy database: an overwiew of mutation typesand paradoxical cases that confirm the reading-frame rule. Muscle Nerve 2006;34:135-144.

Aartsma-Rus A, van Vliet L, Hirschi m, et al. Guidelines for antisense oligo-nucleotide design and insight into splice-modulating mechanisms. Mol Ther 2009,17:548-53.

Balaban B, Matthews DJ, Clayton GH, et al. Corticosteroid treatment and functional improvement in Duchenne muscular dystrophy: long-term effect. Am J Phys Med Rehabil. 2005;84:843–850.

Bewick GS, Nicholson LV, Young C, et al. Diffferent distributions of dystrophin and related proteins at nerve-muscle junctions. Neuroreport. 1992;3;857–860.

Biggar WD, Gingras M, Fehlings DL, et al. Deflazacort treatment of Duchenne muscular dystrophy. J Pediatr. 2001;138:45–50.

Biggar WD, Harris VA, Eliasoph L, et al. Long-term benefits of deflazacort treatment for boys with Duchenne muscular dystrophy in their second decade. Neuromuscul Disord. 2006;16:249–255.

Billard C, Gillet P, Signoret JL, et al. Cognitive function in Duchenne muscular dystrophy and spinal muscular atrophy. Neuromuscul Disord. 1992;2:371–378.

Blake DJ, Weir A, Newey SE, Davies KE. Function and genetics of dystrophin and dystrophin-related proteins in muscle. Physiol Rev. 2002;82:291–329

Blau HM, Webster C, Pavlath GK, Chiu CP. Evidence for defective myoblasts in Duchenne muscular dystrophy. Adv Exp Med Biol 1985;182:85-110.

Bremmer-Bout M, Aartsma-Rus A, de Meijer EK, Kaman WE, Janson AA, Vossen RH, van Ommen GJ, den Dunnen JT, van Deutekom JC. Targeted exon skipping in transgenic hDMD mice: a model for direct preclinical screening of human-specific antisense oligonucleotides. Mol Ther 2004;10:232-40.

Bresolin N, Castelli E, Comi GP, et al. Cognitive impairment in Duchenne muscular dystrophy. Neuromuscul Disord. 1994;4:359–369.

Brown Jr RH. Dystrophin associated proteins and the muscular dystrophy. Annu Rev Med. 1997;48:457–466.

Burdzinska A, Gala K Paczek L. Myogenic stem cells. Folia Histochem Cytobiol. 2008;46(4):401-12.

Camirand G, Rousseau J, Ducharme ME, Rothstein DM, Tremblay JP. Novel Duchenne muscular dystrophy treatment through myoblast transplantation tolerance with anti-CD45RB, anti-CD154 and mixed chimerism. Am J Transplant. 2004;4(8):1255-65.

Chan J, O'Donoghue K, Gavina M et. al. Galectin-1 induces skeletal muscle differentiation in human fetal mesenchymal stem cells and increases muscle regeneration. Stem Cells. 2006;24:1879-1891.

Cooper RN, Butler-Browne GS, Mouly V. Human muscle stem cells. Curr Opin Pharmacol. 2006;6(3):295-300.

Corrado K, Mills PL, Chamberlain JS. Deletion analysis of the dystrophin-actin binding domain. FEBS Lett. 1994;344:255–260.

Cossu G, Bianco P. Mesoangioblasts vascular progenitors for extravascular mesodermal tissues. Curr Opin Genet Dev. 2003;13(5):537-42.

Cousins JC, Woodward KJ, Gross JG, Partridge TA, Morgan JE. Regeneration of skeletal muscle from transplanted immortalised myoblasts is oligoclonal. J Cell Sci. 2004;117(Pt 15):3259-69.

Dellavalle A, Sampaolesi M, Tonlorenzi R, Tagliafico E, Sacchetti B, Perani L, Innocenzi A, Galvez BG, Messina G, Morosetti R, Li S, Belicchi M, Peretti G, Chamberlain JS, Wright WE, Torrente Y, Ferrari S, Bianco P, Cossu G. Pericytes of human skeletal muscle are myogenic precursors distinct from satellite cells. Nat Cell Biol. 2007;9(3):255-67

Demoule A, Divangahi M, Danialou G, Gvozdic D, Larkin G, Bao W, Petrof BJ. Expression and regulation of CC class chemokines in the dystrophic (mdx) diaphragm. Am J Respir Cell Mol Biol. 2005;33(2):178-85.

Denti MA, Rosa A, D'Antona G, Sthandier O, De Angelis FG, Nicoletti C, Allocca M, Pansarasa O, Parente V, Musarò A, Auricchio A, Bottinelli R, Bozzoni I. Chimeric adeno-associated virus/antisense U1 small nuclear RNA effectively rescues dystrophin synthesis and muscle function by local treatment of mdx mice. Hum Gene Ther. 2006;17(5):565-74

DeSilva S, Drachman DB, Mellits D, et al. Prednisone treatment in Duchenne muscular dystrophy: Long term benefit. Arch Neurol. 1987;44:818–822.

Dezawa M, Ishikawa H, Itokazu Y et. al. Bone marrow stromal cells generate muscle cells and repair muscle degeneration. Science. 2005;309:314-317.

Di Rocco G, Iachininoto MG, Tritarelli A, Straino S, Zacheo A, Germani A, Crea F, Capogrossi MC. Myogenic potential of adipose-tissue-derived cells. J Cell Sci. 2006;119(Pt 14):2945-52.

Díaz-Manera J, Touvier T, Dellavalle A, Tonlorenzi R, Tedesco FS, Messina G, Meregalli M, Navarro C, Perani L, Bonfanti C, Illa I, Torrente Y, Cossu G. Partial dysferlin reconstitution by adult murine mesoangioblasts is sufficient for full functional recovery in a murine model of dysferlinopathy. Cell Death Dis. 2010 Aug 5;1:e61.

Dubowitz V, Kinali M, Main M, et al. Remission of clinical signs in early Duchenne muscular dystrophy on intermittent low-dosage prednisolone therapy. Eur J Paediatr Neurol. 2002;6:153-159.

Dubowitz V. Neuromuscular disorders in childhood. Old dogmas, new concepts. Arch Dis Child. 1975;50:335-346.

El Fahime E, Torrente Y, Caron NJ, Bresolin MD, Tremblay JP. In vivo migration of transplanted myoblasts requires matrix metalloproteinase activity. Exp Cell Res. 2000;258(2):279-87.

Emery AE. Duchenne Muscular Dystrophy, 2nd edition. Cary, NC: Oxford University Press, 1993.

Fan Y, Maley M, Beilharz M, Grounds M. Rapid death of injected myoblasts in myoblast transfer therapy. Muscle Nerve. 1996;19(7):853-60.

Farini A, Razini P, Erratico S, Torrente Y, Meregalli M. Cell based therapy for Duchenne muscular dystrophy. J Cell Physiol. 2009;221(3):526-34.

Fukuhara S, Tomita S, Yamashiro S et. al. Direct cell-cell interaction of cardiomyocytes is key for bone marrow stromal cells to go into cardiac lineage in vitro. J Thorac Cardiovasc Surg. 2003;125:1470-14

Floyd SS Jr, Clemens PR, Ontell MR, Kochanek S, Day CS, Yang J, Hauschka SD, Balkir L, Morgan J, Moreland MS, Feero GW, Epperly M, Huard J. Ex vivo gene transfer using adenovirus-mediated full-length dystrophin delivery to dystrophic muscles. Gene Ther. 1998;5(1):19-30.

Gavina M, Belicchi M, Rossi B, Ottoboni L, Colombo F, Meregalli M, Battistelli M, Forzenigo L, Biondetti P, Pisati F, Parolini D, Farini A, Issekutz AC, Bresolin N, Rustichelli F, Constantin G, Torrente Y. VCAM-1 expression on dystrophic muscle vessels has a critical role in the recruitment of human blood-derived CD133+ stem cells after intra-arterial transplantation. Blood. 2006;108(8):2857-66.

Goemans NM, Tulinius M, van den Akker JT, Burm BE, Ekhart PF, Heuvelmans N, Holling T, Janson AA, Platenburg GJ, Sipkens JA, Sitsen JM, Aartsma-Rus A, van Ommen GJ, Buyse G, Darin N, Verschuuren JJ, Campion GV, de Kimpe SJ, van Deutekom JC. Systemic administration of PRO051 in Duchenne's muscular dystrophy. N Engl J Med. 2011 Apr 21;364(16):1513-22. Epub 2011 Mar 23.

Goncalves MA, de Vries AA, Holkers M, van de Watering MJ, van der Velde I, van Nierop GP, Valerio D, Knaän-Shanzer S. Human mesenchymal stem cells ectopically expressing full-length dystrophin can complement Duchenne muscular dystrophy myotubes by cell fusion. Hum Mol Genet. 2006a;15(2):213-21.

Gonçalves MA, Holkers M, Cudré-Mauroux C, van Nierop GP, Knaän-Shanzer S, van der Velde I, Valerio D, de Vries AA. Transduction of myogenic cells by retargeted dual high-capacity hybrid viral vectors: robust dystrophin synthesis in duchenne muscular dystrophy muscle cells. Mol Ther. 2006b;13(5):976-86.

Gosselin LE, McCormick KM. Targeting the immune system to improve ventilator function in muscular dystrophy. Med Sci Sports Exerc. 2004;36:44-51.

Goyenvalle A, Vulin A, Fougerousse F, Leturcq F, Kaplan JC, Garcia L, Danos O. Rescue of dystrophic muscle through U7 snRNA-mediated exon skipping. Science. 2004;306(5702):1796-9.

Griggs RC, Griggs RC, Moxley RT 3rd, et al. Duchenne dystrophy: randomized, controlled trial of prednisone (18 months) and azathioprine (12 months). Neurology. 1993;43:520-527.

Guérette B, Asselin I, Skuk D, Entman M, Tremblay JP. Control of inflammatory damage by anti-LFA-1: increase success of myoblast transplantation. Cell Transplant. 1997;6(2):101-7.

Guérette B, Asselin I, Vilquin JT, Roy R, Tremblay JP. Lymphocyte infiltration following allo- and xenomyoblast transplantation in mice. Transplant Proc. 1994;26(6):3461-2.

Gussoni, E, Pavlath GK, Lanctot AM, Sharma KR, Miller RG, Steinman L, Blau HM. Normal dystrophin transcripts detected in Duchenne muscular dystrophy patients after myoblast transplantation. Nature. 1992;356(6368):435-8.

Hall ZW, Sanes JR. Synaptic structure and development: The neuromuscular junction. Cell. 1993;72 (Suppl):99-121.

Hardiman OR, Sklar M, Brown RH Jr. Direct effects of cyclosporin A and cyclophosphamide on differentiation of normal human myoblasts in culture. Neurology. 1993;43(7):1432-4.

Hawke TJ, Garry DJ. Myogenic satellite cells: physiology to molecular biology. J Appl Physiol 2001;91:534-51.

Heemskerk H, de Winter C, van Kuik P, et al. Preclinical PK and PD studies on 2'-O-methyl-phosphorothioate RNA antisense oligonucleotides in the mdx mouse model. Mol Ther 2010;18:1210-7.

Heemskerk H, de Winter Cl, de Kimpe SJ, van Kuik-Romeijn P, Heuvelmans N, Platenburg GJ, van Ommen GJ, van Deutekom JC, Aartsma-Rus A. in vivo comparison of 2'-O-methyl phosphorothioate and mopholino antisense oligonucleotides for Duchenne muscular dystrophy exon skipping. J Gene Med 2009;11:257-66.

Helderman-van den Enden AT, Straathof CS, Aartsma-Rus A, et al. Becker muscular dystrophy patients with deletions around exon 51: a promising outlook for xon skipping therapy in Duchenne patients. Neuromuscul Disord 2010;20:251-4.

Henry MD, Campbell KP. A role for dystroglican in basement membrane assembly. Cell. 1998;95:859-870.

Henry MD, Campbell KP. Dystroglican inside and out. Curr Opin Cell Biol. 1999;11:602-607.

Hoffman EP, Brown Jr RH, Kunkel LM. Dystrophin: The protein product of the Duchenne muscular dystrophy locus. Cell. 1987;51:919–928.

Hoffman EP, Dressman D. Molecular pathophysiology and targeted therapeutics for muscular dystrophy. Trends Pharmacol Sci 2001;22: 465–70

Hohenester E, Tisi D, Talts JF, et al. The crystal structure of a laminin G-like module reveals the molecular basis of alpha-destroglycan binding to laminins, perlecan, and agrin. Mol Cell. 1999;4:783–792.

Hong, F, Lee J, Song JW, Lee SJ, Ahn H, Cho JJ, Ha J, Kim SS. Cyclosporin A blocks muscle differentiation by inducing oxidative stress and inhibiting the peptidyl-prolyl-cis-trans isomerase activity of cyclophilin A: cyclophilin A protects myoblasts from cyclosporin A-induced cytotoxicity. Faseb J. 2002;16(12):1633-5.

Houde S, Filiatrault M, Fournier A, et al. Deflazacort use in Duchenne muscular dystrophy: an 8-year follow-up. Pediatr Neurol. 2008;38:200–206.

Huang X, Poy F, Zhang E, et al. Structure of a WW domain containing fragment of dystrophin in complex with beta-dystroglican. Nat Struct Biol. 2000;7:634–638.

Huard J, Acsadi G, Jani A, Massie B, Karpati G. Gene transfer into skeletal muscles by isogenic myoblasts. Hum Gene Ther. 1994;5(8):949-58.

Huard J, Bouchard JP, Roy R, Labrecque C, Dansereau G, Lemieux B, Tremblay JP. Myoblast transplantation produced dystrophin-positive muscle fibres in a 16-year-old patient with Duchenne muscular dystrophy. Clin Sci (Lond). 1991;81(2):287-8.

Huard J, Bouchard JP, Roy R, Malouin F, Dansereau G, Labrecque C, Albert N, Richards CL, Lemieux B, Tremblay JP. Human myoblast transplantation: preliminary results of 4 cases. Muscle Nerve. 1992;15(5):550-60.

Iannitti T, Capone S, Feder D, Palmieri B. Clinical use of immunosuppressants in duchenne muscular dystrophy. J Clin Neuromuscul Dis. 2010;12(1):1-21.

Ichim TE, Alexandrescu DT, Solano F, Lara F, Campion Rde N, Paris E, Woods EJ, Murphy MP, Dasanu CA, Patel AN, Marleau AM, Leal A, Riordan NH. Mesenchymal stem cells as anti-inflammatories: implications for treatment of Duchenne muscular dystrophy. Cell Immunol. 2010;260(2):75-82.

Jazedje T, Secco M, Vieira NM, Zucconi E, Gollop TR, Vainzof M, Zatz M. Stem cells from umbilical cord blood do have myogenic potential, with and without differentiation induction in vitro. J Transl Med. 2009;14; 7:6.

Jennekens FG, ten Kate LP, de Visser M et al. Diagnostic criteria for Duchenne and Becker muscular dystrophy and myotonic dystrophy. Neuromuscul Disord. 1991;1:389–391.

Jung D, Yang B, Meyer J, et al. Identification and characterizion of the dystrophin anchoring site on betadystroglican. J Biol Chem. 1995;270:27305-27310.

Karpati, G, Ajdukovic D, Arnold D, Gledhill RB, Guttmann R, Holland P, Koch PA, Shoubridge E, Spence D, Vanasse M. Myoblast transfer in Duchenne muscular dystrophy. Ann Neurol. 1993;34(1):8-17.

Kemaladewi DU, Hoogaars WM, van Heiningen SH, Terlouw S, de Gorter DJ, den Dunnen JT, van Ommen GJ, Aartsma-Rus A, Ten Dijke P, 't Hoen PA. Dual exon skipping in myostatin and dystrophin for Duchenne muscular dystrophy. BMC Med Genomics. 2011;4:36.

Kinali M, Arechavala-Gomeza V, Feng L, Cirak S, Hunt D, Adkin C, Guglieri M, Ashton E, Abbs S, Nihoyannopoulos P, Garralda ME, Rutherford M, McCulley C, Popplewell L, Graham IR, Dickson G, Wood MJ, Wells DJ, Wilton SD, Kole R, Straub V, Bushby K, Sewry C, Morgan JE, Muntoni F. Local restoration of dystrophin expression with the morpholino oligomer AVI-4658 in Duchenne muscular dystrophy: a single-blind, placebo-controlled, dose-escalation, proof-of-concept study. Lancet Neurol. 2009 Oct;8(10):918-28. Epub 2009 Aug 25. Erratum in: Lancet Neurol. 2009 Dec;8(12):1083.

Kinoshita I, Roy R, Dugré FJ, Gravel C, Roy B, Goulet M, Asselin I, Tremblay JP. Myoblast transplantation in monkeys: control of immune response by FK506. J Neuropathol Exp Neurol. 1996;55(6):687-97.

Kinoshita I, Vilquin JT, Guérette B, Asselin I, Roy R, Tremblay JP. Very efficient myoblast allotransplantation in mice under FK506 immunosuppression. Muscle Nerve. 1994;17(12):1407-15.

Kirschner J, Schessl J, Ihorst G, et al; Muskeldystrophie Netzwerk MD-NET. Treatment of Duchenne muscular dystrophy with cyclosporin A—a randomized, double-blind, placebo controlled trial. Neuropediatrics. 2008;44:39.

Koenig M, Monaco AP, Kunkel LM. The complete sequence of dystrophin predicts a rod-shaped cytoskeletal protein. Cell. 1988;53:219–226.

Krause DS, Theise ND, Collector MI, Henegariu O, Hwang S, Gardner R, Neutzel S, Sharkis SJ. Multi-organ, multi-lineage engraftment by a single bone marrow-derived stem cell. Cell. 2001;105(3):369-77.

Kunkel LM. Analysis of deletions in DNA from patients with Becker and Duchenne muscular dystrophy. Nature. 1986;622:73–77.

Law PK, Goodwin TG, Fang Q, Duggirala V, Larkin C, Florendo JA, Kirby DS, Deering MB, Li HJ, Chen M. Feasibility, safety, and efficacy of myoblast transfer therapy on Duchenne muscular dystrophy boys. Cell Transplant. 1992;1(2-3):235-44.

Le Grand F, Rudnicki M. Satellite and stem cells in muscle growth and repair. Development. 2007a;134(22):3953-7.

Le Grand F, Rudnicki M. Skeletal muscle satellite cells and adult myogenesis. Curr Opin Cell Biol. 2007b;19(6):628-33.

Lee-Pullen TF, Grounds MD. Muscle-derived stem cells: implications for effective myoblast transfer therapy. IUBMB Life. 2005;57(11):731-6.

Lee JH, Kosinski PA, Kemp DM. Contribution of human bone marrow stem cells to individual skeletal myotubes followed by myogenic gene activation. Exp Cell Res. 2005;307:174-182.

Liu Y, Song J, Liu W, Wan Y, Chen X, Hu C. Growth and differentiation of rat bone marrow stromal cells: does 5-azacytidine trigger their cardiomyogenic differentiation? Cardiovasc Res. 2003;58:460-468.

Lodi D, Iannitti T, Palmieri B. Stem cells in clinical practice: applications and warnings. J Exp Clin Cancer Res. 2011;30:9.

Mann CJ, Honeyman K, McClorey G, Fletcher S, Wilton SD. Improved antisense oligonucleotide induced exon skipping in the mdx mouse model of muscular dystrophy. J Gene Med 2002;4:644-54.

Manzur AY, Muntoni F. Diagnosis and new treatments in muscular dystrophies. J Neurol Neurosurg Psychiatry 2009;80:706-14.

Markham LW, Spicer RL, Khoury PR, et al. Steroid therapy and cardiac function in Duchenne muscular dystrophy. Pediatr Cardiol. 2005;26:768–771.

Mavrogeni S, Papavasiliou A, Douskou M, Kolovou G, Papadopoulou E, Cokkinos DV. Effect of deflazacort on cardiac and sternocleidomastoid muscles in Duchenne musculardystrophy: a magnetic resonance imaging study. Eur J Paediatr Neurol. 2009 Jan;13(1):34-40. Epub 2008 Apr 11.

Melis MA, Cau M, Muntoni F, et al. Elevation of serum creatine kinase as the only manifestation of an intragenic dletion of the dystrophin gene in three unrelated families. Eur J Paediatr neurol 1998; 2:255-61.

Mendell JR, Kissel JT, Amato AA, King W, Signore L, Prior TW, Sahenk Z, Benson S, McAndrew PE, Rice R. Myoblast transfer in the treatment of Duchenne's muscular dystrophy. N Engl J Med. 1995;333(13):832-8

Mezey E, Chandross KJ, Harta G, Maki RA, McKercher SR. Turning blood into brain: cells bearing neuronal antigens generated in vivo from bone marrow. Science. 2000;290(5497):1779-82.

Miller RG, Sharma KR, Pavlath GK, Gussoni E, Mynhier M, Lanctot AM, Greco CM, Steinman L, Blau HM. Myoblast implantation in Duchenne muscular dystrophy: the San Francisco study. Muscle Nerve. 1997;20(4):469-78.

Monaco AP, Bertelson CJ, Liechti-gallati S, Moser H, Kunkel LM. An explanation for the phenotypic differences between patients bearing partial deletions of the DMD locus. Genomics 1988;2:90-95.

Muntoni F, Torelli S, Ferlini A. Dystrophin and mutations: one gene, several proteins, multiple phenotypes. Lancet Neurol. 2003;2:731–740.

Naesens M, Kuypers DR, Sarwal M. Calcineurin inhibitor nephrotoxicity. Clin J Am Soc Nephrol. 2009;4:481–508.

Nassiri SM, Khaki Z, Soleimani M, Ahmadi SH, Jahanzad I, Rabbani S, Sahebjam M, Ardalan FA, Fathollahi MS. The similar effect of transplantation of marrow-derived mesenchymal stem cells with or without prior differentiation induction in experimental myocardial infarction. J Biomed Sci. 2007 Nov;14(6):745-55. Epub 2007 Jul 1.

Newey SE, Benson MA, Pointing CP, et al. Alternative splicing of dystrobrevin regulates the stoichiometry of syntrophin binding to the dystrophin protein complex. Curr Biol. 2000;10:1295–1298.

Norwood FL, Sutherland-Smith AJ, Keep NH, et al. The structure of the N-terminal actin-binding domain of human dystrophin and how mutations in this domain maybe cause Duchenne or Becker muscular dystrophy. Structure Fold Des. 2000;8:481–491.

Nunes VA, Cavaçana N, Canovas M, Strauss BE, Zatz M. Stem cells from umbilical cord blood differentiate into myotubes and express dystrophin in vitro only after exposure to in vivo muscle environment. Biol Cell. 2007;99(4):185-96.

Otto A, Collins-Hooper H, Patel K. The origin, molecular regulation and therapeutic potential of myogenic stem cell populations. J Anat. 2009;215(5):477-97.

Palmieri B, Sblendorio V. Duchenne Muscular Dystrophy: An Update, Part I. Journal of Clinical Neromuscular Disease 8 (2) 2006.

Palmieri B, Tremblay JP, Daniele L. Past, present and future of myoblast transplantation in the treatment of Duchenne muscular dystrophy. Pediatr Transplant. 2010;14(7):813-9.

Peault B, Rudnicki M, Torrente Y, Cossu G, Tremblay JP, Partridge T, Gussoni E, Kunkel LM, Huard J. Stem and progenitor cells in skeletal muscle development, maintenance, and therapy. Mol Ther. 2007;15(5):867-77.

Petrof BJ. Molecular pathophysiology of myofiber injury in deficiencies of the dystrophin-glycoprotein complex. Am. J. Phys. Med. Rehabil. 2002;81, S162-S174.

Pittenger MF, Mackay AM, Beck SC, Jaiswal RK, Douglas R, Mosca JD, Moorman MA, Simonetti DW, Craig S, Marshak DR. Multilineage potential of adult human mesenchymal stem cells. Science. 1999;284(5411):143-7.

Prockop DJ. Marrow stromal cells as stem cells for nonhematopoietic tissues. Science. 1997;276(5309):71-4.

Quenneville SP, Chapdelaine P, Skuk D, Paradis M, Goulet M, Rousseau J, Xiao X, Garcia L, Tremblay JP. Autologous transplantation of muscle precursor cells modified with a lentivirus for muscular dystrophy: human cells and primate models. Mol Ther. 2007;15(2):431-8.

Rivière C, Danos O, Douar AM. Long-term expression and repeated administration of AAV type 1, 2 and 5 vectors in skeletal muscle of immunocompetent adult mice. Gene Ther. 2006;13(17):1300-8

Roberts RG, Bobrow M. Dystrophins in vertebrates and invertebrates. Hum Mol Genet. 1998;7:589–595.

Sampaolesi M, Blot S, D'Antona G, Granger N, Tonlorenzi R, Innocenzi A, Mognol P, Thibaud JL, Galvez BG, Barthélémy I, Perani L, Mantero S, Guttinger M, Pansarasa O, Rinaldi C, Cusella De Angelis MG, Torrente Y, Bordignon C, Bottinelli R, Cossu G. Mesoangioblast stem cells ameliorate muscle function in dystrophic dogs. Nature. 2006 Nov 30;444(7119):574-9. Epub 2006 Nov 15.

Sampaolesi M, Torrente Y, Innocenzi A, Tonlorenzi R, D'Antona G, Pellegrino MA, Barresi R, Bresolin N, De Angelis MG, Campbell KP, Bottinelli R, Cossu G. Cell therapy of alpha-sarcoglycan null dystrophic mice through intra-arterial delivery of mesoangioblasts. Science. 2003 Jul 25;301(5632):487-92. Epub 2003 Jul 10.

Sanes JR, Lichtam JW. Development of the vertebrate neuromuscular junction. Ann Rev Neurosci. 1999;22:389–442.

Sarig, R, Baruchi Z, Fuchs O, Nudel U, Yaffe D. Regeneration and transdifferentiation potential of muscle-derived stem cells propagated as myospheres. Stem Cells. 2006;24(7):1769-78.

Sealock R, Butler MH, Kramarcy NR, et al. Localization of dystrophin relative to acetylcholine receptor domains in electric tissue and adult and cultured skeletal muscle. J Cell Biol. 1991;113:1133–1144.

Sharma KR, Mynhier MA, Miller RG. Cyclosporine increases muscular force generation in Duchenne muscular dystrophy. Neurology. 1993;43:527–532.

Shi D., Reinecke H, Murry CE, Torok-Storb B. Myogenic fusion of human bone marrow stromal cells, but not hematopoiecti cells. Blood. 2004;104:290-294.

Sigesmund DA, Weleber RG, Pillers DA, et al. Characterization of the ocular phenotype of Duchenne and Becker muscular dystrophy. Ophthalmology. 1994;101:856–865.

Skuk D, Goulet M, Roy B, Chapdelaine P, Bouchard JP, Roy R, Dugré FJ, Sylvain M, Lachance JG, Deschênes L, Senay H, Tremblay JP. Dystrophin expression in muscles of duchenne muscular dystrophy patients after high-density injections of normal myogenic cells. J Neuropathol Exp Neurol. 2006;65(4):371-86.

Skuk D, Goulet M, Roy B, Piette V, Côté CH, Chapdelaine P, Hogrel JY, Paradis M, Bouchard JP, Sylvain M, Lachance JG, Tremblay JP. First test of a "high-density injection" protocol for myogenic cell transplantation throughout large volumes of muscles in a Duchenne muscular dystrophy patient: eighteen months follow-up. Neuromuscul Disord. 2007;17(1):38-46.

Skuk D, Roy B, Goulet M, Chapdelaine P, Bouchard JP, Roy R, Dugré FJ, Lachance JG, Deschênes L, Hélène S, Sylvain M, Tremblay JP Dystrophin expression in myofibers of Duchenne muscular dystrophy patients following intramuscular injections of normal myogenic cells. Mol Ther. 2004;9(3):475-82.

Skuk D, Roy B, Goulet M, Tremblay JP. Successful myoblast transplantation in primates depends on appropriate cell delivery and induction of regeneration in the host muscle. Exp Neurol. 1999;155(1):22-30.

Smythe GM, Grounds MD. Absence of MyoD increases donor myoblast migration into host muscle. Exp Cell Res. 2001;267(2):267-74.

Stephan L, Pichavant C, Bouchentouf M, Mills P, Camirand G, Tagmouti S, Rothstein D, Tremblay JP. Induction of tolerance across fully mismatched barriers by a nonmyeloablative treatment excluding antibodies or irradiation use. Cell Transplant. 2006;15(8-9):835-46.

Straathof CS, Overweg-Plandsoen WC, van den Burg GJ, van der Kooi AJ, Verschuuren JJ, de Groot IJ. Prednisone 10 days on/10 days off in patients with Duchenne muscular dystrophy. J Neurol. 2009 May;256(5):768-73. Epub 2009 Mar 22.

Tennyson CN, Dally GY, Ray PN, et al. Expression of the dystrophin isoform Dp71 in differentiating human fetal myogenic cultures. Hum Mol Genet. 1996;5:1559-1566.

Torrente Y, Belicchi M, Marchesi C, Dantona G, Cogiamanian F, Pisati F, Gavina M, Giordano R, Tonlorenzi R, Fagiolari G, Lamperti C, Porretti L, Lopa R, Sampaolesi M, Vicentini L, Grimoldi N, Tiberio F, Songa V, Baratta P, Prelle A, Forzenigo L, Guglieri M, Pansarasa O, Rinaldi C, Mouly V, Butler-Browne GS, Comi GP, Biondetti P, Moggio M, Gaini SM, Stocchetti N, Priori A, D'Angelo MG, Turconi A, Bottinelli R, Cossu G, Rebulla P, Bresolin N. Autologous transplantation of muscle-derived CD133+ stem cells in Duchenne muscle patients. Cell Transplant. 2007;16(6):563-77.

Torrente Y, Belicchi M, Sampaolesi M, Pisati F, Meregalli M, D'Antona G, Tonlorenzi R, Porretti L, Gavina M, Mamchaoui K, Pellegrino MA, Furling D, Mouly V, Butler-Browne GS, Bottinelli R, Cossu G, Bresolin N. Human circulating AC133(+) stem cells restore dystrophin expression and ameliorate function in dystrophic skeletal muscle. J Clin Invest. 2004;114(2):182-95.

Tremblay JP, Malouin F, Roy R, Huard J, Bouchard JP, Satoh A, Richards CL. Results of a triple blind clinical study of myoblast transplantations without immunosuppressive treatment in young boys with Duchenne muscular dystrophy. Cell Transplant. 1993;2(2):99-112.

Trollet C, Athanasopoulos T, Popplewell L, Malerba A, Dickson G. Gene therapy for muscular dystrophy: current progress and future prospects. Expert Opinion on Biologicla Therapy 2009; 9:849-66.

van Deutekom JC, Janson AA, Ginjaar IB, Frankhuizen WS, Aartsma-Rus A, Bremmer-Bout M, den Dunnen JT, Koop K, van der Kooi AJ, Goemans NM, de Kimpe SJ, Ekhart PF, Venneker EH, Platenburg GJ, Verschuuren JJ, van Ommen GJ. Local dystrophin restoration with antisense oligonucleotide PRO051. N Engl J Med. 2007 Dec 27;357(26):2677-86.

van Ommen GJ, van Deutekom J, Aartsma-Rus A. The therapeutic potential of antisense-mediated exon skiping. Curr Opin Mol Ther 2008,10:140-9.

Way M, Pope B, Cross RA, et al. Expression of the N-terminal domain of dystrophin in E. Coli and demonstration of binding of F-actin. FEBS Lett. 1992;301:243-245.

Whitehead NP, Yeung EW, Allen DG. Muscle damage in mdx (dystrophic) mice: role of calcium and reactive oxygen species. Clin Exp Pharmacol Physiol. 2006;33:657-662.

Wognum AW, Eaves AC, Thomas TE. Identification and isolation of hematopoietic stem cells. Arch Med Res. 2003;34(6):461-75.

Xiong, F, Zhang C, Xiao SB, Li MS, Wang SH, Yu MJ, Shang YC. Construction of recombinant adenovirus including microdystrophin and expression in the mesenchymal cells of mdx mice. Sheng Wu Gong Cheng Xue Bao. 2007;23(1):27-32.

Yang B, Jung D, Rafael JA, et al. Identification of alpha-syntrophin binding to syntrophin triplet, dystrophin, and utrophin. J Biol Chem. 1995;270:4975-4978.

Yoshida N, Yoshida S, Koishi K, Masuda K, Nabeshima Y. Cell heterogeneity upon myogenic differentiation: down-regulation of MyoD and Myf-5 generates 'reverse cells'. J Cell Sci 1998;111:769-79.

4

Stem Cell Based Therapy for Muscular Dystrophies: Cell Types and Environmental Factors Influencing Their Efficacy

Jennifer Morgan[1] and Hala Alameddine[2]
[1]The Dubowitz Neuromuscular Centre, UCL Institute of Child Health, London,
[2]UMRS 974, UMR7215, Institut de Myologie, Paris
[1]UK
[2]France

1. Introduction

Muscular dystrophies are inherited disorders in which muscle fibers are unusually susceptible to damage, leading to progressive loss of muscle structure and function. Some types of muscular dystrophy affect heart muscles, other involuntary muscles and other organs. The most common form of muscular dystrophy, Duchenne Muscular Dystrophy (DMD), is due to genetic deficiency of the protein dystrophin (Monaco et al., 1985). This protein is one of several partners that interact to link intracellular cytoskeleton to extracellular matrix (ECM) hence consolidating the scaffold necessary for maintaining structural integrity of skeletal muscle fibers. Dystrophin deficiency destabilizes muscle fibers, which become less resistant to contractions leading to muscle fiber necrosis and subsequent regeneration.

Skeletal muscle repair, maintenance and regeneration are mediated by muscle-specific stem cells: the satellite cells (Mauro, 1961), located underneath basal lamina of muscle fibers. In DMD muscles, fat and connective tissue often replace muscle fibers in the late stages of muscular dystrophy, indicating that muscle regeneration does not keep up with fiber loss. Defective muscle regeneration could be due to exhaustion of proliferative capacity of satellite cells (Blau et al., 1983; Webster & Blau, 1990) or to environmental factors that are not conducive to their function. The healing process usually includes sequential and overlapping events of muscle fiber degeneration, inflammatory reaction, regeneration and remodeling of ECM components that require tightly regulated orchestration of the interactive cross-talk that conditions the outcome of the regenerative process. Uncontrolled wound-healing, in response to chronic injury and inflammation, results in tissue fibrosis and scarring which impacts on the efficiency of muscle regeneration, hence contributing to the degradation of muscle function.

At present, we still have no cure for any form of muscular dystrophy, but medications and therapy can slow the course of the disease to allow people with muscular dystrophy to remain mobile for as long as possible. Nevertheless, experimental therapeutic strategies have been initiated in light of basic and technical advances of skeletal muscle biology and pathophysiology. The description of the muscle regeneration process and the identification of the cells responsible for myofiber regeneration led to stem cell therapy being considered as a potential strategy to alleviate muscle deficiency in DMD patients. Alternatively, the identification of gene defects and the sophistication of molecular biology technologies have opened perspectives for gene therapy, either by providing the deficient gene, or by restoring gene function. Other strategies combining both approaches have been considered and imply the correction of patients' own stem cells before grafting them into the diseased muscles. These promising strategies have been challenged in animal models of muscular dystrophies and although they achieved a certain success, they also identified a number of limitations. Moreover, the failure of myogenic cell grafting to improve muscle function and to restore dystrophin expression in clinical trials of DMD patients, underscored the need to improve the efficiency of cell therapy. Cell environment, which comprises ECM and extracellular matrix deposited factors such as growth factors, cytokines and chemokines, regulate diverse cellular functions. These molecules are metabolized by Matrix MetalloProteinases (MMPs) that play a central role as regulators of tissue microenvironment. In normal situations, precise spatiotemporal repertoires of MMPs balanced by inhibitors, among which are the four Tissue Inhibitors of MatrixmetalloProteinases (TIMPs), regulate extracellular signaling networks and maintain tissue homeostasis. On the contrary, increased MMPs expression or activity has been demonstrated in various disease situations including, practically every known inflammatory disease (Manicone & McGuire, 2008). Such disruption of the dynamic equilibrium between MMPs and TIMPs may affect diverse cellular functions including cell proliferation, migration, adhesion and apoptosis (Holmbeck et al., 2005; Hulboy et al., 1997; Vu & Werb, 2000). In DMD, for example, inflammation and fibrosis are major hurdles in the path of therapeutic strategies (Wells et al., 2002) and their resolution is expected to positively impact on the efficiency of any form of therapy, but more specifically, on the efficiency of cell therapy. Indeed, myogenic stem cells have limited migratory capacity, which is further aggravated by excessive proliferation of connective tissue. Therefore, improving the efficiency of cell therapy could be achieved either by myogenic cells better able to digest accumulated ECM components or, alternatively, by other types of stem cells that can be recruited from a resident or circulating pool and are capable of migrating through one or several tissue barriers to home into skeletal muscles. In this chapter, we consider the use of stem cell therapy to treat muscular dystrophies. By going through the different cell types that have been used, we will try to define the best cell type to use, how to handle and expand these cells before transplantation and the best route of delivery. Moreover, the possibility of using genetically-modified autologous stem cells for transplantation will be presented. This would only be possible if the stem cell had not been deleteriously affected by the dystrophic environment. Finally, we will consider the host environment as a modulator of cell behaviour and the dual role MMPs play in the control of this environment and their impact on transplanted cells migration, differentiation and self-renewal.

2. Potential therapies for duchenne muscular dystrophy

Muscular dystrophies are a heterogeneous group of inherited neuromuscular disorders, including X-linked recessive as in DMD, autosomal recessive as in limb–girdle muscular dystophy type 2, or autosomal dominant as in facioscapulohumeral muscular dystophy, myotonic dystrophy, and limb–girdle muscular dystophy type 1 (Emery, 2002). In the last two decades, different types of dystrophies have been genetically characterized. The most frequent and most severe form, DMD, is a progressive, incurable X-linked recessive disorder that affects 1 in 3500 newborn boys and leads to death in the second or third decade of life (Bushby et al., 2010). DMD patients lack the protein dystrophin while in-frame mutations of the same gene led to expression of a partially functional protein, resulting in the milder Becker muscular dystrophies (BMD). As a result of the absence of dystrophin, muscle fibers of DMD patients undergo necrosis followed by regeneration which, in the long run, fails to keep up with the recurrent cycles of degeneration-regeneration and muscle fibers are lost and replaced by fibro-fatty tissue. Interruption of these cycles can be achieved by dystrophin restoration to the muscle fiber membrane (Meng et al., 2011a). Several strategies can now be used to restore dystrophin to the muscle fibers of affected patients. They include virally-mediated gene therapy, read-through of stop codons, up-regulation of compensatory genes, or skipping of mutated dystrophin exons to give rise to a shorter, but still functional dystrophin protein. However, all of these have possible drawbacks (reviewed (Goyenvalle & Davies, 2011; Guglieri & Bushby, 2010; Hoffman et al., 2011; Sugita & Takeda, 2010)). Either gene therapy, or application of antisense oligonucleotides to skip mutated dystrophin exons, requires that the patient has sufficient muscle fibers remaining for treatment. In addition, exon skipping is mutation-dependent and not all patients have mutations amenable to this approach.

3. Stem cell therapy for the treatment of DMD

The concept of a cell-based therapy to alleviate loss of muscle structure and function in muscular dystrophy originated with the observation of the intrinsic ability of myogenic stem cells to fuse either with each other to form multinucleated myofibers, or with necrotic muscle fibers to form mosaic fibers. In theory, functional correction could be achieved in DMD by the generation of either hybrid muscle fibers where the donor nuclei provide the missing gene product and/or the regeneration of normal myofibers from the fusion of normal donor cells to replace lost muscle fibers. Cell therapy was the first biologically based approach applied for the treatment of DMD and required the use of animal models to explore the beneficial effects of this therapy. The ability of cultured myogenic cells to regenerate new muscle fibers, that reconstitute the same architectural organization of the original muscle and induce functional recovery, has been validated using an experimental model of irreversible injury to adult rodent muscle associating auto-transplantation of skeletal muscle to X-irradiation (Alameddine et al., 1989; Alameddine et al., 1991; Alameddine et al., 1994).

3.1 Stem cells

Stem cells are defined as cells that can both self-renew and give rise to more differentiated cell type, whereas precursor cells do not have the ability to self-renew. Both cell types present a great advantage for the treatment of muscular dystrophies as they could repair segmental necrosis and also give rise to regenerated muscle fibers to replace those that are lost as a consequence of the dystrophy. They could therefore be effective at later stages of the dystrophy, when muscle fibers have already been lost. Donor cells derived from a normal individual will automatically express dystrophin when they differentiate into a muscle fiber, but the quantity and distribution of dystrophin within the fiber will depend on the number of donor myonuclei and the size of segments of the fiber to which they contribute. However, the recipient and donor will need to be HLA-matched, so that stem cells from one normal donor could not be used to treat all patients.

Although many different stem or precursor cells have been shown to contribute to muscle regeneration in animal models, many of these give rise to only limited amount of muscle, for example haematopoietic stem cells (Ferrari et al., 1998) and mesenchymal stem cells (Chan et al., 2006; Meng et al., 2010). Satellite cells are the archetypal skeletal muscle stem cell, but they are by definition quiescent cells underneath the basal lamina of muscle fibers and it would be impossible to obtain enough of them for therapeutic application. However, the progeny of satellite cells, muscle precursor cells or myoblasts, could be prepared in sufficient quantity for transplantation. In this review, therefore, we will focus on cells that can be expanded in culture and that have been shown to contribute to muscle regeneration-myoblasts, cells derived from blood-vessel associated pericytes (termed mesoangioblasts) and skeletal muscle-derived AC133+ cells. There are several recent reviews on stem cells to treat muscular dystrophies, which cover most of the cell types that have been studied (Meng et al., 2011a; Negroni et al., 2011; Palmieri et al., 2010; Skuk & Tremblay, 2011; Tedesco et al., 2010).

3.2 Models and markers

To investigate the potential contribution of a particular cell type to muscle regeneration, the standard experiment is to graft the cells into an animal model of DMD and measure their contribution to skeletal muscle fibers, which may be quantified by either counting the number of dystrophin-positive fibers, or measuring the amount of dystrophin on western blot. Several animal models of DMD exist but the most widely-used is the dystrophin-deficient *mdx* mouse (Bulfield et al., 1984) used in 1,940 pubmed publications, as of 21 July 2011. Other models of DMD include the golden retriever muscular dystrophy (GRMD also known as Canine X-linked Muscular Dystrophy CXMD) dog and zebrafish (reviewed (Banks & Chamberlain, 2008; Collins & Morgan, 2003)). Mouse and dog models have been used to investigate different potential therapies for DMD, including precursor/stem cell transplantation (Nakamura & Takeda, 2011). However, when grafting cells from one donor to another, the host must either be immunodeficient or immunosuppressed. Therefore, *mdx* mice with different types of immunodeficiency have been used as hosts in cell transplantation experiments, including *mdx* nu/nu (Boldrin et al., 2009; Collins et al., 2005; Partridge et al., 1989), SCID *mdx* (Benchaouir et al., 2007; Dellavalle et al., 2007; Torrente et al., 2004), Rag-/- *mdx* (Gerard et al., 2011), or *mdx* mice immunosuppressed with FK506 (Kinoshita et al., 1994b), but to what extent these different hosts are comparable, being on different genetic backgrounds and having different mechanisms and degrees of immunodeficiency, has not been ascertained (reviewed (Meng et al., 2011b)). Immunodeficient mice are more convenient to work with than mice that have to be immunosuppressed and seem to permit greater donor-myoblast-derived muscle regeneration (Partridge et al., 1989). However, it is important to consider the effect of the immunological system on donor-derived muscle regeneration, as DMD patients will not be immunodeficient. Non-dystrophic mice or monkeys, whose muscles have been injured to mimic the degeneration and regeneration that occurs in dystrophic muscles, have also been used as recipients to test cell transplantation (Cooper et al., 2001; Morgan et al., 2002; Sacco et al., 2008; Skuk et al., 1999), as have mice that model different types of dystrophy, e.g. sarcoglycan (Sampaolesi et al., 2003) and dysferlin-deficient mice (Diaz-Manera et al., 2010).

A major consideration when using both dystrophic and non-dystrophic animal models to test stem cells is that the host muscle usually has to be injured in some way to enhance donor cell engraftment. This is surprising, as the muscle fiber degeneration and regeneration that is already occurring in dystrophic muscle would be thought to be sufficient to promote donor stem cells to contribute to muscle regeneration. However, muscle fiber necrosis is often focal and only cells located nearby contribute to regeneration (Yokota et al., 2006). Therefore, if the transplanted stem cell is located a distance away, it may not either receive the correct signals, or be able to migrate to the damaged fibers. As many of these injury regimes are very severe, for example, cryoinjury (Brimah et al., 2004; Irintchev et al., 1997; Negroni et al., 2009) or use of snake venoms (Lefaucheur & Sebille, 1995; Silva-Barbosa et al., 2005) to induce degeneration and regeneration in host muscles, they could not be used in patients. Even in dystrophin-deficient *mdx* nu/nu host mice, satellite cells contribute little, if any, to muscle regeneration (Boldrin et al., 2009; Collins et al., 2005) although myoblasts contribute to muscle regeneration to a greater extent (Morgan et al., 2002; Partridge et al., 1989). This poor contribution of donor cells to muscle regeneration is likely to be due to the fact that *mdx* mouse muscles, in contrast to those of DMD patients, regenerate very well. We therefore blocked muscle regeneration in *mdx* muscles by applying local high doses of radiation, to obtain a model more similar to DMD, in which the muscle degenerates and atrophies but does not regenerate (Morgan et al., 1990; Pagel & Partridge, 1999; Wakeford et al., 1991). If host muscle is irradiated with 18 Gy before donor cell grafting, satellite cell and myoblast contribution to muscle regeneration is significantly augmented (Boldrin et al., 2009; Collins et al., 2005; Morgan et al., 2002). This may be due to prevention of competition from local host stem or satellite cells, as irradiated *mdx* muscles do not regenerate (Pagel & Partridge, 1999; Wakeford et al., 1991) unless a severe injury, e.g. injection of snake venom notexin, is imposed on them, which evokes rare radiation-resistant stem cells to regenerate (Gross & Morgan, 1999; Heslop et al., 2000). Other models that could be used to test whether a wholly or partially emptied satellite cell niche is necessary for efficient donor muscle stem cell engraftment include Pax7 knockout mice (Seale et al., 2000) that lack satellite cells, or the *mdx* mouse that also lacks telomerase (mTR) activity and therefore shows a reduction in the regenerative capacity of myogenic stem cells (Sacco et al., 2010).

Another important consideration is the marker(s) to be used to assess the contribution of donor cells to regenerated muscle fibers and/or satellite cells (reviewed (Meng et al., 2011a)). As the aim is to produce dystrophin in host muscle fibers, it is sensible to quantify dystrophin restoration in the host muscles (Partridge et al., 1989). Because "revertant" fibers that spontaneously express dystrophin are present in animal models of DMD (Hoffman et al., 1990) and in DMD patients (Arechavala-Gomeza et al., 2010) and because clusters of revertant fibers increase in number with time (Hoffman et al., 1990; Yokota et al., 2006), revertant fibers must be controlled for, particularly if dystrophin is being used alone as a marker of donor-derived muscle fibers and especially in time course studies. If grafting human cells into mouse, a human-specific dystrophin antibody (e.g. Novocastra Dys3 (Brimah et al., 2004)) may be used, that will not identify mouse revertant fibers. Because of the existence of revertant fibers, many groups use a second marker of either muscle fibers or cells of donor origin, e.g. by using donor cells from genetically-modified mice, e.g. myosin 3f nLacZ-E, that is expressed in myonuclei of donor origin, Myf5 nLacZ/$^+$ that is expressed in satellite cells of donor origin (Collins et al., 2005), or ubiquitously (Morgan et al., 2002) or muscle-specifically (Kinoshita et al., 1994a) expressed β-gal or GFP. Donor cells may alternatively be marked in culture with constructs expressing a marker protein (Blaveri et al., 1999; Cousins et al., 2004; Diaz-Manera et al., 2010; Morgan et al., 2002). However, caution should be used in interpreting results, as GFP is notoriously difficult to use in skeletal muscle (Jackson et al., 2004), some markers spread further along a mosaic muscle fiber than others (Blaveri et al., 1999) and others are switched off in vivo (Boldrin et al.,2009).

3.3 Contribution of locally-delivered donor stem cells to muscle regeneration.

A large body of evidence can be found in the literature to illustrate the contribution of myoblasts to skeletal muscle regeneration, although the number of donor-derived muscle fibers is limited (Figure 1). However, the host muscle environment that permits regeneration from myoblasts of mouse and human origin appears to be different, although a comparative experiment to establish this point has not been performed: human myoblasts form more muscle within host muscles that have been cryoinjured prior to grafting (Brimah et al., 2004), whereas mouse myoblasts form significantly more muscle in irradiated host muscles (Boldrin and Morgan, manuscript in preparation).

Different muscle injury models used for intra-muscular grafting of putative muscle stem cells may also give rise to discrepancies between groups. Some groups have grafted cells into muscles of non-dystrophic mice that had been cryo-injured immediately prior to grafting (Brimah et al., 2004; Cooper et al., 2001; Ehrhardt et al., 2007), but others grafted cells into muscles of *mdx* SCID mice that had been injected 48 hours previously with cardiotoxin, (Dellavalle et al., 2007) or into cryo–injured muscles of immunodeficient Rag2-/- gamma chain-non-dystrophic mice (Pisani et al., 2010). Vauchez et al. grafted into muscles of non-dystrophic SCID mice, injuring the muscles prior to grafting by a combination of irradiation and notexin (Vauchez et al., 2009); Zheng et al. grafted cells into muscles of SCID mice that had been injured by cardiotoxin one day previously (Zheng et al., 2007). How these different injury regimes mimic the dystrophic muscle environment and to what extent the local environment, genetic background and immunological status of the host mouse affect muscle stem cell behavior are important to determine, for the identification of robust methodologies which could reliably be used for therapeutic trials in muscular dystrophies.

Interestingly, although they contributed to much muscle regeneration after intra-arterial injection, pericytes only gave rise to very small numbers of muscle fibers after intra-muscular transplantation: CD56+/ALP- cells (satellite-cell derived myoblasts) gave rise to more muscle than CD56+/ALP+ cells (pericytes), but CD56-/ALP- cells, taken to be fibroblasts, made very few donor muscle fibers (Dellavalle et al., 2007). Meng et al. also found that both CD56+ and CD56- skeletal muscle-derived cells contributed to muscle regeneration, CD56+ cells making significantly more muscle than either CD56-, or non-fractionated cells after intra-muscular transplantation. CD56+ cells contributed predominantly to nuclei inside the basal lamina of muscle fibers, i.e. within muscle fibers and/or satellite cells. But CD56- or non-sorted cells contributed to significantly more nuclei outside the basal lamina, confirming that there were more non-myogenic cells within CD56- cell population (Meng et al., 2011b). Zheng et al showed that human skeletal muscle-derived CD56+ cells that also expressed CD34 and CD144 (myoendothelial cells) contributed to more muscle regeneration than did CD56+/CD34-/CD144- cells (myoblasts) (Zheng et al., 2007) in contrast to the findings of Meng suggesting that pericytes, rather than endothelial cells, are the major CD56- contributor to muscle regeneration (Meng et al., 2011b)

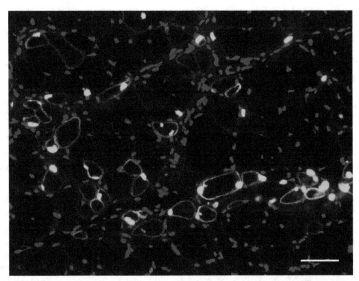

Fig. 1. 7 μm transverse cryosection of *mdx* nu/nu host *tibialis anterior* muscle, that had been cryoinjured and grafted with 5 x 10⁵ human skeletal muscle-derived stem cells 4 weeks previously. Stained with antibodies to human spectrin and human specific lamin a/c, that recognise muscle fibers and nuclei of human origin respectively. Counterstained with DAPI. Bar= 50 μm. (Courtesy of Dr Jinhong Meng).

3.4 Contribution of systemically-delivered donor stem cells to muscle regeneration

The contribution of blood vessel-derived cells (both from skeletal muscle and embryonic dorsal aorta) to skeletal muscle regeneration *in vivo* after their systemic delivery has been demonstrated in several publications (Dellavalle et al., 2007; Sampaolesi et al., 2003; Sampaolesi et al., 2006)(reviewed (Sancricca et al., 2010)), however these promising findings could not be replicated by others (Meng et al., 2011b). For long-term efficacy, it would be useful to know whether a grafted pericyte self-renews to give more functional pericytes and if so, what contribution these have to further muscle regeneration. Another stem cell that is promising for systemic delivery to skeletal muscle is the AC133+ cell, derived from either blood (Torrente et al., 2004), or skeletal muscle (Benchaouir et al., 2007).

3.5 Death and proliferation of grafted cells

Donor myoblasts die on intra-muscular grafting (Beauchamp et al., 1999; Skuk et al., 2002; Smythe et al., 2000) possibly as a result of one or a combination of various factors: cell dissociation, trophic factor withdrawal, oxidative stress, excito-toxicity, hypoxia and, possibly, anoikis (reviewed (Gerard et al., 2011; Skuk & Tremblay, 2011)) and much effort has been expended to prevent this death (reviewed (Skuk & Tremblay, 2011)). Recent experiments have indicated that the number and density of cells transplanted into one site intra-muscularly may also be critical factors influencing their survival and proliferation (Pellegrini & Beilharz, 2011) and that more cells may not give rise to more muscle fibers of donor origin (Pellegrini & Beilharz, 2011; Praud et al., 2003; Rando & Blau, 1994), possibly because cells in the centre of dense pellets undergo more apoptosis. But another theory is that the cells that die are irrelevant, as those that survive proliferate extensively under appropriate environmental conditions, to reconstitute the host muscle (Beauchamp et al., 1999). It is however unclear whether other types of muscle stem cell undergo death after transplantation, or if they proliferate within the grafted muscles.

3.6 Signals inducing muscle stem cells to contribute to muscle regeneration

Intra-arterial injection of mesoangioblasts has shown that only a very small percentage reach downstream skeletal muscles, most being trapped in the filter organs. To enable cells to exit blood vessels, the vessels must express the appropriate adhesion molecules for that cell type. Molecules that have been shown to be important for mesangioblast extravasation into skeletal muscle include HMGB1, SDF-1 and TNF-α (Palumbo et al., 2004). Expression of the adhesion molecules L-selectin and alpha 4 integrin on mesoangioblasts improved their migration into skeletal muscle (Galvez et al., 2006). Pre-treatment with nitric oxide was shown to augment the positive effects of TNF-α, TGF-β and VEGF on mesangioblast migration (Sciorati et al., 2006).

Once the donor stem cells have entered the muscles, they must migrate to sites of injury, proliferate to give a pool of muscle precursor cells and then differentiate to form muscle fibers, either by fusing with each other or by repairing necrotic segments of dystrophic fibers. This will require them to respond to a new series of signals, which might be more appropriate for satellite cells than for stem cells.

In order to have long term benefit, the donor stem cells muscle repopulate a stem cell niche within the muscle and must retain the properties of a functional muscle stem cell within this niche. It is not clear if pericytes within their niche contribute to muscle regeneration, so the best niche to occupy would be the satellite cell niche. However, efficient repopulation of any niche, for example, the satellite cell niche, would only be possible if it were emptied as a consequence of the dystrophy and if the niche environment remains permissive for donor-derived stem cell function. As satellite cell of donor origin are most commonly found on fibers containing myonuclei of donor origin, they may not be called upon to regenerate, as the fiber on which they are situated will already have been strengthened by the new dystrophin and may not undergo further necrosis, at least at the sites where dystrophin is expressed. A means of activating these cells and drawing them towards more distant areas of injury is therefore required to enable them to respond to future muscle fiber necrosis elsewhere within the muscle.

3.7 Autologous cell transplantation

An attractive proposition for treating muscular dystrophies is to use genetically-corrected autologous stem cells. The use of autologous stem cells should circumvent the need for immunosuppression, although tissue culture components or expression of novel protein isotypes *in vivo* may evoke an immunological reaction. But, if the stem cells are skeletal-muscle derived, their function may be impaired by either the primary genetic defect, or secondary environmental consequences of the primary defect.

In some muscular dystrophies, the gene responsible is not expressed in satellite cells (reviewed (Morgan & Zammit, 2010)); for example, dystrophin is not expressed in satellite cells (or other types of muscle stem cell), so satellite cells in DMD muscles would therefore be expected to have normal function. However, the satellite cells may have undergone many divisions in their previous attempts to repair the dystrophic fibers and could therefore be close to senescence (Decary et al., 1996; Decary et al., 1997; Webster & Blau, 1990). They would consequently be of little use for autologous therapy, as they would undergo insufficient divisions *in vitro* to be genetically modified and then to proliferate following transplantation. But although human myoblasts are exhausted in DMD (Decary et al., 1996; Decary et al., 1997; Webster & Blau, 1990), *mdx* satellite cells do not appear to suffer the same consequence of dystrophin deficiency (Bockhold et al., 1998). Recent evidence has indicated that *mdx* satellite cells are highly functional following transplantation into irradiated *mdx* nu/nu muscles (Boldrin and Morgan, unpublished observations). So although satellite cells may not be lost in DMD (reviewed (Boldrin et al., 2010)), their function is compromised, which may be due to telomere shortening leading to reduced proliferative capacity, or a change in the timing or extent of differentiation. However, caution must be taken when comparing *mdx* and DMD cells, as there are differences in telomere biology between mice and humans: inbred mouse strains have extremely long telomeres (20–150 kilobases) compared with humans (up to 15 kilobases) (Bekaert et al., 2005) and telomerase activity is lower in human compared to mouse cells (reviewed (Mather et al., 2011)).

It is unclear whether skeletal muscle-resident cells other than satellite cells contribute to muscle regeneration in muscular dystrophies, or even to maintenance and repair of normal muscle. If they had not actively contributed to the cycles of degeneration and regeneration that occur in DMD, they would be capable of many more divisions than the satellite-cell derived myoblasts and therefore be a more attractive candidate for autologous therapy. However, if they do not contribute to muscle regeneration in DMD, why do they not do so? And why would they be effective after transplantation, if they are not functional *in situ*? Possibly they are not recruited to muscle fiber maintenance and regeneration when they are in their natural niche *in vivo*, but do so after they encounter the site of muscle damage after either intra-muscular or systemic injection.

An ideal autologous stem cell would be derived non-invasively, e.g. from the peripheral blood, or a skin biopsy. However, to date there is only one report of blood-derived stem cells that make reasonable amounts of muscle after their systemic delivery (Torrente et al., 2004).

3.7.1 Genetic modification of autologous cells.

Genetic correction of autologous stem cells has been successfully used as a therapeutic option in other conditions and encouraging preclinical results have also been recently obtained in animal models of DMD (Meregalli et al., 2008). However key questions that need to be resolved before this approach could be used in DMD include the optimal vector configuration and the safety profile of the gene delivery methodology. Lentiviral vectors efficiently infect quiescent cells, including stem cells (S. Li et al., 2005) and give long-term, heritable, gene expression because they integrate into the host genome. Drawbacks with lentiviral vectors include possible gene silencing, or mutagenesis (Wilson & Cichutek, 2009), due to the site at which the virus inserts into the host genome. Although lentiviruses integrate preferentially into active transcription sites (Ciuffi, 2008) the development of third generation lentiviruses with advanced SIN design (Bokhoven et al. 2009), physiological promoters and cell-specific envelope proteins (Rahim et al., 2009) and enhancer-less regulatory elements, e.g. the ubiquitously acting chromatin opening element (UCOE) (Montini et al., 2006; Zhang et al., 2007) should circumvent these problems.

A lentiviral vector has been used to insert a 6.8 kb dystrophin mini gene (S. Li et al., 2005), to give rise to a shorter dystrophin protein in regenerated muscle fibers. While these engineered mini-dystrophins appear to retain most of the functional properties of full-length dystrophin, they nevertheless miss important domains, such as the nitric oxide synthase anchoring domain (Lai et al., 2009). Considering the cloning capacity of lentiviral vectors (up to 10kb (M. Kumar et al., 2001)), it should be possible to further optimise a vector so that it accommodates most of the functionally relevant coding region of dystrophin. An optimal dystrophin construct in a lentiviral vector could be used to treat patients with different mutations, in contrast to the U7 constructs, which, although they can be placed in a lentiviral vector and induce dystrophin expression in stem cells *in vitro* and following their transplantation *in vivo* (Quenneville et al., 2007), are mutation-specific.

4. Matrix Metalloproteinases: modulators of microenvironment and cell function in skeletal muscles

The Matrix Metalloproteinases (MMPs) are a large group of zinc-dependent extracellular endopeptidase proteinases within the Metzincin superfamily of protease that also includes a disintegrin and metalloproteinases (ADAM) and ADAM with thrombospondin motifs (ADAMTS). MMPs family comprises 23 members in humans that share common modular domains and form 5 main sub-groups based on their structure and substrate: collagenases, gelatinases, matrilysins, stromelysins and membrane-type (Figure 2). With the exception of membrane bound MMPs, the other members of the group are secreted in the extracellular space where they are present in latent forms and become activated by other proteases or in response to signaling events. Their activity is regulated at the transcriptional and post-transcriptional levels as well as by their physiological inhibitors, Tissue Inhibitors of Matrix Metalloproteinases (TIMPs). Collectively, they are able to degrade all components of the ECM. Initially confined to the degradation of ECM, their function has progressively evolved and they are now regarded as major regulators of tissue environment and cell functions (Murphy, 2010; Rodriguez et al., 2010). They modulate cell proliferation, adhesion, migration and signaling (Fanjul-Fernandez et al., 2010).

4.1 Matrix Metalloproteinases in remodeling muscles

The adult skeletal muscle is a very stable tissue yet it is endowed with a high capacity to adapt to modification of functional demands, trauma or disease. In normal situations, the dynamic equilibrium between MMPs and TIMPs maintains homeostasis of ECM that provides a dynamic support and stores a number of growth factors that are liberated during ECM remodeling. In response to remodeling situations, dysregulation of this balance occurs in favor of MMPs, to allow necessary hydrolysis of ECM which results in the liberation of neo-epitopes from basement membrane components, as well as various growth factors and signaling molecules that modulate cell response to environmental modifications. Such imbalance may be temporary and the equilibrium is restored upon the disappearance of remodeling stimuli.

MMP Member	Common Name	Cellular Localization
MMP 1	Collagenase-1/Interstial collagenase	
MMP 8	Collagenase-2/Neutrophil collagenase	
MMP 13	Collagenase-3	
MMP 2	Gelatinase-2/72kDa gelatinase	
MMP 9	Gelatinase-9/92kDa gelatinase	
MMP 12	Macrophage metalloelastase	
MMP 7	Matrilysin-1/Uterine	Secreted
MMP 26	Matrilysin-2/Endometase	
MMP 3	Stromelysin-1/Progelatinase	
MMP 10	Stromelysin-2	
MMP 11	Stromelysin-3	
MMP 28	Epilysin	
MMP 18	Collagenase 4	
MMP 19	RASI-1	
MMP 20	Enamelysin	
MMP 27		
MMP 21	MMP-23A	
MMP 14	MT1-MMP	
MMP 15	MT2-MMP	
MMP 16	MT3-MMP	TM Type I
MMP 24	MT5-MMP	
MMP 17	MT4-MMP	
MMP 25	MT6-MMP/Leukolysin	
MMP 22	MMP-23B	TM Type II

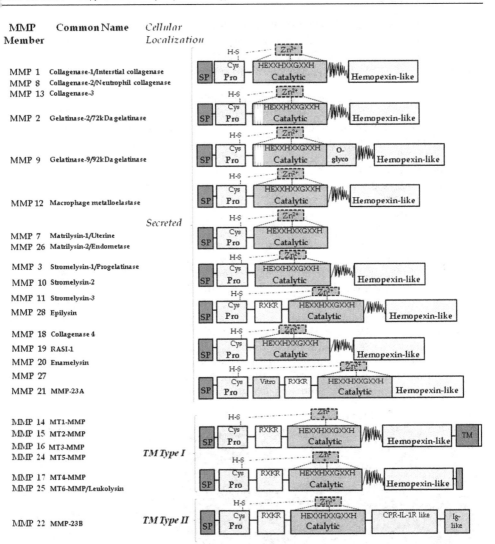

Fig. 2. Structural domains and nomenclature of the matrix metalloproteinases, A: Schematic representation of modular domains composing MMPs which are translated as inactive zymogens with an amino terminal signal peptide (SP), a pro-domain which folds over the zinc ion, in the catalytic site, to maintain latency (Pro), a catalytic domain that carries zinc at the active site, a hemopexin that confers the specificity to and interaction with the substrates or inhibitors (TIMPs) and presents the substrate to the catalytic site via a highly flexible hinge domain. Membrane-type (MT-) MMPs are anchored to the membrane either with a hydrophobic domain and a short cytoplasmic tail (Type I transmembrane protein) or with a glycosyl-phosphatidyl-inositol (GPI) domain. Gelatinases A and B also contain three collagen-binding fibronectin type II repeats within the catalytic domain and MMP-9 has an additional Serine-Threonine and proline rich O-Glycosylated domain. Some MMP have a furin-like motif

between the pro- and catalytic domains that allow their activation before they are secreted or localize to the membrane. MMP- 22 has a cysteine/proline rich, interleukin-1R domain and an Immunoglobulin–like domain. Compiled from (Bourboulia & Stetler-Stevenson, 2010; Fanjul-Fernandez et al., 2010; Rosenberg, 2009; Sternlicht & Werb, 2001).

In skeletal muscles, normal muscle development, limb immobilisation, electrical stimulation and muscle injury are all remodeling situations characterized by MMPs/TIMPs dysregulation. However, the nature of MMPs that is upregulated and the time frame of this upregulation depend, a great deal, on the model used. Immobilization or unloading, that result in muscle fiber atrophy, induce upregulation of both MMP-2 and MMP-9 and downregulation of TIMPs (Berthon et al., 2007; Giannelli et al., 2005; Reznick et al., 2003; Stevenson et al., 2003; Wittwer et al., 2002) (Berthon et al., 2007; Giannelli et al., 2005; Reznick et al., 2003; Stevenson et al., 2003; Wittwer et al., 2002) but only MMP-2 is active (Liu et al., 2010). Whereas a single bout of degeneration-regeneration, induced by experimental injury to the muscle, also results in upregulation of these two proteases but the time frame and intensity differ according to the type/extent of injury (Ferre et al., 2007; Frisdal et al., 2000; Kherif et al., 1999). In a cardiotoxin injury model that induced massive myofiber necrosis, gelatinase activity progressively increased and peaked at day 7, when muscle fiber formation was the most active. It then returned to normal at later stages. This increase was due to simultaneous and consecutive steps of gelatinases regulation- both expression and activation. Within hours after tissue injury, MMP-9 was induced in the tissue that expressed only MMP-2 in the normal situation. It correlated with inflammatory cells infiltration of necrotic muscle fibers that exhibit high gelatinase intracellularly, in contrast to pericellular localization of gelatinase in normal muscles (Figure 3). Simultaneously, MMP-2 expression and activation decreased within the first 24 hours and was followed by a progressive reconstitution of these forms afterwards. MMP-9 transcripts localized to

Normal   **CTX Day 3**

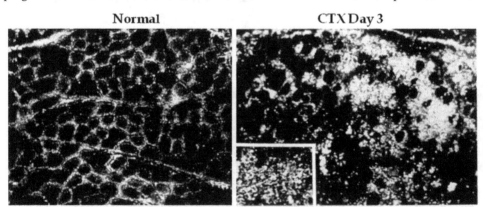

Fig. 3. *In situ* zymography of normal and cardiotoxin injured muscle 3 days after injury. In normal muscles, gelatinase activity (shown in white) localized to the endomysium and mononucleated cells present at the vicinity of muscle fibers. In injured muscles, gelatinase activity localizes to inflammatory cells. At early time points when necrotic muscle fibers are invaded by inflammatory cells, gelatinase activity is detected within degenerating muscle fibers that are invaded by inflammatory cells. Original magnification, X40 (Alameddine, Unpublished results).

inflammatory cells and mononucleated cells at satellite cell position (Kherif et al., 1999). The possibility that myogenic cells upregulate MMP-9 has been confirmed recently. When exposed to debris of damaged myotubes, the myogenic cells upregulated MMP-9, monocyte chemoattractant protein (MCP)-1 and other factors necessary for angiogenesis, tissue regeneration, and phagocyte recruitment (Dehne et al., 2011). Latent MT1-MMP (63kDA), which contributes with TIMP-2 to MMP-2 activation, is processed to its active (50kDa) form that retained its ability to process MMP-2 and was preceded by TIMP-2 decrease (Barnes et al., 2009). MMP-3 and TIMP-1 transcripts were also shown to be upregulated within the first 24 hours following cold injury. TIMP-1 started to decrease 72 hours post injury and early increase was followed by a decrease of active MMP-3 (Urso et al., 2010).

4.2 Matrix Metalloproteinases in dystrophic muscles

In dystrophic *mdx* and CXMD muscles, MMP-2 and MMP-9 are found in muscle extracts whereas only MMP-2 is found in normal muscles (Fukushima et al., 2007; Kherif et al., 1999). MMP-9 is upregulated in both muscles and serum of *mdx* mice (H. Li et al., 2009) throughout their lifespan (Alameddine et al., unpublished results). MT1-MMP, TIMP-1 and TIMP-2 are also upregulated in CXMD muscles and gelatinase activity localized to necrotic fibers and endomysium, demonstrated by *in situ* zymography (Fukushima et al., 2007). Differences in MMP expression and activity patterns detected in different adult *mdx* muscles - gastrocnemius, soleus and diaphragm- led Bani (Bani et al., 2008) to hypothesize that the microenvironment of distinct skeletal muscles may influence a particular kinetic pattern of MMP activity, which ultimately favors persistent inflammation and myofiber regeneration at different stages of the myopathy in *mdx* mice. Gene array analysis revealed profound modification of mRNA levels of several MMPs and other associated proteins in gastrocnemius and *tibialis anterior* muscles of *mdx* mice. MMP-3, -8, -9,-10,-12, -14 and -15 Adamts2 and Timp-1 mRNA levels are increased, MMP-11 as well as Adamts1, Adamts5, Adamts8 and Timp-2 and Timp-3 were downregulated (A. Kumar et al., 2010).

In DMD muscles, TIMP-1, TIMP-2 and MMP-2 transcripts are upregulated and MMP-2 activity is increased (von Moers et al., 2005). TIMP-1 levels, usually increased in the serum and plasma of patients with fibrotic diseases, are elevated in serum, plasma, and muscle extracts of muscular dystrophy patients and animal models. It correlated with TGFβ1 levels in DMD and in congenital muscular dystrophy (CMD) patients but not with Becker muscular dystrophy patients (Sun et al., 2010). In muscle tissue from dystrophin deficient and LAMA2-mutated muscular dystrophy patients, pro-fibrotic TGF-β1 is increased partly through a positive autocrine feedback loop and is released from decorin that is degraded by MMP-2. DMD fibroblasts have been shown to produce more soluble collagen, biglycan, decorin, TGF-β1 and MMP-7 and less MMP-1 than normal fibroblasts. TGF-β1 is known to modulate the ability of cells to synthesize various ECM components and was shown to modify the protein pattern produced by DMD fibroblasts upon their transformation to myofibroblasts. It increased MMP-7 thought to contribute to fibrosis (Fadic et al., 2006; Simona Zanotti et al., 2010; S. Zanotti et al., 2007).

In Emery-Dreifuss muscular dystrophy, screening of MMP-2, MMP-9 and MT1-MMP levels in the serum showed an increase of MMP-2 levels in both the autosomal and X- linked forms, suggesting it may serve as biomarker for the detection of cardiac involvement in patients with no subjective cardiac symptoms (Niebroj-Dobosz et al., 2009).

4.3 MMPs and inflammation in the development of fibrosis

End-stage DMD muscles are characterized by an almost complete disappearance of muscle fibers and their replacement by fibro-fatty tissue. Although DMD is not a fibrotic disease *per se*, their muscle biopsies are generally characterized by excessive production, deposition, and contraction of extracellular matrix. This accumulation results from factors, produced in diseased muscles, that influence the normal balance between production and/or hydrolysis of ECM components. Clearly, structural and functional changes of tissue microenvironment in dystrophic muscles are not equivalent to those that accompany normal muscle development. The permanent induction of wound–healing response with its inflammatory component may be essential contributors to the development of fibrosis in dystrophic muscles. Acute or chronic inflammation includes exudation of plasma proteins, recruitment of leukocytes and activation of cell and plasma derived inflammatory mediators as well as increased expression of MMPs (Manicone & McGuire, 2008). When inflammation is continuous or excessive, it is thought to contribute to tissue injury, organ dysfunction or chronic disease states. Inversely, decrease of MMP activity has been incriminated in the development of fibrotic conditions. Decreased MMP activity may result from dysregulation of the balance between MMPs and TIMPs. Upregulation of MMPs or downregulation of TIMPs activity could be applied for resolution of tissue fibrosis (reviewed (Hemmann et al., 2007)).

Experimental evidence shows that inflammatory cells such as macrophages, eosinophiles and T lymphocytes, the major infiltrating cell types, contribute to increased fibrosis (J. Morrison et al., 2000). Inflammatory cells produce cytokines/chemokines that regulate MMPs expression. In their turn, MMPs modulate the activities of cytokines and their receptors at the cell surface. The list of validated ECM components, growth factors (receptors and binding proteins) and cytokines/chemokines substrates is compiled in table 1.

Studies using gene microarrays have demonstrated that dystrophic muscles are characterized by an inflammatory "molecular signature", in which CC chemokines are prominent (Y. W. Chen et al., 2000; Y. W. Chen et al., 2005; Porter et al., 2003; Porter et al., 2002). Similarly, CC chemokines are greatly upregulated in normal skeletal muscles after experimental injury (Hirata et al., 2003). CC chemokine receptors (CCRs 1, 2, 3, 5) and ligands (macrophage inflammatory protein-1α, RANTES) are expressed at higher levels in dystrophic than in wild-type muscles across age groups (6, 12, and 24 wk). Moreover, chemokine ligand expression and muscle inflammation are significantly higher in dystrophic diaphragms than in limb muscles of the same animals. *In vitro*, CCR1 is constitutively expressed by myotubes formed from primary myoblasts derived from diaphragm muscles. Stimulation of myotubes by proinflammatory cytokines (tumor necrosis factor-α, interleukin-1α, interferon-γ) found within the *in vivo* dystrophic muscle environment, upregulates CCR1 in *mdx* and wild-type myoblast cultures, and also increases expression of its ligand RANTES to a significantly greater degree (Demoule et al., 2005).

In damaged muscles, various cytokines and growth factors are also released during necrosis and regeneration of muscle fibers. The most widely documented pro-fibrotic agent that is over-expressed in dystrophic muscles is TGF-β. It is upregulated in dystrophic muscles, after invasion of the damaged muscle by inflammatory cells (Y. W. Chen et al., 2005; Zhou et al., 2006) that were shown to express TGF-β mRNA although these cells may not be the sole contributors to its production (Bernasconi et al., 1999; Gosselin et al., 2004).

Enzyme	Enzymes ECM substrates	Growth factors & Cytokines/Chemokines
Secreted-type MMP **Collagenases**		
Interstitial collagenase MMP-1	Aggrecan; Collagens I,- III, VII, VIII, X, XI; Entactin; Fn; Gelatins; Ln; Link protein; Tenascin; Vn; Perlecan;	CTGF; IL1-β; IGFBPs; MCP-1, MCP-2, MCP-3, MCP-4; TNF-α
Neutrophil collagenase MMP-8	Aggrecan; Collagens I- III; Gelatins; link protein	LIX/CXCL5
Collagenase-3 MMP-13	Aggrecan; Collagens I-III,VI, IX, X, XIV; Fibrillin; Fn; Gelatins; Osteonectin; Ln; Perlecan	CTGF; MCP-3/CCL7, TGF-β; SDF-1/CXCL12
Collagenase-4 MMP-18	Collagen I	
Gelatinases		
Gelatinase A MMP-2	Aggrecan; Collagens I, III-V, VII, X- XI; Decorin; Elastin; Entactin; Fibrillin; Fn; Fibulins; Gelatins; Ln; Link protein; Osteonectin; Tenascin;	CTGF; FGFR1; CX$_3$CL1; IL1-β; IGFBPs; MCP-3/CCL7; TGF-β; TNF-α; SDF-1/CXCL12
Gelatinase B MMP-9	Aggrecan; Collagens III, IV-V, XI; Decorin; Elastin; Entactin; Fibrillin; Gelatins; Ln; Link protein; Osteonectin; N-telopeptide of collagen I; Vn	MCP-3; CCL11; CCL17; Fractalkine; GRO-alpha; IGFBP-3; IL1-β; IL-2Rα; IL-8/CXCL8; Kit-L; LIF; TGF-β; TNF-α; SDF-1/CXCL12; VEGF
Stromelysins		
Stromelysin-1 MMP-3	Aggrecan; Collagens III-V, VII, IX- XI; Decorin; Elastin; Entactin; Fibrillin; Fn; Gelatins;Ln; link protein; Osteonectin; Perlecan; Tenascin; Vn;	CTGF; HB-EGF; IL1-β; IGFBPs; MCP-1, MCP-2, MCP-3, MCP-4; IL-1β; TGF-β1; TNF-α; SDF-1/CXCL12;
Stromelysin-2 MMP-10	Aggrecan; Collagens III-V; Elastin; Fn; Gelatin; Link protein	
Matrilysins		
Matrilysin-1 (MMP-7)	Aggrecan; Collagens I, IV; Decorin; Elastin; Entactin; Fn; Fibulins; Gelatins; Ln; Link protein; Osteonectin; Osteopontin; Tenascin; Vn; Syndecan-1,	CTGF; Fas-L; HB-EGF; IGFBP-3; TNF-α; RANKL
Matrilysin-2 MMP-26	Collagen IV; Fn; Fibrinogen; Gelatin; Vn	

Furin-activated MMP		
Stromelysin-3 MMP-11	Aggrecan; Fn; Gelatins; Ln;	IGFBP-1
Epilysin MMP-28	Unknown	
Other secreted-type MMP		
Metalloelastase MMP-12	Aggrecan; Collagen I, IV; Elastin; Entactin; Fibrillin; Fn; Gelatin; Ln; Osteonectin; Vn;	TNF-α
RASI-1 (MMP-19)	Aggrecan; Collagen I, IV; COMP; Fn; Gelatin; Ln; Tenascin;	IGFBP-3
Enamelysin (MMP-20)	Aggrecan; Amelogenin; COMP; Gelatin;	Unknown
MMP-21	Unknown	Unknown
MMP-27	Unknown	Unknown
Membrane-anchored MMP		
Type I transmembrane-type MMP		
MT1-MMP MMP-14	Aggrecan; Collagens I-III, VI; Entactin; Fibrillin; Fn; Gelatins; Ln; Osteonectin; Vn;	CTGF; IL-8; MCP-3/CCL7; TNF-α
MT2-MMP MMP-15	Aggrecan; Entactin	
MT3-MMP MMP-16	Collagen III; Fn; Gelatins	
MT5-MMP MMP-24	PG	
GPI-linked MMP		
MT4-MMP MMP-17	Gelatin;	
MT6-MMP MMP-25	collagen IV; Fibrin; Fn; Gelatin; Ln	
Type II transmembrane-type MMP	Gelatins	
MMP-23		

CCL11, CC chemokine ligand 11; CCL17, CC chemokine ligand 17, COMP, cartilage oligomeric matrix protein; CTGF, connective tissue growth factor; Fas-L, Fas ligand; FGF, Fibroblast Growth Factor;, FGFR1, Fibroblast growth factor receptor 1; Fn, fibronectin; HB-EGF, heparin-binding epidermal growth factor like growth factor; IGFBP, insulin-like growth factor binding proteins; IL1-β, interleukin-1β; IL-2Rα, Interleukin 2 receptor; IL-8, interleukin 8; Kit-L, kit ligand; Ln, laminin; LIF, Leukimia inhibitory factor; LIX-CXL, lipopolysaccharide induced CXC chemokine, MCP-, monocyte chemotactic protein-; PCPE, Procollagen C protein enhancer; PG, proteoglycan; Pro, proteinase type; SDF-1/CXCL12, Stromal cell derived factor, TNF-α, tumor necrosis factor-α; TGF-β, transforming growth factor β; RASI-1, rheumatoid arthritis synovium inflamed-1; RANKL, receptor activator for nuclear factor κ B ligand.

Table 1. Validated MMPs substrates that include ECM and non-ECM proteins. Of the long list of non-ECM substrates, only growth factors, receptors and cytokines/chemokines have been extracted because of the role they play in the modification of tissue environment and the modulation of cell functions (Manicone & McGuire, 2008; C. J. Morrison et al., 2009; Shiomi et al., 2010; Sternlicht & Werb, 2001).

TGF-β is thought to play a prominent role in the pathogenesis of muscle fibrosis. Its short-term neutralization by decorin administration resulted in a 40% decline in type I collagen mRNA expression in *mdx* mice. *In vitro*, it stimulates collagen synthesis and inhibits collagen degradation in fibroblasts (Grande et al., 1997; Ignotz & Massague, 1986; Sharma & Ziyadeh, 1994)}. Myoblast stimulation by TGF-β1 induced autocrine production of TGF-β1, downregulation of myogenic proteins, production of fibrosis-related proteins and phenotypic transformation of myogenic cells to fibrobroblast/myofibroblast cell types *in vitro* (Yong Li et al., 2004). TGF-β treatment of myogenic cells also upregulated Connective Tissue Growth Factor (CTGF) (Maeda et al., 2005) incriminated in various fibrotic diseases. CTGF is overexpressed in dystrophic muscles and is thought to contribute, with TGF-β, to the development of fibrosis (Sun et al., 2008). Interestingly, both factors are validated MMPs substrates and could be modulated through MMPs action.

Tumor necrosis factor-(TNF-α), also upregulated in muscular dystrophy (Porreca et al., 1999) may exert direct adverse effects on skeletal muscle function and regeneration potential. Blockade of TNF-α by inhibitory antibodies reduced necrosis and contractile dysfunction in response to eccentric exercise (Piers et al., 2011; Radley et al., 2008). *In vitro* TNF-α has been shown to stimulate collagen synthesis in fibroblasts (Lurton et al., 1999) hence contributing directly to muscle fibrosis. *In vivo*, short-term pharmacological blockade of TNF-α in *mdx* mice significantly reduced the level of both TGF-β1 and type I collagen mRNA (Gosselin et al., 2004). Whether TNF-α mediates muscle fibrosis directly or indirectly (by upregulating the expression of TGF-β1) remains an open question. However, TNF-α induces MMP-9 upregulation in myogenic cells (Torrente et al., 2003).

Concomitance between inflammation and upregulation of MMPs in mouse models or human diseases with inflammatory conditions, led several groups to propose MMPs as potential therapeutic targets in pathological conditions with aberrant MMP expression and activity (reviewed (Clutterbuck et al., 2009)). Inhibition of MMPs has been recently investigated in *mdx* mice. MMP-9 inhibition either by the administration of nuclear factor-kappa B inhibitory peptide, gene deletion or by L-arginine treatment was reported to reduce muscle injury, inflammation, fibrosis and decrease pro-inflammatory cytokine release (Hnia et al., 2008; A. Kumar et al., 2010; H. Li et al., 2009). However, whether this inhibition is acting directly on the development of fibrosis or through prevention of muscle fibers necrosis and tissue scarring remains an open question.

Extreme precaution has to be taken into consideration regarding MMPs inhibition in muscular dystrophy particularly as animal models of MMP gain- or loss- of function and clinical trials of MMP inhibition in cancer patients have unraveled the dual role an individual MMP could exert, depending on tissue type or stage of the disease (protective/detrimental) (reviewed (Fanjul-Fernandez et al., 2010). In skeletal muscles, the beneficial effect of certain MMPs has been documented, underscoring the necessity for better knowledge of the role MMPs are playing in muscle diseases (Alameddine manuscript in preparation). Indeed, Mmp-2 gene ablation has been shown to impair the growth of muscle fibers by downregulating VEGF and nNOS (Miyazaki et al., 2011). Moreover, proteinases upregulation, during satellite cells activation, is essential for dismantling the satellite cells niche (Pallafacchina et al., 2010) and MMP-1 has been shown to reduce muscle fibrosis (Kaar et al., 2008).

4.4 MMPs favor cell migration

Myogenic cells have been reported to express various MMPs -MMP-1, -2, -3, -7, -9, -10, -14 and -16, either constitutively or after treatment with growth factors, cytokines or phorbol esters (Balcerzak et al., 2001; Caron et al., 1999; El Fahime et al., 2000; Guérin & Holland, 1995; Kherif et al., 1999; Lewis et al., 2000; Lluri & Jaworski, 2005; Nishimura et al., 2008; Ohtake et al., 2006). Cytokines and growth factors differentially modulate MMPs expression in myogenic cells. Treatment of adult mouse myoblasts by soluble serum fibronectin, PDGF-BB, TGF-β or IGF-1 had no effect on the expression of MMP-9 expression, whereas TNF-α and b-FGF reproducibly induced the expression of MMP-9 expression 30- and 10-folds. Other MMPs, such as MMP-1 and MMP-2, were not significantly affected by any of these growth factors (Allen et al., 2003; Torrente et al., 2003).

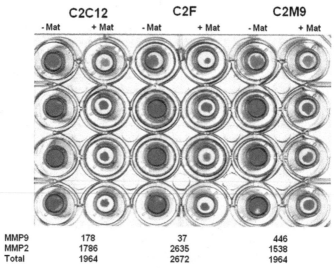

	C2C12		C2F		C2M9	
	- Mat	+ Mat	- Mat	+ Mat	- Mat	+ Mat
MMP9		178		37		446
MMP2		1786		2635		1538
Total		1964		2672		1964

Fig. 4. Invasion assay establishing the correlation between migratory capacity of myogenic cells and MMP-9 expression levels. Three different cell types, C2C12 and 2 variant clones, expressing different levels of MMP-2 and MMP-9, that were quantified in the same zymography gels with Image J, were assayed in a two chamber migration assay with (+Mat) or without (–Mat) growth factor reduced Matrigel as substrate. The invasive capacity is measured by the ratio between cells that migrated through Matrigel and those diffused through the porous membrane. MMP-2, MMP-9 and total gelatinase values are expressed in arbitrary units. Invasive capacity of C2M9 was > to C2C12>C2F cells.

The role MMPs/TIMPs play in myogenic cells migration and potentially in cell fusion has been confirmed by overexpression and inhibition studies. Myoblasts overexpressing MMP-7 had a higher propensity to form myotubes than parental controls and generated more fibers when transplanted into a single site (Caron et al., 1999). MMP-1 enhanced C2C12 myoblast migration in a wound healing assay *in vitro* by increasing the expression of migration related marker proteins such as N-cadherin, β-catenin, latent MMP-2 and TIMP-1 (Wang et al., 2009). C2C12 cells stably transfected with MMP-2 and MMP-14 cDNA significantly increased the number of myonuclei without affecting the number of myotubes formed (Echizenya et al.,

2005). MT1-MMP has been proposed as a major MMP checkpoint regulator of myotube formation, as shMT1-MMP partly inhibited muscle cell fusion at a specific stage (Ohtake et al., 2006). MMP-9 and TIMP-1 have also been suspected to play a role in myogenesis *in vitro*. MMP-9 expression in human myogenic cells favored their migration on fibronectin and its inhibition by a blocking antibody decreased two dimensional cell migration (Lewis et al., 2000). Cells overexpressing MMP-9 have also better three dimensional migratory capacities (Figure 4). They exhibit higher migration when seeded on top of a Matrigel gel that better mimics ECM and their migration is inhibited in the presence of a specific MMP-9 inhibitor (Morgan et al., 2010). Of relevance to this review is that these cells have also higher engraftment capacities. Upon transplantation in a single site in irradiated and non-irradiated muscles of *mdx* nu/nu mice, they formed more dystrophin positive muscle fibers over larger areas, indicating they migrated better in a dystrophic environment (Morgan et al., 2010).

5. Conclusion

Although promising, there are several challenges to be overcome before stem or precursor cells could be used to treat muscular dystrophies. Apart from reliably and reproducibly identifying and purifying the cells of interest, their characteristics have to be maintained on expansion in culture: attempts at re-creating the niche *in vitro* may facilitate the retention of stem cell characteristics (Cosgrove et al., 2009; Gilbert et al., 2010). Encouraging results from one laboratory should be independently confirmed, before any particular stem cell is considered for therapeutic application.

Systemic delivery would involve turning a cell into a leukocyte to cross the blood vessel endothelium (Springer, 1994) and then switching on survival, migration, proliferative and myogenic regulatory factors once the cells are within the muscle. Even if it does not prove possible to treat muscles body-wide, transplanting stem cells locally into a small, vital, muscle, e.g. in the finger, may prove more practicable and although not life-saving, would improve the quality of life of DMD patients.

But for successful local as well as systemic delivery of stem cells to skeletal muscle, the inhospitable muscle environment remains a major hurdle. Studies on the factors and signaling pathways that hinder donor cell survival, proliferation and migration within both normal and dystrophic muscle and how these may be modified to augment the regenerative capacity of transplanted cells, remain vital for the successful use of stem cells in neuromuscular diseases. More importantly, elucidation of the role MMPs in general and individual MMPs in particular, play in the modulation of the dystrophic microenvironment and stem cell response to this environment warrants further study. In light of our present knowledge, it is tempting to propose that MMPs are temporally upregulated to permit migration and fusion of stem cells, then down-regulated, after donor-derived muscle has been formed, to reduce inflammation and fibrosis and thus improve muscle function. However, it is not clear whether the presence of either stem cells of normal origin, or muscle fibers expressing dystrophin, are sufficient to prevent the uncontrolled wound healing response that occurs in dystrophic muscles.

6. Acknowledgments

J.E.M is funded by a Wellcome Trust University award, the Muscular Dystrophy Campaign, the Duchenne Parent Project (Netherlands), the International Collaborative Effort for

Duchenne muscular dystrophy, and the Medical Research Council. H.S.A is funded by Association Institut de Myologie/Association Française contre les Myopathies and by INSERM (France).

7. References

Alameddine, H.S.; Dehaupas, M. & Fardeau, M. (1989). Regeneration of skeletal muscle fibers from autologous satellite cells multiplied in vitro. An experimental model for testing cultured cell myogenicity. *Muscle Nerve*, Vol.12, No.7, (Jul), pp. 544-55, ISSN 0148-639X

Alameddine, H.S.; Hantaï D.; Dehaupas, M.; & Fardeau, M. (1991). Role of persisting basement membrane in the reorganization of myofibres originating from myogenic cell grafts in the rat. *Neuromuscular Disorders*, Vol.1, No.2, pp. 143-52, ISSN 0960-8966

Alameddine, H.S.; Louboutin,J.P.; Dehaupas, M.; Sebille,A. & Fardeau, M. (1994). Functional recovery induced by satellite cell grafts in irreversibly injured muscles. *Cell Transplantation*, Vol.3, No.1, (Jan-Feb), pp. 3-14, ISSN 0963-6897

Allen, D.L.; Teitelbaum, D.H. & Kurachi, K. (2003). Growth factor stimulation of matrix metalloproteinase expression and myoblast migration and invasion in vitro. *American Journal of Physiology - Cell Physiology*, Vol.284, No.4, (Apr 1), pp. C805-C815,

Arechavala-Gomeza, V.; Kinali, M.; Feng, L.; Guglieri, M.; Edge, G.; Main, M.; Hunt, D.; Lehovsky, J.; Straub, V.; Bushby, K.; Sewry, C.A.; Morgan, J.E. & Muntoni, F. (2010). Revertant fibres and dystrophin traces in Duchenne muscular dystrophy: implication for clinical trials. *Neuromuscular Disorders*, Vol.20, No.5, (May), pp. 295-301, ISSN 1873-2364

Balcerzak, D.; Querengesser, L.; Dixon, W.T. & Baracos, V.E. (2001). Coordinated expression of matrix-degrading proteinases and their activators and inhibitors in bovine skeletal muscle. *Journal Animal Sciences*, Vol.79, No.1, (Jan 1), pp. 94-107,

Bani, C.; Lagrota-Candido, J.; Pinheiro, D.F.; Leite, P.E.; Salimena, M.C.; Henriques-Pons, A. & Quirico-Santos, T. (2008). Pattern of metalloprotease activity and myofiber regeneration in skeletal muscles of mdx mice. *Muscle Nerve*, Vol.37, No.5, (May), pp. 583-92, ISSN 0148-639X

Banks, G.B. & Chamberlain, J.S. (2008). The value of mammalian models for Duchenne muscular dystrophy in developing therapeutic strategies. *Current Topics in Developmental Biology*, Vol.84, pp. 431-53,

Barnes, B.R.; Szelenyi,E.R.; Warren, G.L. & Urso, M.L. (2009). Alterations in mRNA and protein levels of metalloproteinases-2, -9, and -14 and tissue inhibitor of metalloproteinase-2 responses to traumatic skeletal muscle injury. *American Journal of Physiology – Cell Physiology*, Vol.297, No.6, (Dec), pp. C1501-8, ISSN 1522-1563

Beauchamp, J.R.; Morgan, J.E.; Pagel, C.N. & Partridge, T.A. (1999). Dynamics of myoblast transplantation reveal a discrete minority of precursors with stem cell-like properties as the myogenic source. *The Journal of Cell Biology*, Vol.144, No.6, (Mar 22), pp. 1113-22,

Bekaert, S.; De Meyer, T. & Van Oostveldt, P. (2005). Telomere attrition as ageing biomarker. *Anticancer Research*, Vol.25, No.4, (Jul-Aug), pp. 3011-21, ISSN 0250-7005

Benchaouir, R.; Meregalli, M.; Farini ,A.; D'Antona, G.; Belicchi, M.; Goyenvalle, A.; Battistelli, M.; Bresolin, N.; Bottinelli, R.; Garcia, L. & Torrente, Y. (2007). Restoration of human dystrophin following transplantation of exon-skipping-engineered DMD patient stem cells into dystrophic mice. *Cell Stem Cell*, Vol.1, No.6, (Dec 13), pp. 646-57,

Bernasconi, P.; Di Blasi, C.; Mora, M.; Morandi, L.; Galbiati, S.; Confalonieri, P.; Cornelio, F.& Mantegazza, R. (1999). Transforming growth factor-[beta]1 and fibrosis in congenital muscular dystrophies. *Neuromuscular Disorders*, Vol.9, No.1, (Jan 1), pp. 28-33,

Berthon, P.; Duguez, S.; Favier, F.B.; Amirouche, A.; Feasson, L.; Vico, L.; Denis, C. & Freyssenet, D. (2007). Regulation of ubiquitin-proteasome system, caspase enzyme activities, and extracellular proteinases in rat soleus muscle in response to unloading. *Pflügers Archives*, Vol.454, No.4, (Jul), pp. 625-33, ISSN 0031-6768

Blau, H.M.; Webster, C. & Pavlath, G.K. (1983). Defective myoblasts identified in Duchenne muscular dystrophy. *Proceedings of the National Academy of Science USA*, Vol.80, No.15, (Aug), pp. 4856-60, ISSN 0027-8424

Blaveri, K.; Heslop, L.; Yu, D.S.; Rosenblatt, J.D.; Gross, J.G.; Partridge, T.A. & Morgan, J.E. (1999). Patterns of repair of dystrophic mouse muscle: studies on isolated fibers. *Developmental Dynamics*, Vol.216, No.3, pp. 244-56., ISSN

Bockhold, K.J.; Rosenblatt J.D. & Partridge, T.A. (1998). Aging normal and dystrophic mouse muscle: analysis of myogenicity in cultures of living single fibers. *Muscle Nerve*, Vol.21, No.2, (Feb), pp. 173-83,

Bokhoven, M.; Stephen, S.L.; Knight, S.; Gevers, E.F.; Robinson, I.C.; Takeuchi, Y. & Collins, M.K. (2009). Insertional gene activation by lentiviral and gammaretroviral vectors. *Journal of Virology*, Vol.83, No.1, (Jan), pp. 283-94,

Boldrin, L.; Muntoni, F. & Morgan, J.E. (2010). Are human and mouse satellite cells really the same? *Journal of Histochemistry & Cytochemistry*, Vol.58, No.11, (Nov), pp. 941-55, ISSN 1551-5044

Boldrin, L.; Zammit, P.S.; Muntoni, F. & Morgan, J.E. (2009). Mature adult dystrophic mouse muscle environment does not impede efficient engrafted satellite cell regeneration and self-renewal. *Stem Cells*, Vol.27, No.10, pp. 2478-2487, ISSN 1549-4918

Bourboulia, D. & Stetler-Stevenson, W.G. (2010). Matrix metalloproteinases (MMPs) and tissue inhibitors of metalloproteinases (TIMPs): Positive and negative regulators in tumor cell adhesion. *Seminars in Cancer Biology*, Vol.15, No.11, (Nov), pp. 1109-24,

Brimah, K.; Ehrhardt, J.; Mouly, V.; Butler-Browne, G.S.; Partridge, T.A. & Morgan, J.E. (2004). Human muscle precursor cell regeneration in the mouse host is enhanced by growth factors. *Human Gene Therapy*, Vol.15, No.11, (Nov), pp. 1109-24,

Bulfield, G.; Siller, W.G.; Wight, P.A. & Moore, K.J. (1984). X chromosome-linked muscular dystrophy (mdx) in the mouse. *Proceedings of the National Academy of Science USA*,Vol.81, No.4, (Feb), pp. 1189-92,

Bushby, K.; Finkel, R.; Birnkrant, D.J.; Case, L.E.; Clemens, P.R.; Cripe, L.; Kaul, A.; Kinnett, K.; McDonald, C.; Pandya, S.; Poysky, J.; Shapiro, F.; Tomezsko, J. & Constantin, C. (2010). Diagnosis and management of Duchenne muscular dystrophy, part 1: diagnosis, and pharmacological and psychosocial management. *Lancet Neurology*, Vol.9, No.1, (Jan), pp. 77-93, ISSN 1474-4465

Caron, N.J.; Asselin, I.; Morel, G. & Tremblay, J.P. (1999). Increased myogenic potential and fusion of matrilysin-expressing myoblasts transplanted in mice. *Cell Transplantation,* Vol.8, No.5, (Sep-Oct), pp. 465-76, ISSN 0963-6897

Chan, J.; O'Donoghue, K.; Gavina, M.; Torrente, Y.; Kennea, N.; Mehmet, H.; Stewart, H.; Watt ,D.J.; Morgan, J.E. & Fisk, N.M. (2006). Galectin-1 induces skeletal muscle differentiation in human fetal mesenchymal stem cells and increases muscle regeneration. *Stem Cells,* Vol.24, No.8, (Aug), pp. 1879-91,

Chen, Y.W.; Zhao, P.; Borup, R. & Hoffman, E. (2000). Expression profiling in the muscular dystrophies: identification of novel aspects of molecular pathophysiology. *The Journal of Cell Biology,* Vol.151, pp. 1321–36,

Chen, Y.W.; Nagaraju, K.; Bakay, M.; McIntyre, O.; Rawat, R.; Shi, R. & Hoffman, E.P. (2005). Early onset of inflammation and later involvement of TGF{beta} in Duchenne muscular dystrophy. *Neurology,* Vol.65, No.6, (Sep 27), pp. 826-834,

Ciuffi, A. (2008). Mechanisms governing lentivirus integration site selection. *Current Gene Therapy,* Vol.8, No.6, (Dec), pp. 419-29,

Clutterbuck, A.L.; Asplin, K.E.; Harris, P.; Allaway, D. & Mobasheri, A. (2009). Targeting matrix metalloproteinases in inflammatory conditions. *Current Drug Targets,* Vol.10, No.12, (Dec), pp. 1245-54, ISSN 1873-5592

Collins, C.A. & Morgan, J.E. (2003). Duchenne's muscular dystrophy: animal models used to investigate pathogenesis and develop therapeutic strategies. *International Journal of Experimental Pathology,* Vol.84, No.4, (Aug), pp. 165-72,

Collins, C.A.; Olsen, I.; Zammit, P.S.; Heslop, L.; Petrie, A.; Partridge T.A. & Morgan,. J.E. (2005). Stem cell function, self-renewal, and behavioral heterogeneity of cells from the adult muscle satellite cell niche. *Cell,* Vol.122, No.2, pp. 289-301,

Cooper, R.N.; Irintchev, A.; Di Santo, J.P.; Zweyer, M.; Morgan, J.E.; Partridge, T.A.; Butler-Browne, G.S.; Mouly, V. & Wernig, A. (2001). A new immunodeficient mouse model for human myoblast transplantation. *Human Gene Therapy,* Vol.12, No.7, (May 1), pp. 823-31,

Cosgrove, B.D.; Sacco, A.; Gilbert, P.M. & Blau, H.M. (2009). A home away from home: challenges and opportunities in engineering in vitro muscle satellite cell niches. *Differentiation,* Vol.78, No.2-3, (Sep-Oct), pp. 185-94, ISSN 1432-0436

Cousins, J.C.; Woodward, K.J.; Gross, J.G.; Partridge, T.A. & Morgan, J.E. (2004). Regeneration of skeletal muscle from transplanted immortalised myoblasts is oligoclonal. *Journal of Cell Science,* Vol.117, No.15, (Jul 1), pp. 3259-3269,

Decary, S.; Mouly, V. & Butler-Browne, G.S. (1996). Telomere length as a tool to monitor satellite cell amplification for cell-mediated gene therapy. *Human Gene Therapy,* Vol.7, No.11, (Jul 10), pp. 1347-50,

Decary, S.; Mouly, V.; Hamida, C.B.; Sautet, A.; Barbet, J.P. & Butler-Browne, G.S. (1997). Replicative potential and telomere length in human skeletal muscle: implications for satellite cell-mediated gene therapy. *Human Gene Therapy,* Vol.8, No.12, (Aug 10), pp. 1429-38,

Dehne, N.; Kerkweg, U.; Flohe, S.B.; Brune, B. & Fandrey, J. (2011). Activation of HIF-1 in skeletal muscle cells after exposure to damaged muscle cell debris. *Shock,* Vol. 35, No.6, (Jun), pp. 632-8., ISSN 1073-2322

Dellavalle, A.; Sampaolesi, M.; Tonlorenzi, R.; Tagliafico, E.; Sacchetti, B.; Perani, L.; Innocenzi, A.; Galvez, B.G.; Messina, G.; Morosetti, R.; Li, S.; Belicchi, M.; Peretti,

G.; Chamberlain, J.S.; Wright, W.E.; Torrente, Y.; Ferrari, S.; Bianco P. & Cossu, G. (2007). Pericytes of human skeletal muscle are myogenic precursors distinct from satellite cells. *Nature Cell Biology*, Vol.9, No.3, (Mar), pp. 255-67,

Demoule, A.; Divangahi, M.; Danialou, G.; Gvozdic, D.; Larkin, G.; Bao; W.& Petrof, B.J. (2005). Expression and regulation of CC class chemokines in the dystrophic (mdx) diaphragm. *American Journal of Respiratory Cell and Molecular Biology*, Vol.33, No.2, (Aug), pp. 178-185,

Diaz-Manera, J.; Touvier, T.; Dellavalle, A.; Tonlorenzi, R.; Tedesco, F.S.; Messina, G.; Meregalli, M.; Navarro, C.; Perani, L.; Bonfanti, C.; Illa, I.; Torrente, Y.& Cossu, G. (2010). Partial dysferlin reconstitution by adult murine mesoangioblasts is sufficient for full functional recovery in a murine model of dysferlinopathy. *Cell death & disease*, Vol.1, pp. e61, ISSN 2041-4889

Echizenya, M.; Kondo, S.; Takahashi, R.; Oh, J.; Kawashima, S.; Kitayama, H.; Takahashi, C. & Noda, M. (2005). The membrane-anchored MMP-regulator RECK is a target of myogenic regulatory factors. *Oncogene*, Vol.24, No.38, pp. 5850-5857,

Ehrhardt, J.; Brimah, K.; Adkin, C.; Partridge, T. & Morgan, J. (2007). Human muscle precursor cells give rise to functional satellite cells in vivo. *Neuromuscular Disorders*, Vol.17, No.8, (Aug), pp. 631-8,

El Fahime, E.; Torrente, Y.; Caron, N.J.; Bresolin, M.D. & Tremblay, J.P. (2000). In vivo migration of transplanted myoblasts requires Matrix Metalloproteinase activity. *Experimental Cell Research*, Vol.258, No.2, (Aug), pp. 279-287,

Emery, A.E. (2002). The muscular dystrophies. *Lancet*, Vol.359, No.9307, (Feb 23), pp. 687-95, ISSN 0140-6736

Fadic, R.; Mezzano, V.; Alvarez, K.; Cabrera, D.; Holmgren, J. & Brandan, E. (2006). Increase in decorin and biglycan in Duchenne Muscular Dystrophy: role of fibroblasts as cell source of these proteoglycans in the disease. *Journal of Cellular and molecular medicine*, Vol.10, No.3, (Jul-Sep), pp. 758-69, ISSN 1582-1838

Fanjul-Fernandez, M.; Folgueras, A.R.; Cabrera, S. & Lopez-Otin, C. (2010). Matrix metalloproteinases: evolution, gene regulation and functional analysis in mouse models. *Biochimica Biophysica Acta*,Vol.1803, No.1, (Jan), pp. 3-19, ISSN 0006-3002

Ferrari, G.; Cusella-De Angelis, G.; Coletta, M.; Paolucci, E.; Stornaiuolo, A.; Cossu, G. & Mavilio, F. (1998). Muscle regeneration by bone marrow-derived myogenic progenitors. *Science*, Vol.279, No.5356, (Mar 6), pp. 1528-30,

Ferre, P.J.; Liaubet, L.; Concordet, D.; SanCristobal, M.; Uro-Coste, E.; Tosser-Klopp, G.; Bonnet, A.; Toutain, P.L.; Hatey, F. & Lefebvre, H.P. (2007). Longitudinal analysis of gene expression in porcine skeletal muscle after post-injection local injury. *Pharmaceutical Research*, Vol.24, No.8, (Aug), pp. 1480-9, ISSN 0724-8741

Frisdal, E.; Teiger, E.; Lefaucheur, J.P.; Adnot, S.; Planus, E.; Lafuma, C.& D'Ortho, M. P.. (2000). Increased expression of gelatinases and alteration of basement membrane in rat soleus muscle following femoral artery ligation. *Neuropathology and Applied Neurobiology*, Vol.26, No.1, (Feb), pp. 11-21, ISSN 0305-1846

Fukushima, K.; Nakamura, A.; Ueda, H.; Yuasa, K.; Yoshida, K.; Takeda, S. & Ikeda, S. (2007). Activation and localization of matrix metalloproteinase-2 and -9 in the skeletal muscle of the muscular dystrophy dog (CXMDJ). *BMC Musculoskeletal Disorders*, Vol.8, pp. 54, ISSN 1471-2474

Galvez, B.G.; Sampaolesi, M.; Brunelli, S.; Covarello, D.; Gavina, M.; Rossi, B.; Constantin, G.; Torrente, Y. & Cossu, G. (2006). Complete repair of dystrophic skeletal muscle by mesoangioblasts with enhanced migration ability. *The Journal of Cell Biology,* Vol.174, No.2, (Jul 17), pp. 231-43,

Gerard, C.; Forest, M.A.; Beauregard, G.; Skuk, D. & Tremblay, J.P.. (2011). Fibrin gel improves the survival of transplanted myoblasts. *Cell Transplantation,* Vol.20, No.5, (Apr 29), pp. ISSN 1555-3892

Giannelli, G.; De Marzo, A.; Marinosci, F. & Antonaci, S. (2005). Matrix metalloproteinase imbalance in muscle disuse atrophy. *Histology & Histopathology,* Vol.20, No.1, (Jan), pp. 99-106, ISSN 0213-3911

Gilbert, P.M.; Havenstrite, K.L.; Magnusson, K.E.; Sacco, A.; Leonardi, N.A.; Kraft, P.; Nguyen, N.K.; Thrun, S.; Lutolf, M.P. & Blau, H.M. (2010). Substrate elasticity regulates skeletal muscle stem cell self-renewal in culture. *Science,* Vol.329, No.5995, (Aug 27), pp. 1078-81, ISSN 1095-9203

Gosselin, L.E.; Williams, J.E.; Deering, M.; Brazeau, D.; Koury, S. & Martinez, D.A. (2004). Localization and early time course of TGF-β1 mRNA expression in dystrophic muscle. *Muscle Nerve,* Vol.30, No.5, pp. 645-653, ISSN 1097-4598

Goyenvalle, A. & Davies, K.E. (2011). Challenges to oligonucleotides-based therapeutics for Duchenne muscular dystrophy. *Skeletal muscle,* Vol.1, No.1, pp. 8, ISSN 2044-5040

Grande, J.P.; Melder, D.C. & Zinsmeister, A.R. (1997). Modulation of collagen gene expression by cytokines: stimulatory effect of transforming growth factor-beta1, with divergent effects of epidermal growth factor and tumor necrosis factor-alpha on collagen type I and collagen type IV. *Journal of Laboratory and Clinical Medicine,* Vol.130, pp. 476–486.,

Gross, J.G. & Morgan, J.E. (1999). Muscle precursor cells injected into irradiated mdx mouse muscle persist after serial injury. *Muscle Nerve,* Vol.22, No.2, pp. 174-85.,

Guérin, C.W. & Holland, P.C. (1995). Synthesis and secretion of matrix-degrading metalloproteases by human skeletal muscle satellite cells. *Developmental Dynamics,* Vol.202, No.1, (Jan), pp. 91-99,

Guglieri, M. & Bushby, K. (2010). Molecular treatments in Duchenne muscular dystrophy. *Current Opinion in Pharmacology,* Vol.10, No.3, (Jun), pp. 331-7, ISSN 1471-4973

Hemmann, S.; Graf, J.; Roderfeld, M. & Roeb, E. (2007). Expression of MMPs and TIMPs in liver fibrosis - a systematic review with special emphasis on anti-fibrotic strategies. *Journal of Hepatology,* Vol.46, No.5, pp. 955-975,

Heslop, L.; Morgan, J.E. & Partridge, T.A. (2000). Evidence for a myogenic stem cell that is exhausted in dystrophic muscle. *Journal of Cell Science,* Vol.113 (Pt 12), (Jun), pp. 2299-308,

Hirata, A.; Masuda, S.; Tamura, T.; Kai, K.; Ojima, K.; Fukase, A.; Motoyoshi, K.; Kamakura, K.; Miyagoe-Suzuki, Y. & Takeda, S. (2003). Expression profiling of cytokines and related genes in regenerating skeletal muscle after cardiotoxin injection: a role for osteopontin. *American Journal of Pathology,* Vol.163, pp. 203–15,

Hnia, K.; Gayraud, J.; Hugon, G.; Ramonatxo, M.; De La Porte, S.; Matecki, S.& Mornet, D. (2008). L-arginine decreases inflammation and modulates the nuclear factor-kappaB/matrix metalloproteinase cascade in mdx muscle fibers. *American Journal of Pathology,* Vol.172, No.6, (Jun), pp. 1509-19, ISSN 1525-2191

Hoffman, E.P.; Morgan, J.E.; Watkins, S.C. & Partridge, T.A. (1990). Somatic reversion/suppression of the mouse mdx phenotype in vivo. *Journal of the Neurological Sciences* , Vol.99, No.1, (Oct), pp. 9-25,

Hoffman, E.P.; Bronson, A.; Levin, A.A.; Takeda, S.; Yokota, T.;. Baudy, A.R & Connor, E.M. (2011). Restoring dystrophin expression in duchenne muscular dystrophy muscle progress in exon skipping and stop codon read through. *American Journal of Pathology,* Vol.179, No.1, (Jul), pp. 12-22, ISSN 1525-2191

Holmbeck, K.; Bianco, P.; Pidoux, I.; Inoue, S.; Billinghurst, R.C.; Wu, W.; Chrysovergis, K.; Yamada, S.; Birkedal-Hansen, H.& Poole, A.R. (2005). The metalloproteinase MT1-MMP is required for normal development and maintenance of osteocyte processes in bone. *Journal of Cell Science,* Vol.118, No.Pt 1, (Jan 1), pp. 147-56, ISSN 0021-9533

Hulboy, D.L.; Rudolph, L.A. & Matrisian, L.M. (1997). Matrix metalloproteinases as mediators of reproductive function. *Molecular Human Reproduction,* Vol.3, No.1, (Jan), pp. 27-45, ISSN 1360-9947

Ignotz, R.A. & Massague, J. (1986). Transforming growth factor-beta stimulates the expression of fibronectin and collagen and their incorporation into the extracellular matrix. *Journal of Biological Chemistry,* Vol.261, pp. 4337–4345.,

Irintchev, A.; Langer, M.; Zweyer, M.; Theisen R. & Wernig, A. (1997). Functional improvement of damaged adult mouse muscle by implantation of primary myoblasts. *Journal of Physiology,* Vol.500 (Pt 3), (May 1), pp. 775-85,

Jackson, K.A.; Snyder, D.S. & Goodell, M.A. (2004). Skeletal muscle fiber-specific green autofluorescence: potential for stem cell engraftment artifacts. *Stem Cells,* Vol.22, No.2, pp. 180-7, ISSN 1066-5099

Kaar, J.L.; Li, Y.; Blair, H.C.; Asche, G.; Koepsel, R.R.; Huard, J. & Russell, A.J. (2008). Matrix metalloproteinase-1 treatment of muscle fibrosis. *Acta Biomaterialia,* Vol.4, No.5, (Sep), pp. 1411-20, ISSN 1742-7061

Kherif, S.; Lafuma, C.; Dehaupas, M.; Lachkar, S.; Fournier, J.G.; Verdiere-Sahuque, M.; Fardeau, M. & Alameddine, H.S. (1999). Expression of matrix metalloproteinases 2 and 9 in regenerating skeletal muscle: a study in experimentally injured and mdx muscles. *Developmental Biology,* Vol.205, No.1, (Jan 1), pp. 158-70, ISSN 0012-1606

Kinoshita, I.; Huard J. & Tremblay, J.P. (1994a). Utilization of myoblasts from transgenic mice to evaluate the efficacy of myoblast transplantation. *Muscle Nerve,* Vol.17, No.9, (Sep), pp. 975-80, ISSN 0148-639X

Kinoshita, I.; Vilquin, J.T.; Guerette, B.; Asselin, I.; Roy, R.; Lille S. & Tremblay, J.P. (1994b). Immunosuppression with FK 506 insures good success of myoblast transplantation in mdx mice. *Transplantation Proceedings,* Vol.26, No.6, (Dec), pp. 3518, ISSN 0041-1345

Kumar, A.; Bhatnagar, S. & Kumar, A. (2010). Matrix metalloproteinase inhibitor batimastat alleviates pathology and improves skeletal muscle function in dystrophin-deficient mdx mice. *American Journal of Pathology,* Vol.177, No.1, (Jul), pp. 248-60, ISSN 1525-2191

Kumar, M.; Keller, B.; Makalou, N. & Sutton, R.E. (2001). Systematic determination of the packaging limit of lentiviral vectors. *Human Gene Therapy,* Vol.12, No.15, (Oct 10), pp. 1893-905,

Lai, Y.; Thomas, G.D.; Yue, Y.; Yang, H.T.; Li, D.; Long, C.; Judge, L.; Bostick, B.; Chamberlain, J.S.; Terjung, R.L. & Duan, D. (2009). Dystrophins carrying spectrin-like repeats 16 and 17 anchor nNOS to the sarcolemma and enhance exercise performance in a mouse model of muscular dystrophy. *The Journal of Clinical Investigation*, Vol.119, No.3, (Mar), pp. 624-35,

Lefaucheur, J.P. & Sebille, A. (1995). Basic fibroblast growth factor promotes in vivo muscle regeneration in murine muscular dystrophy. *Neuroscience Letters*, Vol.202, No.1-2, (Dec 29), pp. 121-4,

Lewis, M.P.; Tippett, H.L.; Sinanan, A.C.; Morgan, M.J. & Hunt, N.P. (2000). Gelatinase-B (matrix metalloproteinase-9; MMP-9) secretion is involved in the migratory phase of human and murine muscle cell cultures. *Journal of Muscle Research and Cell Motility*, Vol.21, No.3, pp. 223-233,

Li, H.; Mittal, A.; Makonchuk, D.Y.; Bhatnagar, S. & Kumar, A. (2009). Matrix metalloproteinase-9 inhibition ameliorates pathogenesis and improves skeletal muscle regeneration in muscular dystrophy. *Human Molecular Genetics*, Vol.18, No.14, (Jul 15), pp. 2584-98, ISSN 1460-2083

Li, S.; Kimura, E.; Fall, B.M.; Reyes, M.; Angello, J.C.; Welikson, R.; Hauschka, S.D. & Chamberlain, J.S. (2005). Stable transduction of myogenic cells with lentiviral vectors expressing a minidystrophin. *Gene Therapy* , Vol.12, No.14, (Jul), pp. 1099-108,

Li, Y.; Foster, W.; Deasy, B.M.; Chan, Y.; Prisk, V.; Tang ,Y.; Cummins, J. & Huard, J. (2004). Transforming Growth Factor-{beta}1 induces the differentiation of myogenic cells into fibrotic cells in injured skeletal muscle: A key event in muscle fibrogenesis. *American Journal of Pathology*, Vol.164, No.3, (March 1, 2004), pp. 1007-1019,

Liu, X.; Lee, D.J.; Skittone, L.K.; Natsuhara, K. & Kim, H.T. (2010). Role of gelatinases in disuse-induced skeletal muscle atrophy. *Muscle Nerve*, Vol.41, No.2, (Feb), pp. 174-8, ISSN 1097-4598

Lluri, G. & Jaworski, D.M. (2005). Regulation of TIMP-2, MT1-MMP, and MMP-2 expression during C2C12 differentiation. *Muscle Nerve*, Vol.32, No.4, (Oct), pp. 492-9, ISSN 0148-639X

Lurton, J.; Soto, H.; Narayanan, A. & Raghu, G. (1999). Regulation of human lung fibroblast C1q-receptors by transforming growth factor-beta and tumor necrosis factor-alpha. *Experimental Lung Research*, Vol.25, pp. 151–164,

Maeda, N.; Kanda, F.; Okuda, S.; Ishihara, H. & Chihara, K. (2005). Transforming growth factor-beta enhances connective tissue growth factor expression in L6 rat skeletal myotubes. *Neuromuscular Disorders*, Vol.15, No.11, (Nov), pp. 790-3,

Manicone, A.M. & McGuire, J.K. (2008). Matrix metalloproteinases as modulators of inflammation. *Seminars of Cell and Developmental Biology*, Vol.19, No.1, (Feb), pp. 34-41, ISSN 1084-9521

Mather, K.A.; Jorm, A.F.; Parslow, R.A. & Christensen, H. (2011). Is telomere length a biomarker of aging? A review. *The Journals of Gerontology. Series A, Biological sciences and medical sciences*, Vol.66, No.2, (Feb), pp. 202-13, ISSN 1758-535X

Mauro, A. (1961). Satellite cell of skeletal muscle fibers. *Journal of Biophysical and Biochemical Cytology*, Vol.9, (Feb), pp. 493-5, ISSN 0095-9901

Meng, J.; Muntoni, F.& Morgan, J.E. (2011a). Stem cells to treat muscular dystrophies - where are we? *Neuromuscular Disorders*, Vol.21, No.1, (Jan), pp. 4-12, ISSN 1873-2364

Meng, J.; Adkin, C.F.; Xu, S.W.; Muntoni, F. & Morgan, J.E. (2011b). Contribution of human muscle-derived cells to skeletal muscle regeneration in dystrophic host mice. *PloS One*, Vol.6, No.3, pp. e17454, ISSN 1932-6203

Meng, J.; Adkin, C.F.; Arechavala-Gomeza, V.; Boldrin, L.; Muntoni, F. & Morgan, J.E. (2010). The contribution of human synovial stem cells to skeletal muscle regeneration. *Neuromuscular Disorders*, Vol.20, No.1, (Jan), pp. 6-15, ISSN 1873-2364

Meregalli, M.; Farini, A. & Torrente, Y. (2008). Combining stem cells and exon skipping strategy to treat muscular dystrophy. *Expert Opinion in Biological Therapy*, Vol.8, No.8, (Aug), pp. 1051-61,

Miyazaki, D.; Nakamura, A.; Fukushima, K.; Yoshida, K.; Takeda, S. & Ikeda, S.I. (2011). Matrix metalloproteinase-2 ablation in dystrophin-deficient mdx muscles reduces angiogenesis resulting in impaired growth of regenerated muscle fibers. *Human Molecular Genetics*, Vol.20, No.9, (May 1), pp. 1787-99., ISSN 1460-2083

Monaco, A.P.; Bertelson, C.J.; Middlesworth, W.; Colletti, C.A.; Aldridge, J.; Fischbeck, K.H.; Bartlett, R.; Pericak-Vance, M.A.; Roses, A.D. & Kunkel, L.M. (1985). Detection of deletions spanning the Duchenne muscular dystrophy locus using a tightly linked DNA segment. *Nature*, Vol.316, No.6031, (Aug 29-Sep 4), pp. 842-5, ISSN 0028-0836

Montini, E.; Cesana, D.; Schmidt, M.; Sanvito, F.; Ponzoni, M.; Bartholomae, C.; Sergi Sergi, L.; Benedicenti, F.; Ambrosi, A.; Di Serio, C.; Doglioni, C.; von Kalle, C. & Naldini, L. (2006). Hematopoietic stem cell gene transfer in a tumor-prone mouse model uncovers low genotoxicity of lentiviral vector integration. *Nature Biotechnology*, Vol.24, No.6, (Jun), pp. 687-96,

Morgan, J.; Rouche, A.; Bausero, P.; Houssaini, A.; Gross, J.; Fiszman, M.Y. & Alameddine,H.S. (2010). MMP-9 overexpression improves myogenic cell migration and engraftment. *Muscle Nerve*, Vol.42, No.4, (Oct), pp. 584-95, ISSN 1097-4598

Morgan, J.E. & P.S. Zammit. (2010). Direct effects of the pathogenic mutation on satellite cell function in muscular dystrophy. *Experimental Cell Research*, Vol.316, No.18, pp. 3100-3108, ISSN 1090-2422

Morgan, J.E.; Hoffman, E.P. & Partridge, T.A. (1990). Normal myogenic cells from newborn mice restore normal histology to degenerating muscles of the mdx mouse. *The Journal of Cell Biology*, Vol.111, No.6 Pt 1, pp. 2437-49.,

Morgan, J.E.; Gross, J.G.; Pagel, C.N.; Beauchamp, J.R.; Fassati, A.; Thrasher, A.J.; Di Santo, J.P.; Fisher, I.B.; Shiwen, X.; Abraham, D.J.& Partridge,T.A. (2002). Myogenic cell proliferation and generation of a reversible tumorigenic phenotype are triggered by preirradiation of the recipient site. *The Journal of Cell Biology*, Vol.157, No.4, pp. 693-702, ISSN 0021-9525

Morrison, C.J.; Butler, G.S.; Rodriguez, D. & Overall, C.M. (2009). Matrix metalloproteinase proteomics: substrates, targets, and therapy. *Current Opinion in Cell Biology*, Vol.21, No.5, (Oct), pp. 645-53, ISSN 1879-0410

Morrison, J.; Lu, Q.L.; Pastoret, C.; Partridge T. & Bou-Gharios, G. (2000). T-cell-dependent fibrosis in the mdx dystrophic mouse. *Laboratory Investigation*, Vol.80, No.6, pp. 881-91.,

Murphy, G. (2010). Fell-Muir Lecture: Metalloproteinases: from demolition squad to master regulators. *International Journal of Experimental Pathology*, Vol.91, No.4, (Aug), pp. 303-13, ISSN 1365-2613

Nakamura, A. & Takeda, S. (2011). Mammalian models of Duchenne Muscular Dystrophy: pathological characteristics and therapeutic applications. *Journal of Biomedicine & Biotechnology,*Vol.2011, pp. 184393, ISSN 1110-7251

Negroni, E.; Vallese, D.; Vilquin, J.T.; Butler-Browne, G.; Mouly, V. & Trollet, C. (2011). Current advances in cell therapy strategies for muscular dystrophies. *Expert Opinion on Biological Therapy*, Vol.11, No.2, (Feb), pp. 157-76, ISSN 1744-7682

Negroni, E.; Riederer, I.; Chaouch, S.; Belicchi, M.; Razini, P.; Di Santo, J.; Torrente, Y.; Butler-Browne, G.S. & Mouly, V. (2009). In vivo myogenic potential of human CD133+ muscle-derived stem cells: a quantitative study. *Molecular Therapy*, Vol.17, No.10, (Oct), pp. 1771-8, ISSN 1525-0024

Niebroj-Dobosz, I.; Madej-Pilarczyk, A.; Marchel, M.; Sokolowska, B. & Hausmanowa-Petrusewicz, I. (2009). Matrix metalloproteinases in serum of Emery-Dreifuss muscular dystrophy patients. *Acta Biochimica Polonica*, Vol.56, No.4, pp. 717-22, ISSN 1734-154X

Nishimura, T.; Nakamura, K.; Kishioka, Y.; Kato-Mori, Y.; Wakamatsu, J. & Hattori, A. (2008). Inhibition of matrix metalloproteinases suppresses the migration of skeletal muscle cells. *Journal of Muscle Research and Cell Motility*, Vol.29, No.1, pp. 37-44, ISSN 0142-4319

Ohtake, Y.; Tojo, H. & Seiki, M. (2006). Multifunctional roles of MT1-MMP in myofiber formation and morphostatic maintenance of skeletal muscle. *Journal of Cell Science*, Vol.119, No Pt 18, (Sep 15), pp. 3822-32, ISSN 0021-9533

Pagel, C.N. & Partridge, T.A. (1999). Covert persistence of mdx mouse myopathy is revealed by acute and chronic effects of irradiation. *Journal of Neurological Science*, Vol.164, No.2, (Apr 1), pp. 103-16,

Pallafacchina, G.; Francois, S.; Regnault, B.; Czarny, B.; Dive, V.; Cumano, A.; Montarras, D. & Buckingham, M. (2010). An adult tissue-specific stem cell in its niche: a gene profiling analysis of in vivo quiescent and activated muscle satellite cells. *Stem Cell Research*, Vol.4, No.2, (Mar), pp. 77-91, ISSN 1876-7753

Palmieri, B.; Tremblay, J.P. & Daniele, L. (2010). Past, present and future of myoblast transplantation in the treatment of Duchenne muscular dystrophy. *Pediatric transplantation*, Vol.14, No.7, (Nov), pp. 813-9, ISSN 1399-3046

Palumbo, R.; Sampaolesi, M.; De Marchis, F.; Tonlorenzi, R.; Colombetti, S.; Mondino, A.; Cossu G. & Bianchi, M.E. (2004). Extracellular HMGB1, a signal of tissue damage, induces mesoangioblast migration and proliferation. *The Journal of Cell Biology*, Vol.164, No.3, (Feb 2), pp. 441-9, ISSN 0021-9525

Partridge, T.A.; Morgan, J.E.; Coulton, G.R.; Hoffman, E.P. & Kunkel, L.M. (1989). Conversion of mdx myofibers from dystrophin-negative to-positive by injection of normal myoblasts. *Nature*, Vol.337, pp. 176-179,

Pellegrini, K.L. & Beilharz, M.W. (2011). The survival of myoblasts after intramuscular transplantation is improved when fewer cells are injected. *Transplantation*, Vol.91, No.5, (Mar 15), pp. 522-6, ISSN 1534-6080

Piers, A.T.; Lavin, T.; Radley-Crabb, H.G.; Bakker, A.J.; Grounds ,M.D. & Pinniger, G.J. (2011). Blockade of TNF in vivo using cV1q antibody reduces contractile dysfunction of skeletal muscle in response to eccentric exercise in dystrophic mdx and normal mice. *Neuromuscular Disorders*, Vol.21, No.2, (Feb), pp. 132-41, ISSN 1873-2364

Pisani, D.F.; Clement, N.; Loubat, A.; Plaisant, M.; Sacconi, S.; Kurzenne, J.Y.; Desnuelle, C.; Dani C. &Dechesne, C.A. (2010). Hierarchization of myogenic and adipogenic progenitors within human skeletal muscle. *Stem Cells*, Vol.28, No.12, (Dec), pp. 2182-94, ISSN 1549-4918

Porreca, E.; Guglielmi, M.; Uncini, A.; Di Gregorio, P.; Angelini, A.; Di Febbo, C.; Pierdomenico, S.; Baccante G. & Cuccurullo,. F. (1999). Haemostatic abnormalities, cardiac involvement and serum tumor necrosis factor levels in X-linked dystrophic patients. *Thrombosis Haemostasis*, Vol.81, pp. 543-546.,

Porter, J.D.; Guo, W.; Merriam, A.P.; Khanna, S.; Cheng, G.; Zhou, X.; Andrade, F.H.; Richmonds, C. & Kaminski, H.J. (2003). Persistent over-expression of specific CC class chemokines correlates with macrophage and T-cell recruitment in mdx skeletal muscle. *Neuromuscular Disorders*, Vol.13, pp. 223-35,

Porter, J.D.; Khanna, S.; Kaminski, H.J.; Rao, J.S.; Merriam, A.; Richmonds, C.R.; Leahy, P.; Li, J.; Guo, W. & Andrade, F.H. (2002). A chronic inflammatory response dominates the skeletal muscle molecular signature in dystrophin-deficient mdx mice. *Human Molecular Genetics*, Vol.11, pp. 263-72,

Praud, C.; Montarras, D.; Pinset,C. & Sebille, A. (2003). Dose effect relationship between the number of normal progenitor muscle cells grafted in mdx mouse skeletal striated muscle and the number of dystrophin-positive fibres. *Neuroscience Letters*, Vol.352, No.1, (Nov 27), pp. 70-2,

Quenneville, S.P.; Chapdelaine, P.; Skuk, D.; Paradis, M.; Goulet, M.; Rousseau, J.; Xiao, X.; Garcia, L. & Tremblay, J.P. (2007). Autologous transplantation of muscle precursor cells modified with a lentivirus for muscular dystrophy: human cells and primate models. *Molecular Therapy*, Vol.15, No.2, (Feb), pp. 431-8,

Radley, H.G.; Davies, M.J. & Grounds,M.D. (2008). Reduced muscle necrosis and long-term benefits in dystrophic mdx mice after cV1q (blockade of TNF) treatment. *Neuromuscular Disorders*, Vol.18, No.3, (Mar), pp. 227-38, ISSN 0960-8966

Rahim, A.A.; Wong, A.M.; Howe, S.J.; Buckley, S.M.; Acosta-Saltos, A.D.; Elston, K.E.; Ward, N.J.; Philpott, N.J.; Cooper, J.D.; Anderson, P.N.; Waddington, S.N.; Thrashe, A.J. & Raivich,G. (2009). Efficient gene delivery to the adult and fetal CNS using pseudotyped non-integrating lentiviral vectors. *Gene Therapy*, Vol.16, No. 4, (Apr), pp. 509-20, ISSN 0969-7128

Rando, T.A. &Blau, H.M. (1994). Primary mouse myoblast purification, characterization, and transplantation for cell-mediated gene therapy. *The Journal of Cell Biology*, Vol.125, No.6, (Jun), pp. 1275-87, ISSN 0021-9525

Reznick, A.Z.; Menashe, O.; Bar-Shai, M.; Coleman, R. & Carmeli, E. (2003). Expression of matrix metalloproteinases, inhibitor, and acid phosphatase in muscles of immobilized hindlimbs of rats. *Muscle Nerve*, Vol.27, No.1, (Jan), pp. 51-9, ISSN 0148-639X

Rodriguez, D.; Morrison, C.J. & Overall, C.M. (2010). Matrix metalloproteinases: what do they not do? New substrates and biological roles identified by murine models and proteomics. *Biochimica Biophysica Acta*, Vol.1803, No.1, (Jan), pp. 39-54, ISSN 0006-3002

Rosenberg, G.A. (2009). Matrix metalloproteinases and their multiple roles in neurodegenerative diseases. *The Lancet Neurology*, Vol.8, No.2, pp. 205-216,

Sacco, A.; Doyonnas, R.; Kraft, P.; Vitorovic, S. & Blau,H.M. (2008). Self-renewal and expansion of single transplanted muscle stem cells. *Nature*, Vol.456, No.7221, (Nov 27), pp. 502-6,

Sacco, A.; Mourkioti, F.; Tran, R.; Choi, J.; Llewellyn, M.; Kraft, P.; Shkreli, M.; Delp, S.; Pomerantz, J.H.; Artandi, S.E. & Blau, H.M. (2010). Short telomeres and stem cell exhaustion model Duchenne muscular dystrophy in mdx/mTR mice. *Cell*, Vol.143, No.7, (Dec 23), pp. 1059-71, ISSN 1097-4172

Sampaolesi, M.; Torrente, Y.; Innocenzi, A.; Tonlorenzi, R.; D'Antona, G.; Pellegrino, M.A.; Barresi, R.; Bresolin, N.; De Angelis, M.G.; Campbell, K.P.; Bottinelli, R. & Cossu, G. (2003). Cell therapy of alpha-sarcoglycan null dystrophic mice through intra-arterial delivery of mesoangioblasts. *Science*, Vol.301, No.5632, (Jul 25), pp. 487-92, ISSN 1095-9203

Sampaolesi, M.; Blot, S.; D'Antona, G.; Granger, N.; Tonlorenzi,R.; Innocenzi, A.; Mognol, P.; Thibaud, J.L.; Galvez ,B.G.; Barthelemy, I.; Perani, L.; Mantero, S.; Guttinger, M.; Pansarasa, O.; Rinaldi, C.; Cusella De Angelis, M.G.; Torrente, Y.; Bordignon, C.; Bottinelli, R. & Cossu, G. (2006). Mesoangioblast stem cells ameliorate muscle function in dystrophic dogs. *Nature*, Vol.444, No.7119, (Nov 30), pp. 574-9,

Sancricca, C.; Mirabella, M.; Gliubizzi, C.; Broccolini, A.; Gidaro, T. & Morosetti, R. (2010). Vessel-associated stem cells from skeletal muscle: From biology to future uses in cell therapy. *World Journal of Stem Cells*, Vol.2, No.3, (Jun 26), pp. 39-49, ISSN 1948-0210

Sciorati, C.; Galvez, B.G.; Brunelli, S.; Tagliafico, E.; Ferrari, S.; Cossu G.& Clementi, E. (2006). Ex vivo treatment with nitric oxide increases mesoangioblast therapeutic efficacy in muscular dystrophy. *Journal of Cell Science*, Vol.119,.Pt 24, (Dec 15), pp. 5114-23,

Seale, P.;. Sabourin, L.A; Girgis-Gabardo, A.; Mansouri, A.; Gruss, P. & Rudnicki, M.A. (2000). Pax7 is required for the specification of myogenic satellite cells. *Cell*, Vol.102, No.6, (Sep 15), pp. 777-86,

Sharma, K. & Ziyadeh,F.N. (1994). The emerging role of transforming growth factor-beta in kidney diseases. *American Journal of Physiology Renal Physiology*, Vol.266, pp. F829-F842.,

Shiomi, T.; Lemaitre, V.; D'Armiento, J. & Okada, Y. (2010). Matrix metalloproteinases, a disintegrin and metalloproteinases, and a disintegrin and metalloproteinases with thrombospondin motifs in non-neoplastic diseases. *Pathology International*, Vol.60, No.7, (Jul), pp. 477-96, ISSN 1440-1827

Silva-Barbosa, S.D.; Butler-Browne, G.S.; Di Santo, J.P. & Mouly, V. (2005). Comparative analysis of genetically engineered immunodeficient mouse strains as recipients for human myoblast transplantation. *Cell Transplantation*, Vol.14, No.7, pp. 457-67,

Skuk, D. & Tremblay, J.P. (2011). Intramuscular cell transplantation as a potential treatment of myopathies: clinical and preclinical relevant data. *Expert Opinion on Biological Therapy*, Vol.11, No.3, (Mar), pp. 359-74, ISSN 1744-7682

Skuk, D.; Roy, B.; Goulet, M. & Tremblay, J.P. (1999). Successful myoblast transplantation in primates depends on appropriate cell delivery and induction of regeneration in the host muscle. *Experimental Neurology*, Vol.155, No.1, (Jan), pp. 22-30, ISSN 0014-4886

Skuk, D.; Caron, N.; Goulet, M.; Roy, B.; Espinosa, F. & Tremblay, J.P. (2002). Dynamics of the early immune cellular reactions after myogenic cell transplantation. *Cell Transplantation*, Vol.11, No.7, pp. 671-81,

Smythe, G.M.; Fan, Y. & Grounds, M.D. (2000). Enhanced migration and fusion of donor myoblasts in dystrophic and normal host muscle. *Muscle Nerve,* Vol.23, No.4, (Apr), pp. 560-74, ISSN 0148-639X

Springer, T.A. (1994). Traffic signals for lymphocyte recirculation and leukocyte emigration: the multistep paradigm. *Cell,* Vol.76, No.2, (Jan 28), pp. 301-14, ISSN 0092-8674

Sternlicht, M.D. & Werb, Z. (2001). How matrix metalloproteinases regulate cell behavior. *Annual Review of Cell and Developmental Biology,* Vol.17, pp. 463-516, ISSN 1081-0706

Stevenson, E.J.; Giresi, P.G.; Koncarevic, A. & Kandarian, S.C. (2003). Global analysis of gene expression patterns during disuse atrophy in rat skeletal muscle. *Journal of Physiology,* Vol.551, Pt 1, (Aug 15), pp. 33-48, ISSN 0022-3751

Sugita, H. & Takeda, S. (2010). Progress in muscular dystrophy research with special emphasis on gene therapy. *Proceedings of the Japan Academy. Series B, Physical and Biological sciences,* Vol.86, No.7, pp. 748-56, ISSN 1349-2896

Sun, G.; Haginoya, K.; Chiba, Y.; Uematsu, M.; Hino-Fukuyo, N.; Tanaka, S.; Onuma, A.; Iinuma, K. & Tsuchiya,S. (2010). Elevated plasma levels of tissue inhibitors of metalloproteinase-1 and their overexpression in muscle in human and mouse muscular dystrophy. *Journal of the Neurological Sciences,* Vol.297, No.1-2, pp. 19-28,

Sun, G.; Haginoya, K.; Wu, Y.; Chiba, Y.; Nakanishi, T.; Onuma, A.; Sato, Y.; Takigawa, M.; Iinuma, K. & Tsuchiya, S. (2008). Connective tissue growth factor is overexpressed in muscles of human muscular dystrophy. *Journal of Neurological Sciences,* Vol.267, No.1, (04/15), pp. 48-56,

Tedesco, F.S.; Dellavalle, A.; Diaz-Manera, J.; Messina G. & Cossu, G. (2010). Repairing skeletal muscle: regenerative potential of skeletal muscle stem cells. *The Journal of Clinical Investigation,* Vol.120, No.1, (Jan 4), pp. 11-9, ISSN 1558-8238

Torrente, Y.; El Fahime, E.; Caron, N.J.; Del Bo, R.; Belicchi, M.; Pisati, F.; Tremblay, J.P. & Bresolin, N. (2003). Tumor necrosis factor-alpha (TNF-alpha) stimulates chemotactic response in mouse myogenic cells. *Cell Transplantation,* Vol.12, No.1, pp. 91-100, ISSN 0963-6897

Torrente, Y.; Belicchi, M.; Sampaolesi, M.; Pisati, F.; Meregalli, M.; D'Antona, G.; Tonlorenzi, R.; Porretti, L.; Gavina, M.; Mamchaoui, K.; Pellegrino, M.A.; Furling, D.; Mouly, V.; Butler-Browne, G.S.; Bottinelli, R.; Cossu, G. & Bresolin, N. (2004). Human circulating AC133(+) stem cells restore dystrophin expression and ameliorate function in dystrophic skeletal muscle. *The Journal of Clinical Investigation,* Vol.114, No.2, (Jul), pp. 182-95,

Urso, M.L.; Szelenyi, E.R.; Warren, G. L. & Barnes, B. R. (2010). Matrix metalloprotease-3 and tissue inhibitor of metalloprotease-1 mRNA and protein levels are altered in response to traumatic skeletal muscle injury. *European Journal Applied Physiology,* Vol.109, No.5, pp. 963-72,

Vauchez, K.; Marolleau, J.P.; Schmid, M.; Khattar, P.; Chapel, A.; Catelain, C.; Lecourt, S.; Larghero, J.; Fiszman, M. & Vilquin, J.T. (2009). Aldehyde dehydrogenase activity identifies a population of human skeletal muscle cells with high myogenic capacities. *Molecular Therapy,* Vol.17, No.11, (Nov), pp. 1948-58, ISSN 1525-0024

Von Moers, A.; Zwirner, A.; Reinhold, A.; Bruckmann, O.; van Landeghem, F.; Stoltenburg-Didinger, G.; Schuppan, D.; Herbst, H. & Schuelke, M.. (2005). Increased mRNA expression of tissue inhibitors of metalloproteinase-1 and -2 in Duchenne muscular dystrophy. *Acta Neuropathologica,* Vol.109, No.3, (Mar), pp. 285-93, ISSN 0001-6322

Vu, T.H. & Werb, Z. (2000). Matrix metalloproteinases: effectors of development and normal physiology. *Genes & Development*, Vol.14, No.17, (Sep 1), pp. 2123-33, ISSN 0890-9369

Wakeford, S.; Watt, D.J. & Partridge, T.A. (1991). X-irradiation improves mdx mouse muscle as a model of myofiber loss in DMD. *Muscle Nerve*, Vol.14, No.1, (Jan), pp. 42-50,

Wang, W.; Pan, H.; Murray, K.; Jefferson, B.S. & Li, Y. (2009). Matrix metalloproteinase-1 promotes muscle cell migration and differentiation. *American Journal of Pathology*, Vol.174, No.2, (Feb), pp. 541-9, ISSN 1525-2191

Webster, C. & Blau, H.M. (1990). Accelerated age-related decline in replicative life-span of Duchenne muscular dystrophy myoblasts: implications for cell and gene therapy. *Somatic Cell Molecular Genetics*, Vol.16, No.6, (Nov), pp. 557-65, ISSN 0740-7750

Wells, D.J.; Ferrer, A. & Wells, K.E. (2002). Immunological hurdles in the path to gene therapy for Duchenne muscular dystrophy. *Expert Review Molecular Medicine*, Vol.4, No.23, (Nov), pp. 1-23, ISSN 1462-3994

Wilson, C.A. & Cichutek, K. (2009). The US and EU regulatory perspectives on the clinical use of hematopoietic stem/progenitor cells genetically modified ex vivo by retroviral vectors. *Methods in Molecular Biology*, Vol.506, pp. 477-88,

Wittwer, M.; Flück, M.; Hoppeler, H.; Müller, S.; Desplanches D. & Billeter, R. (2002). Prolonged unloading of rat soleus muscle causes distinct adaptations of the gene profile. *The FASEB Journal*, Vol.16, pp. 884-886,

Yokota, T.; Lu, Q.L.; Morgan, J.E.; Davies, K.E.; Fisher, R.; Takeda, S. & Partridge, T.A. (2006). Expansion of revertant fibers in dystrophic mdx muscles reflects activity of muscle precursor cells and serves as an index of muscle regeneration. *Journal of Cell Science*, Vol.119, Pt 13, (Jul 1), pp. 2679-87,

Zanotti, S.; Gibertini, S.; & Mora. M. (2010). Altered production of extra-cellular matrix components by muscle-derived Duchenne muscular dystrophy fibroblasts before and after TGF-β1 treatment. *Cell and Tissue Research*, Vol.339, No.2, pp. 397-410,

Zanotti, S.; Saredi, S.; Ruggieri, A.; Fabbri, M.; Blasevich, F.; Romaggi, S.; Morandi, L. & Mora, M. (2007). Altered extracellular matrix transcript expression and protein modulation in primary Duchenne muscular dystrophy myotubes. *Matrix Biology*, Vol.26, No.8, (Oct), pp. 615-24, ISSN 0945-053X

Zhang, F.; Thornhill, S.I.; Howe, S.J.; Ulaganathan, M.; Schambach, A.; Sinclair, J.; Kinnon, C.; Gaspar, H.B.; Antoniou, M. & Thrasher, A.J. (2007). Lentiviral vectors containing an enhancer-less ubiquitously acting chromatin opening element (UCOE) provide highly reproducible and stable transgene expression in hematopoietic cells. *Blood*, Vol.110, No.5, (Sep 1), pp. 1448-57,

Zheng, B.; Cao, B.; Crisan, M.; Sun, B.; Li, G.; Logar, A.; Yap, S.; Pollett, J.B.; Drowley, L.; Cassino, T.; Gharaibeh, B.; Deasy, B.M.; Huard, J. & Peault, B. (2007). Prospective identification of myogenic endothelial cells in human skeletal muscle. *Nature Biotechnology*, Vol.25, No.9, (Sep), pp. 1025-34,

Zhou, L.; Porter, J.D.; Cheng, G.; Gong, B.; Hatala, D.A.; Merriam, A.P.; Zhou, X.; Rafael, J.A. & Kaminski, H.J. (2006). Temporal and spatial mRNA expression patterns of TGF-[beta]1, 2, 3 and T[beta]RI, II, III in skeletal muscles of mdx mice. *Neuromuscular Disorders*, Vol.16, No.1, (Jan), pp. 32-38,

5

Genetic Therapy for Duchenne Muscular Dystrophy: Principles and Progress

Taeyoung Koo, Linda Popplewell,
Alberto Malerba and George Dickson
The Biomedical Sciences, Royal Holloway, University of London, Egham, Surrey,
UK

1. Introduction

This chapter focuses on the gene therapy advances made in relation to Duchenne muscular dystrophy and discusses principles and perspectives of strategies currently being developed. The chapter explains the genetic mutations that cause Duchenne muscular dystrophy (DMD) and Becker muscular dystrophy (BMD) and the differences between the two are discussed in relation to disease severity. The histopathological features of DMD are explained and discussed in the context of available animal models for DMD. There are various genetic therapeutic options available for the treatment of DMD, and the progress of each therapeutic approach is promising. A number of specific areas for the treatment of DMD are comprehensively presented, alongside in-depth description of the genetic biology of muscular dystrophy.

2. Muscular dystrophies

Muscle-related proteins build the structural network of muscle, and disruption of this link can cause muscle wasting and progression of numerous types of muscular dystrophy. Muscular dystrophies are a heterogeneous group of genetic disorders caused by different forms of mutations in various genes related to muscles.

2.1 Duchenne and Becker muscular dystrophy

The most common forms of muscular dystrophy are Duchenne and Becker muscular dystrophy (DMD, BMD). DMD and BMD are X-linked recessive muscle-wasting disorders affecting the skeletal musculature, resulting from mutations in the gene encoding dystrophin, which is a cytoskeletal protein in muscle fibres. Dystrophin protein interacts with the intracellular and extracellular dystrophin associated protein (DAP) complexes. Mutations in dystrophin gene can cause severe muscular wasting.

Different mutation types in exon/ intron regions of dystrophin gene or promoters causes various forms of dystrophinopathies (Giliberto et al., 2004). Dystrophin deficiency leads to disruption of the dystrophin associated protein (DAP) complexes, as do mutations in DAP genes in other forms of congenital and autosomal muscular dystrophy.

DMD affects 1:3500 newborn males worldwide, and patients exhibit severe, progressive muscle weakening. From about the age of 4 years, youngsters affected by DMD suffer bouts of recurrent damage and regeneration of skeletal muscle, leading eventually to muscle wasting and weakness, wheelchair-dependence, and life-threatening cardiac and respiratory complications. This debilitating disease is associated with loss of dystrophin expression caused generally by frameshift gene deletions and duplications, or by nonsense point mutations in the dystrophin gene.

In BMD, muscle pathology is generally milder than in DMD, and can even be virtually asymptomatic. The milder BMD phenotype is caused by the continued expression of truncated but partially functional dystrophin proteins in the affected muscles. This phenotype commonly arises due to mutational events which delete central rod domain elements, but nevertheless maintain the open reading frame upstream and downstream of the mutation boundaries. Thus different mutation types across exon/intron regions of the dystrophin gene can give rise to either DMD or BMD, depending upon the deletion boundaries.

BMD can be related to large in-frame deletions, including examples where up to 46% of the dystrophin-coding sequence has been deleted (Acsadi et al., 1991). Despite the large gene deletion, BMD patients have a mild phenotype due to partial expression of an internally-deleted but highly functional dystrophin protein. Clinical phenotype of BMD pathology is discriminated by mild, intermediate and severe types resulting from different exon deletions (Chao et al., 1996). Around 20% of normal dystrophin expression is seen as the milder BMD phenotype (Beggs et al., 1991).

2.1.1 Histopathological features of DMD

Clinical symptoms of DMD become apparent in patients of three to five years of age, while fetal DMD muscle is histologically normal (Biggar, 2006). The lack of dystrophin causes DAP dissociation, followed by disruption of the transmembrane link between extracellular matrix and the cytoskeleton. This causes severe muscle damage along with progressive fibrosis and muscle fibre loss. Lack of dystrophin in DMD muscles is believed to compromise the integrity of the sarcolemma, leading to calcium influx and myofibre necrosis. Central nucleation and uneven size of fibres are observed in early stages of dystrophinopathies due to the muscle necrosis followed by muscle degeneration and regeneration (Bell et al., 1968, Bradley et al., 1972). In dystrophin-negative muscles, fibres are lost (necrosed) and degeneration of the fibres proceeds, and they are eventually replaced by adipose and fibrous connective tissue, followed by atrophy (**Figure** 1) (Blake et al., 2002).

In addition, an increased number of proteasomes is found in necrotic and regenerative muscles in DMD, leading to muscle fibre degradation (Kumamoto et al., 2000). Muscle membrane becomes abnormally permeable, leading to fragility and leakiness of the muscle cells. The muscle weakness results in loss of independent ambulation, usually by the age of 12 (Emery, 2001). DMD patients eventually die from intercostal muscle weakness and respiratory failure in their early twenties (Emery, 2001). DMD patients also develop cardiac dysfunction with cardiomyopathy, resulting in heart failure and progressive dilated cardiomyopathy (Emery, 2001).

There is also evidence that dystrophin deficiency is associated with aberrant signal transduction from influx of divalent cations such as calcium due to abnormal membrane permeability in DMD muscle cells (Ruegg et al., 2002). Abnormality of calcium homeostasis is found due to structural defects in the ryanodine receptor (RyR) 1, calcium release channel in the sarcoplasmic reticulum, leading to increase of intracellular Ca^{2+} in the dystrophic muscles (Bellinger et al., 2009). Increased intracellular Ca^{2+} can activate calpain, which has a role in proteolysis and increases reactive oxygen species (ROS). Calpain cleaves intracellular proteins including titin, nebulin, desmin, troponin, tropomyosin and many kinases and signalling molecules and it increases protein breakdown (Allen et al., 2005). This can cause protein and membrane damage (Whitehead et al., 2006).

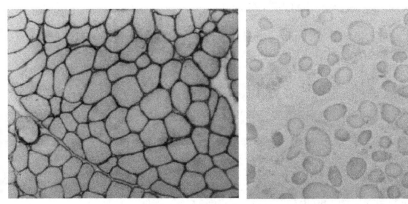

Normal muscle shows even size/diameter distribution of muscle fibres with dystrophin expression localised at the sarcolemma membrane. Lack of dystrophin protein expression in DMD causes muscle damage, which is accelerated by eccentric contraction of the muscle membrane. Eventually, muscle fibres are lost (necrosed) and replaced by adipose and fibrous connective tissue.

Fig. 1. Dystrophin immunohistochemistry in normal (left panel) and DMD muscle (right panel).

Damaged muscle membranes are demonstrated by staining with extracellulary applied labelled endogenous extracellular proteins such as albumin, immunoglobulin (Ig) G and IgM (Blake et al., 2002). The already permeable membrane in DMD becomes more permeable after mechanical stress or electric stimulation. Cardiomyopathies occur as a result of cardiac muscle damage in DMD. Myocardium is replaced by fat and connective tissue in dystrophinopathies. Clinical symptoms of cardiomyopathies appear after 10 years of age in DMD, and are present in all patients over 18 years (Finsterer et al, 2003). It has been currently reported that 20% of BMD and 50% of DMD patients eventually die due to cardiac failure (Finsterer et al., 2003). In the early stages of DMD, focal myofibre necrosis initially leads to muscle stem cell activity and tissue regeneration, via activation of so-called satellite cells. As the disease progresses, however, the capacity to regenerate muscle becomes impaired owing to depletion of stem cells and fibrosis of tissues, leading finally to severe muscle wasting. This leads to inflammation of DMD muscles, as a result of inflammatory cells such as CD4 and CD8, followed by muscle necrosis (Blake et al., 2002).

Creatine kinase (CK) level is one of the indicators for DMD pathology. CK level in DMD in affected boys is elevated at birth, to 50 to 100 times the novel level, and gradually declines in the late stages of the disease (Emery, 2001).

2.1.2 Animal models of DMD

The development of a treatment for any disease relies on the use of appropriate animal models to test the efficacy, deliverability, dosing regimen and toxicology *in vivo* having established the therapeutic potential *in vitro*.

2.1.2.1 Dystrophin deficient *mdx* model

The *mdx* mouse originates from the C57BL/10 colony and does not express the dystrophin protein due to a nonsense mutation (CAA to TAA) in exon 23 of the dystrophin gene (Sicinski et al., 1989). It shows similar pathological symptoms to human DMD patients. However the pathology of *mdx* mice is less severe compared to the human disease, because of effective regeneration of damaged muscles, which has not been observed in human DMD patients (Turk et al., 2005). In *mdx* mice, the event of degeneration/regeneration is ongoing throughout the life of the animal but peaks between the ages of 3-8 weeks (Tanabe et al., 1986). It has been demonstrated that the *mdx* mouse has a reduced life span and progressive dystrophic muscle histopathology compared to the wild-type C57BL/10 mouse (Chamberlain et al., 2007). Moreover, aged *mdx* mice are susceptible to muscle tumours, similar to human alveolar rhabdomyosarcoma (Chamberlain et al., 2007). Inflammatory cells such as CD4 and CD8 are found in dystrophin-deficient muscles followed by muscle necrosis, peaking at 4-8 weeks old of *mdx* mice (Blake et al., 2002). In dystrophic *mdx* mice, elevated CK level was also found in the serum (Bulfield et al., 1984).

2.1.2.2 Canine muscular dystrophy model

The golden retriever muscular dystrophy (*GRMD*) dog was the first characterized canine model of DMD (Cooper et al., 1988, Kornegay et al., 1988, Valentine et al., 1992). It has been reported that *GRMD* dogs eventually die due to cardiomyopathy. *GRMD* has been identified as complete dystrophin deficiency with higher genotypic/phenotypic similarity to human DMD disease than that of the *mdx* mouse model. Complete loss of dystrophin is the result of a nonsense mutation in the 3' consensus splice site of intron 6, leading to skipping of exon 7 and alteration of the reading frame in exon 8, thereby inducing clinical symptoms similar to human DMD (Chamberlain et al., 2007). The Beagle-based *CXMD* canine model was also identified as a DMD model in Japan (Shimatsu et al., 2003). It has been reported that limb muscle abnormality appear after 2 months of age and the dogs eventually die mainly due to cardiomyopathy (Valentine et al., 1988). *CXMD* dog models show longer life span due to slower progression of muscle wasting compared to *GRMD* dogs (Willmann et al., 2009). Progress of cardiomyopathy in the *CXMD* dog is also milder than in *GRMD* (Yugeta et al., 2006).

2.1.2.3 Hypertrophic Feline muscular dystrophy model

Hypertrophic feline muscular dystrophy (*HFMD*) is exhibited in cats (Blake et al., 2002). The creatine kinase (CK) level is increased at the age of 4-5 weeks and development of severe muscle hypertrophy is shown resulting in muscle necrosis and regeneration. However, it is not considered to be a good model for human DMD since it does not induce muscle fibrosis and muscle wasting (Gaschen et al., 1992).

2.2 Other muscular dystrophies

2.2.1 Muscular disorders caused by mutations in membrane proteins

Mutations in integrin have been shown to cause congenital muscular dystrophies. Integrin, membrane protein, binds to laminin. Caveloin-3, which is localised to muscle cell membrane interacts with β-dystroglycan and mutations in Caveloin-3 cause the autosomal dominant form of Limb Girdle muscular dystrophy 1C (LGMD1C), rippling muscle disease and hyper CKemia (Betz et al., 2001, Carbone et al., 2000).

2.2.2 Muscular disorders caused by mutations in extracellular matrix proteins

Mutations in laminin α-2, one of the extracellular matrix proteins, can give rise to congenital muscular dystrophy 1A (MDC1A) (Helbling-Leclerc et al., 1995). α and β form of dystroglycan can interact with laminin and dystrophin, respectively. Mutations in α-dystroglycan have been reported in the muscle-eye-brain disease, Walker-Warburg syndrome (WWS) and a type of congenital MD (Longman et al., 2003). In mice, mutations in the dystroglycan gene can be embryonically lethal (Williamson et al., 1997). Disruption to the transmembrane related sarcoglycan-sarcospan complex leads to various types of LGMD. Sarcoglycan interacts with biglycan, which also binds to α-dystroglycan and as well as to collagen VI. Mutation in collagen VI gives rise to Ullrich syndrome and Bethlem myopathy (Camacho Vanegas et al., 2001).

2.2.3 Muscular disorders caused by mutations in intracellular proteins

Mutation in calpain 3, which is a calcium-dependent protease, gives rise to LGMD 2A. Mutations in several sarcomeric proteins lead to LGMD 2. Heterogeneous chromosomal mutations result in LGMD. There are two types of LGMD called type 1 and type 2, which have autosomal dominant or autosomal recessive mutations, respectively. The symptoms are not as severe as DMD or BMD, but weakness of proximal limb and trunk muscles is exhibited (Lovering et al., 2005). Mutations in syntrophin and dystrobrevin display mild forms of skeletal and cardiac muscle disease.

2.2.4 Muscular disorders caused by mutations in nuclear proteins

Laminopathies are caused by mutations in the LMNA gene, which encodes the inner nuclear envelope proteins lamin A and C, which interact with several proteins in the nucleus and inner nuclear membrane (Worman et al., 2000). Emery-Dreifuss muscular dystrophy (EDMD) has been identified due to a mutation in LMNA gene encoding A-type lamin, or in emerin gene encoding nuclear protein (Bione et al., 1994). Clinical symptoms are related to humero-peroneal weakness and dilated cardiomyopathy with conduction defects (Emery, 2000). Mutations in LMNA gene cause cardiomyocyte nuclear envelope abnormalities, leading to dilated cardiomyopathy in human patients (Gupta et al., 2010) and LGMD 1B (Muchir et al., 2000).

3. Pre-clinical & clinical approaches for DMD

Several pre-clinical research regimes have displayed that DMD pathology can be improved by functional expression of mini-or micro-dystrophin gene variants (Deconinck et al., 1996).

3.1 Recombinant adeno-associated virus vector (rAAV) mediated gene therapy

Gene therapy for DMD aims to compensate for dystrophin loss-of-function by different gene transfer approaches. To prevent muscle degeneration, around 30% of normal levels of dystrophin protein is likely to be required (Neri et al., 2007). Transfer of recombinant genes encoding full-length (~11 kb), mini- (>5 kb) or micro- (<5 kb) dystrophin recombinant gene into DMD-affected muscle is one of the proposed therapies to induce dystrophin protein expression. A Phase I clinical trial has been completed in which a eukaryotic expression plasmid encoding full length human dystrophin was injected directly into the muscles of DMD patients (Fardeau et al., 2005).

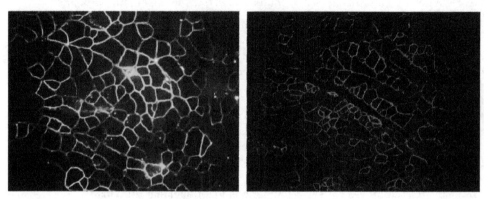

The mdx mice treated with AAV-mediated microdystrophin gene transfer (left-hand panel), or PMO antisense-induced skipping of the mutant exon 23 (right-hand panel) showed dystrophin expression at the sarcolemma in the TA muscle of mdx mouse.

Fig. 2. Dystrophin immunofluorescence staining of muscle.

Dystrophin expression at low levels was shown in all patients without any safety concerns and notably without a detectable immune response to dystrophin. A Phase I/II study is currently in preparation to evaluate this non-viral plasmid-mediated gene therapy using vascular systemic routes of administration to target multiple muscle groups. However, even with the aid of more sophisticated delivery strategies such as electrotransfer or even with enhanced vector configurations such as minicircles and episomes, effective plasmid gene therapy for DMD still has major hurdles to overcome to reach the gene-transfer efficiencies required for effectiveness. Therefore a range of replication-defective viral vectors have been evaluated as attractive delivery systems to mediated dystrophin gene transfer and DMD gene therapy.

In particular, gene transfer into the nuclei of muscle fibres using vectors based on adeno-associated virus (AAV) is one of the most promising delivery approaches for the therapy of muscle disease. AAV is a single-stranded non-pathogenic virus, and derived vectors of various serotypes can efficiently transduce, not only by local muscle injection, but also, notably, by vascular systemic delivery to widespread muscle groups and the heart. The tropism of various AAV vector serotypes for differentiated post-mitotic muscle tissues can be very high, reaching >90%.

However, there is a hurdle to AAV-mediated DMD gene therapy, since the full dystrophin coding sequence spans 14 kb mRNA with an open reading frame of >11 kb, and the packaging capacity of AAV virus vectors is generally thought to be <5 kb. Thus, on the basis of an understanding of the genotype-phenotype correlates in DMD and BMD, and based on structural knowledge of the dystrophin protein, recombinant dystrophin cDNAs have been engineered to produce, partially deleted, but highly functional microdystrophin products in both *mdx* mouse and *CXMD* dog models (Athanasopoulos et al., 2004, Foster et al., 2008, Koo et al., 2011). These genes can be packaged successfully inside AAV vector particles and can be delivered at high efficiency to skeletal muscles to rescue the dystrophin-deficient phenotype in animal models of DMD (**Figure** 2, left hand panel).

The life cycle of AAV vectors results in delayed expression, and it takes several weeks for full transcriptional activity to be established (Ferrari et al., 1996). Recently, self-complementary AAV (scAAV) vectors have been developed for fast expression by bypassing rate-limiting, second-strand DNA synthesis (McCarty 2008). However, scAAV can only retain smaller transgene cassettes compared to single stranded AAV (ssAAV). Moreover, high titres of rAAV are required for systemic delivery (Gregorevic et al., 2004).

AAV-mediated gene therapy has attractive characteristics and some advantages over other vector systems for several reasons. AAV vector particles are very stable and resistant to significant variation in pH and temperature. AAV vectors have an ability of long-term transgene expression without significant immune response. Therefore, it is a promising delivery vehicle for the transfer of therapeutic genes for the treatment of inherited diseases. Recombinant AAV-mediated gene therapy has been approved for use in over 40 clinical trials for various genetic diseases (Mueller at al., 2008). In order to generate recombinant AAV vector for the transfer of therapeutic genes, the genes for the capsid proteins and replication proteins are replaced with the gene of interest and packaged by ITRs. A Phase I clinical trial involving local intramuscular injection of AAV vectors to transfer a microdystrophin variant in DMD patients has been conducted by the groups of Mendel, Xiao and Samulski, in collaboration with Asklepios Biopharmaceuticals. However, microdystrophin expression was only detected in two of six patients treated at very low levels and two patients exhibited pre-existing dystrophin specific T cells (Mendell et al., 2010). Further work to enhance the expression and functionality of microdystrophins is still required due to reported failure of certain microdystrophin variants to protect muscle integrity in larger animal models (Sampaolesi et al., 2006).

3.2 Adenovirus-mediated gene therapy

Adenovirus is another vehicle which can be used to transfer dystrophin genes towards DMD mediated gene delivery applications. Due to the large gene capacity of the adenoviruses, large cDNA cassettes, up to 7 kb for E1/E3 deleted Ad vectors, can be transferred into the muscles. However, adenovirus is highly immunogenic and this may cause loss of transgene expression through immune responses. Moreover, the packaging capacity is still too small for the transfer of full length dystrophin (approximately 11 kb cDNA). To increase the packaging capacity of the viruses, helper dependent adenovirus vectors have been developed (Fisher et al., 1996). These vectors contain only ITR and capsid genes and so increase the packaging genome capacity of adenoviruses up to 36 kb; they are also less immunogenic compared to E1 gene-deleted adenovirus due to the lack of viral genes. Adenovirus-mediated full length dystrophin cDNAs have been successfully transferred to *mdx* mice leading to muscle improvement (Dudley et al., 2004). Cell transplantation of genetically corrected mesenchymal cells (MSCs) by adenovirus carrying microdystrophin gene was attempted and showed successful dystrophin expression in MSCs in *mdx* mice (Xiong et al., 2007).

3.3 Modulation of exon-splicing patterns with antisense oligonucleotides

About 70% of DMD and BMD cases are caused by genomic deletions, leading to the loss of one or more exons (Aartsma-Rus et al., 2006). Frameshift deletions, which juxtapose out-of-phase exons in the dystrophin gene, cause complete loss of expression of dystrophin and a DMD phenotype, whereas juxtaposition of in-phase exons leads to the milder BMD. Inhibition of the splicing of specific exons, by so called exon skipping, using antisense oligonucleotides (AONs) can induce exclusion of targeted exons and skipping of frame-shift exons, leading to restoration of disrupted reading frames and expression of BMD-type dystrophin molecules (**Figure** 2, right hand panel). AONs are designed to hybridize to consensus exon recognition or exonic splicing enhancer (ESE) sequences on dystrophin pre-mRNA, and antisense-induced exon skipping is thought to occur by interfering with binding of serine/arginine-rich (SR) proteins which play crucial roles in recruiting the splicing machinery (**Figure** 3).

AON-induced exon skipping to restore functional but truncated dystrophin protein expression has previously been demonstrated in animal models of DMD both *in vitro* (Graham et al., 2004) and *in vivo* (Yokota et al., 2009), and in DMD patient cells *in vitro* in culture (van Deutekom et al., 2001), and in DMD muscle explants (Arechavala-Gomeza et al., 2007). On the basis of these pre-clinical studies, a number of patient trials, phase I and more recently phase 2, have been undertaken. In the first of these, four DMD patients carrying appropriate deletions received a single intramuscular injection of a high dose of an AON with a 2'O-methylphosphorothioate backbone (PRO051), which targets exon 51. Each patient showed specific exon 51 skipping, myofibre expression of dystrophin protein, which was detectable at 3 to 12% of normal levels four weeks after injection. No clinically adverse events were detected (van Deutekom et al., 2007). In the second trial, the AON AVI-4658, which has a phosphorodiamidate morpholino (PMO) backbone and targets a slightly different intraexonic sequence (+68+95) of exon 51, has been injected intramuscularly in a dose-escalating trial into nine DMD boys. At the higher doses, this PMO AON produced good levels of local dystrophin protein production in treated muscles; the intensity of dystrophin staining was up to 42% of that seen in healthy muscle. The treatment had no adverse effects (Kinali et al., 2009). The clinical evaluation has been extended to 12 week systemic delivery of both exon 51 AONs and results have very recently been reported. Both chemistries showed no adverse effects and dose-dependent restoration of dystrophin production was clearly seen; functionality of this expressed dystrophin protein was established by the detection of other dystrophin-associated proteins at the sarcolemma (for AVI-4658), and by a modest but not statistically significant improvement in the patient six minute walk test after 12 weeks of extended treatment (for PRO051) (Goemans et al., 2011). On the basis of results seen in the mdx model using various dosing regimen over extended periods (Malerba et al., 2011), further clinical studies are required.

PMOs and 2'OMe AONs both have excellent safety profiles (van Deutekom et al., 2007), but PMOs have certain advantages over 2'OMe AONs. They give more sustained, consistent exon skipping in the animal mdx model in vivo (Heemskerk et al., 2009), and in human muscle explants (Arechavala-Gomeza et al., 2007). PMOs can be conjugated to cell-penetrating peptides (PPMO) that improve their deliverability and hence efficacy dramatically (Moulton et al., 2007, Yin et al., 2010).

The drug company AVI BioPharma has performed preclinical studies with AVI-5038 in collaboration with the charity Charley's fund. AVI-5038 is a PPMO targeted to skip exon 50 of the dystrophin gene. Repeated weekly intravenous bolus injection over four weeks at a low dose of this conjugated PMO was shown to be well-tolerated; however higher doses administered weekly for 12 weeks showed significant toxicological effects, particularly in relation to the kidney. As yet this problem has not been resolved, and an unconjugated version of the same PMO (AVI-4038) is being developed for clinical trial. There are a number of alternative peptide conjugates that show promise as enhancers of deliverability and are undergoing rapid pre-clinical development (Yin et al., 2010). The next planned UK phase I trial by the MDEX consortium will involve conjugation of a PPMO developed for the targeted skipping of exon 53 (Popplewell et al., 2010) and is supported by a Wellcome Trust. The Dutch are currently performing a phase I trial using a 2'OMe PS AON for the targeted skipping of exon 45. However, it should be noted that only 8%, 4%, 13% or 18% of DMD patient mutations should be convertible into a BMD phenotype by a single AON exon 45, 50, 51 or 53 skipping, respectively. Personalized molecular medicine for each skippable DMD deletion is necessary and this would require the optimization and clinical trial workup of many specific AONs. It has been suggested that multi-exon skipping, using cocktails of AONs or chemically linked AONs, around deletion hotspots (eg exons 45-55) may have the potential to treat approximately 65% of DMD patients (Adams et al., 2007). Such a strategy has been shown to work in mdx mice, but this has not yet been achieved in DMD patient cells.

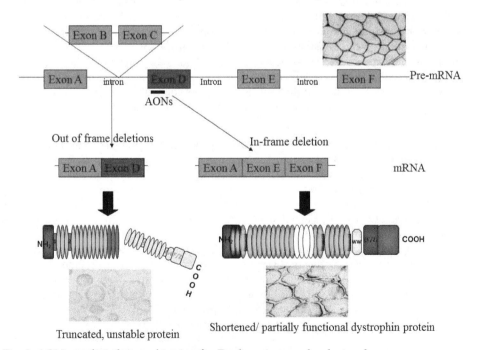

Fig. 3. AONs mediated exon skipping for Duchenne muscular dystrophy.

This gene therapy restores the open reading frame of the disrupted reading frame to allow synthesis of shortened dystrophin. The in-frame transcript contains both the N- and C-terminal domains of dystrophin and is partially functional since these domains have important signalling functions between the extracellular matrix and cytoskeleton. The in-frame transcript of dystrophin produced by AONs exon skipping ameliorates the severe muscle damage seen in *mdx* mice.

There are further obstacles to be overcome for AON-induced exon skipping to be a viable gene therapy for DMD. The cost implications may end up being prohibitive for many patients; since AONs are rapidly cleared from the circulation, regular administrations of high doses of AON would be required for therapeutic effect. Secondly, although deliverability, particularly to the heart, is enhanced with the use of conjugated PMOs, their potential toxicological and immunogenic problems need to be addressed. Lastly, the need for personalized medicine will require the completion of many expensive, lengthy clinical trials of many AONs.

3.4 Cell transplantation therapy

Cell-based gene therapy is another promising approach to treat DMD. Transplantation of genetically modified adult muscle stem cells or healthy wild-type donor cells has great potential to regenerate skeletal muscle cell tissues. For stem cell therapy, adult muscle stem cells, including mesoangioblasts, MDSCs (muscle derived stem cells), adult progenitor cells, AC133+ cells, bone marrow-derived stem cells and side population (SP) cells can be isolated from either muscle biopsies or blood (Farini et al., 2009). Isolated stem cells can be transduced *in vitro* by retroviral or lentiviral vectors to permanently introduce the micro- or mini-dystrophin gene. Retrovirus or lentiviral genome can integrate into the infected cell genome subsequent to cell divisions. Therefore this is a promising vehicle for the correction of muscle satellite stem cells. These genetically modified cells or healthy wild-type donor cells are expanded *ex vivo* and subsequently injected systemically to traffic and target to muscles. If taken from the patient themselves, transplantation of autologous gene-modified stem cells has the advantage to potentially avoid adverse immune responses and cell rejection.

Intramuscular myoblast transplantation in DMD yields dystrophin-positive myofibres at levels of 20-30% up to 18 months after transplantation (Skuk et al., 2007). However, intramuscular myoblasts transfer faces potential limitations in terms of cell migration, lack of systemic whole-body delivery and poor cell survival. There are currently two approaches using a cell transfer platform for systemic delivery of regenerative cell transplants to skeletal musculature, namely the mesoangioblast and the CD133+ stem cell systems. Following lentiviral vector-mediated gene transfer, dystrophin-expressing fibres have been shown in dystrophic dogs after transplantation of genetically modified mesoangioblasts which are vessel-associated progenitor cells. In this study, transplantation efficiency seemed higher in recipients treated with wild-type donor mesoangioblasts compared with autologous gene-modified mesoangioblasts (Sampaolesi et al., 2006), but uncontrolled effects of immune suppression regimes may complicate the interpretation. Even so, a clinical trial of mesoangioblast cells therapy for DMD using tissue –matched wild-type donor cells has been tried (Cossu et al., 2007). CD133+ stem cell therapy is another promising approach introduced recently, making systemic delivery and correction possible. CD133+ cells can be isolated from peripheral blood or skeletal muscle tissue, and differentiated into muscle, hematopoietic and endothelial cell lineages (Peault et al., 2007). A Phase I clinical trial of autologous transplantation of CD133+ stem cells in DMD boys has shown increased potential to contribute to muscle repair without adverse effects (Torrente et al., 2007). However, interaction between satellite cells and stem cells still remains largely unknown to date. Detailed understanding of the biological mechanism of interaction and structure/function relationship between muscle and the multiple components of these therapies can aid the search for an effective cure for DMD and other muscle diseases in the immediate future.

3.5 Muscle augmentation

Neuromuscular disorders, sarcopenia, cancer, AIDS and general insufficient energy intake can decrease the muscle mass with consequent irreversible loss of body weight (Matsakas et al., 2009). Several genetic based strategies have been tried to manipulate expression of specific molecules involved in muscle growth to counteract this muscle loss. One of the most promising approaches is based on the inactivation of the biological activity of myostatin or its receptor, Activin type 2b (ActRIIb). This strategy has a therapeutic potential to treat DMD by inhibiting the severe muscle loss.

3.5.1 Inactivation of Myostatin

Myostatin (named also GDF-8) is a member of transforming growth factor β superfamily of growth factors. Myostatin is initially synthesized as inactive pre-propeptide and it is cleaved to produce a smaller peptide (Thies et al., 2001, Hill et al., 2002) that is biologically active only after further post-translational processing including the formation of a homodimeric protein. Some animals carrying different types of mutations that inactive the functionality of myostatin, present a significant increase in muscle mass (Tobin et al., 2005). In myostatin mutant mice, individual muscles weigh twice as much compared to wild type mice (McPherron et al., 1997) due to hyperplasia and hypertrophy. Other identified mutations of myostatin gene have led to new breeds of cattle (e.g. Belgian blue or Piedmontese (McPherron et al., 1997) and dogs (Mosher et al., 2007). These findings have made myostatin the first target of a genetic approach to silence the gene expression and induce increase in muscle mass as therapeutic treatment for muscle wasting diseases. Indeed, even if the biodistribution of myostatin has not been conclusively clarified, the fact that skeletal muscle is the tissue with the highest expression of myostatin (Sharma et al., 1999, McPherron et al., 1997) means this protein is an appealing target for muscle augmentation strategies. Several strategies aiming to knock down myostatin to induce muscle mass augmentation have been preclinically tested: adeno-associated viral vectors have been used to deliver myostatin propeptide and so inactivate the growth factor by making it unavailable for binding its receptor (Foster et al., 2009; Matsakas et al., 2009). Follistatin-related gene (FLRG) and growth and differentiation factor association protein (GASP-1) are both able to bind to the homodimeric protein myostatin and inhibit its functionality even if the effect is less pronunciated compared to the use of a pro-peptide coded by viral vectors (Thies et al., 2001, Hill et al., 2002). Other strategies to inactivate myostatin are the use of antibodies raised against this growth factor in order to make it unavailable to the receptor. The antibodies JA16 or MYO-029 have been preclinically tested with the latter being also used for a clinical trial in humans where it demonstrated good tolerability and safety (Hill et al., 2002). A recent strategy to knock down myostatin is based on the use of antisense oligonucleotides to bind the pre-mRNA, skip the second exon of myostatin and induce the formation of an out of frame transcript unable of being translated in a functional protein (Kang et al., 2011). The systemic administration of antisense oligonucleotide in mouse showed encouraging results even if the effect was less pronunciated compared to the overexpression of pro-peptide or the myostatin specific antibody administration.

3.5.2 Inactivation of Activin receptor IIb

A second target used to significantly decrease the biological effect of myostatin is to inactivate its binding to the receptor, activin receptor IIb (ActRIIb). The overexpression of myostatin antagonist follistatin, which binds ActRIIb sterically, prevents the binding of myostatin (Rodino-Klapac et al., 2009) and induces an increase in muscle mass. Another study explored the possibility of inhibiting myostatin by using RNAi against ActRIIb and restore quasi dystrophin by AAV-U7 mediated exon skipping in a mouse model of muscular dystrophy (Dumonceaux et al., 2010). Recently in the same animal model the use of soluble ligands of ActRIIb as peptides, including the extracellular portion of the ActRIIb fused to the Fc portion of murine IgG (sActRIIb), has been shown to improve skeletal muscle mass and functional strength (Pistilli et al., 2011).

3.6 Drug-induced read-through of nonsense mutations

Although most DMD cases are caused by large intragenic deletions, 10-15% of DMD mutations are nonsense point mutations which cause premature termination codons (PTCs) in the dystrophin mRNA. PTC 124 is a drug designed to induce translational read through of PTCs, thus inducing expression of dystrophin and reducing nonsense-mediated mRNA decay. Because of the mechanistically structural differences between PTCs and natural stop codons, PTC 124 appears to preferentially recognize mutant nonsense codons without interfering strongly with native termination codons of unrelated genes. PTC 124 has been proven to enhance dystrophin expression in both primary DMD muscle cells and animal models (Welch et al., 2007). A Phase 2b clinical trial in subjects with nonsense-mutation-mediated DMD/BMD has been completed. Unfortunately, PTC 124 did not render any improvement in the six minute walk distance.

4. Conclusion

Preclinical and clinical genetic and cell-based therapy trials are currently progressing rapidly, with the interaction of multiple research units, biotechnology companies and patient groups. Several studies in the clinic are now reporting promising results with restoration of dystrophin expression in local muscle fibres. Future perspectives of the current strategies will be to overcome obstacles in the way of them becoming therapeutic treatments for DMD

5. References

AARTSMA-RUS, A., VAN DEUTEKOM, J.C., FOKKEMA, I.F., VAN OMMEN, G.J. and DEN DUNNEN, J.T. (2006). Entries in the Leiden Duchenne muscular dystrophy mutation database: an overview of mutation types and paradoxical cases that confirm the reading-frame rule. *Muscle & nerve,* 34(2), pp. 135-144.

ACSADI, G., DICKSON, G., LOVE, D.R., JANI, A., WALSH, F.S., GURUSINGHE, A., WOLFF, J.A. and DAVIES, K.E. (1991). Human dystrophin expression in mdx mice after intramuscular injection of DNA constructs. *Nature,* 352(6338), pp. 815-818.

ADAMS, A.M., HARDING, P.L., IVERSEN, P.L., COLEMAN, C., FLETCHER, S. and WILTON, S.D. (2007). Antisense oligonucleotide induced exon skipping and the dystrophin gene transcript: cocktails and chemistries. *BMC molecular biology,* 8, pp. 57.

ALLEN, D.G., WHITEHEAD, N.P. and YEUNG, E.W. (2005). Mechanisms of stretch-induced muscle damage in normal and dystrophic muscle: role of ionic changes. *The Journal of physiology,* 567(Pt 3), pp. 723-735.

ARECHAVALA-GOMEZA, V., GRAHAM, I.R., POPPLEWELL, L.J., ADAMS, A.M., AARTSMA-RUS, A., KINALI, M., MORGAN, J.E., VAN DEUTEKOM, J.C., WILTON, S.D., DICKSON, G. and MUNTONI, F. (2007). Comparative analysis of antisense oligonucleotide sequences for targeted skipping of exon 51 during dystrophin pre-mRNA splicing in human muscle. *Human Gene Therapy,* 18(9), pp. 798-810.

ATHANASOPOULOS, T., GRAHAM, I.R., FOSTER, H. and DICKSON, G. (2004). Recombinant adeno-associated viral (rAAV) vectors as therapeutic tools for Duchenne muscular dystrophy (DMD). *Gene therapy,* 11 Suppl 1, pp. S109-21.

BEGGS, A.H., HOFFMAN, E.P., SNYDER, J.R., ARAHATA, K., SPECHT, L., SHAPIRO, F., ANGELINI, C., SUGITA, H. and KUNKEL, L.M. (1991). Exploring the molecular basis for variability among patients with Becker muscular dystrophy: dystrophin gene and protein studies. *American Journal of Human Genetics,* 49(1), pp. 54-67.

BELL, C.D. and CONEN, P.E. (1968). Histopathological changes in Duchenne muscular dystrophy. *Journal of the neurological sciences,* 7(3), pp. 529-544.

BELLINGER, A.M., REIKEN, S., CARLSON, C., MONGILLO, M., LIU, X., ROTHMAN, L., MATECKI, S., LACAMPAGNE, A. and MARKS, A.R. (2009). Hypernitrosylated ryanodine receptor calcium release channels are leaky in dystrophic muscle. *Nature medicine,* 15(3), pp. 325-330.

BETZ, R.C., SCHOSER, B.G., KASPER, D., RICKER, K., RAMIREZ, A., STEIN, V., TORBERGSEN, T., LEE, Y.A., NOTHEN, M.M., WIENKER, T.F., MALIN, J.P., PROPPING, P., REIS, A., MORTIER, W., JENTSCH, T.J., VORGERD, M. and KUBISCH, C. (2001). Mutations in CAV3 cause mechanical hyperirritability of skeletal muscle in rippling muscle disease. *Nature genetics,* 28(3), pp. 218-219.

BIGGAR, W.D. (2006). Duchenne muscular dystrophy. *Pediatrics in review / American Academy of Pediatrics,* 27(3), pp. 83-88.

BIONE, S., MAESTRINI, E., RIVELLA, S., MANCINI, M., REGIS, S., ROMEO, G. and TONIOLO, D. (1994). Identification of a novel X-linked gene responsible for Emery-Dreifuss muscular dystrophy. *Nature genetics,* 8(4), pp. 323-327.

BLAKE, D.J., WEIR, A., NEWEY, S.E. and DAVIES, K.E. (2002). Function and genetics of dystrophin and dystrophin-related proteins in muscle. *Physiological Reviews,* 82(2), pp. 291-329.

BRADLEY, W.G., HUDGSON, P., LARSON, P.F., PAPAPETROPOULOS, T.A. and JENKISON, M. (1972). Structural changes in the early stages of Duchenne muscular dystrophy. *Journal of neurology, neurosurgery, and psychiatry*, 35(4), pp. 451-455.

BULFIELD, G., SILLER, W.G., WIGHT, P.A. and MOORE, K.J. (1984). X chromosome-linked muscular dystrophy (mdx) in the mouse. *Proceedings of the National Academy of Sciences of the United States of America*, 81(4), pp. 1189-1192.

CAMACHO VANEGAS, O., BERTINI, E., ZHANG, R.Z., PETRINI, S., MINOSSE, C., SABATELLI, P., GIUSTI, B., CHU, M.L. and PEPE, G. (2001). Ullrich scleroatonic muscular dystrophy is caused by recessive mutations in collagen type VI. *Proceedings of the National Academy of Sciences of the United States of America*, 98(13), pp. 7516-7521.

CARBONE, I., BRUNO, C., SOTGIA, F., BADO, M., BRODA, P., MASETTI, E., PANELLA, A., ZARA, F., BRICARELLI, F.D., CORDONE, G., LISANTI, M.P. and MINETTI, C. (2000). Mutation in the CAV3 gene causes partial caveolin-3 deficiency and hyperCKemia. *Neurology*, 54(6), pp. 1373-1376.

CHAMBERLAIN, J.S., METZGER, J., REYES, M., TOWNSEND, D. and FAULKNER, J.A. (2007). Dystrophin-deficient mdx mice display a reduced life span and are susceptible to spontaneous rhabdomyosarcoma. *The FASEB journal : official publication of the Federation of American Societies for Experimental Biology*, 21(9), pp. 2195-2204.

CHAO, D.S., GOROSPE, J.R., BRENMAN, J.E., RAFAEL, J.A., PETERS, M.F., FROEHNER, S.C., HOFFMAN, E.P., CHAMBERLAIN, J.S. and BREDT, D.S. (1996). Selective loss of sarcolemmal nitric oxide synthase in Becker muscular dystrophy. *The Journal of experimental medicine*, 184(2), pp. 609-618.

COOPER, B.J., WINAND, N.J., STEDMAN, H., VALENTINE, B.A., HOFFMAN, E.P., KUNKEL, L.M., SCOTT, M.O., FISCHBECK, K.H., KORNEGAY, J.N. and AVERY, R.J. (1988). The homologue of the Duchenne locus is defective in X-linked muscular dystrophy of dogs. *Nature*, 334(6178), pp. 154-156.

COSSU, G. and SAMPAOLESI, M. (2007). New therapies for Duchenne muscular dystrophy: challenges, prospects and clinical trials. *Trends in molecular medicine*, 13(12), pp. 520-526.

DECONINCK, N., RAGOT, T., MARECHAL, G., PERRICAUDET, M. and GILLIS, J.M. (1996). Functional protection of dystrophic mouse (mdx) muscles after adenovirus-mediated transfer of a dystrophin minigene. *Proceedings of the National Academy of Sciences of the United States of America*, 93(8), pp. 3570-3574.

DUDLEY, R.W., LU, Y., GILBERT, R., MATECKI, S., NALBANTOGLU, J., PETROF, B.J. and KARPATI, G. (2004). Sustained improvement of muscle function one year after full-length dystrophin gene transfer into mdx mice by a gutted helper-dependent adenoviral vector. *Human Gene Therapy*, 15(2), pp. 145-156.

DUMONCEAUX, J., MARIE, S., BELEY, C., TROLLET, C., VIGNAUD, A., FERRY, A., BUTLER-BROWNE, G. and GARCIA, L. (2010). Combination of myostatin pathway interference and dystrophin rescue enhances tetanic and specific force in dystrophic mdx mice. *Molecular therapy : the journal of the American Society of Gene Therapy*, 18(5), pp. 881-887.

EMERY, A.E. (2000). Emery-Dreifuss muscular dystrophy - a 40 year retrospective. *Neuromuscular disorders : NMD*, 10(4-5), pp. 228-232.

EMERY, A.E.H. (2001). *The muscular dystrophies*. Oxford: Oxford University Press.

FARDEAU, M., BRAUN, S., ROMERO, N.B., HOGREL, J.Y., ROUCHE, A., ORTEGA, V., MOUROT, B., SQUIBAN, P., BENVENISTE, O. and HERSON, S. (2005). About a phase I gene therapy clinical trial with a full-length dystrophin gene-plasmid in Duchenne/Becker muscular dystrophy. *Journal de la Societe de biologie*, 199(1), pp. 29-32.

FARINI, A., RAZINI, P., ERRATICO, S., TORRENTE, Y. and MEREGALLI, M. (2009). Cell based therapy for Duchenne muscular dystrophy. *Journal of cellular physiology*, 221(3), pp. 526-534.

FERRARI, F.K., SAMULSKI, T., SHENK, T. and SAMULSKI, R.J. (1996). Second-strand synthesis is a rate-limiting step for efficient transduction by recombinant adeno-associated virus vectors. *Journal of virology*, 70(5), pp. 3227-3234.

FINSTERER, J. and STOLLBERGER, C. (2003). The heart in human dystrophinopathies. *Cardiology*, 99(1), pp. 1-19.

FISHER, K.J., CHOI, H., BURDA, J., CHEN, S.J. and WILSON, J.M. (1996). Recombinant adenovirus deleted of all viral genes for gene therapy of cystic fibrosis. *Virology*, 217(1), pp. 11-22.

FOSTER, H., SHARP, P.S., ATHANASOPOULOS, T., TROLLET, C., GRAHAM, I.R., FOSTER, K., WELLS, D.J. and DICKSON, G. (2008). Codon and mRNA sequence optimization of microdystrophin transgenes improves expression and physiological outcome in dystrophic mdx mice following AAV2/8 gene transfer. *Molecular therapy* 16(11), pp. 1825-1832.

GASCHEN, F.P., HOFFMAN, E.P., GOROSPE, J.R., UHL, E.W., SENIOR, D.F., CARDINET, G.H.,3RD and PEARCE, L.K. (1992). Dystrophin deficiency causes lethal muscle hypertrophy in cats. *Journal of the neurological sciences*, 110(1-2), pp. 149-159.

GILIBERTO, F., FERREIRO, V., DALAMON, V. and SZIJAN, I. (2004). Dystrophin deletions and cognitive impairment in Duchenne/Becker muscular dystrophy. *Neurological research*, 26(1), pp. 83-87.

GOEMANS, N.M., TULINIUS, M., VAN DEN AKKER, J.T., BURM, B.E., EKHART, P.F., HEUVELMANS, N., HOLLING, T., JANSON, A.A., PLATENBURG, G.J., SIPKENS, J.A., SITSEN, J.M., AARTSMA-RUS, A., VAN OMMEN, G.J., BUYSE, G., DARIN, N., VERSCHUUREN, J.J., CAMPION, G.V., DE KIMPE, S.J. and VAN DEUTEKOM, J.C. (2011). Systemic administration of PRO051 in Duchenne's muscular dystrophy. *The New England journal of medicine*, 364(16), pp. 1513-1522.

GRAHAM, I.R., HILL, V.J., MANOHARAN, M., INAMATI, G.B. and DICKSON, G. (2004). Towards a therapeutic inhibition of dystrophin exon 23 splicing in mdx mouse muscle induced by antisense oligoribonucleotides (splicomers): target sequence optimisation using oligonucleotide arrays. *The journal of gene medicine*, 6(10), pp. 1149-1158.

GREGOREVIC, P., BLANKINSHIP, M.J., ALLEN, J.M., CRAWFORD, R.W., MEUSE, L., MILLER, D.G., RUSSELL, D.W. and CHAMBERLAIN, J.S. (2004). Systemic delivery of genes to striated muscles using adeno-associated viral vectors. *Nature medicine*, 10(8), pp. 828-834.

GUPTA, P., BILINSKA, Z.T., SYLVIUS, N., BOUDREAU, E., VEINOT, J.P., LABIB, S., BOLONGO, P.M., HAMZA, A., JACKSON, T., PLOSKI, R., WALSKI, M., GRZYBOWSKI, J., WALCZAK, E., RELIGA, G., FIDZIANSKA, A. and TESSON, F.

(2010). Genetic and ultrastructural studies in dilated cardiomyopathy patients: a large deletion in the lamin A/C gene is associated with cardiomyocyte nuclear envelope disruption. *Basic research in cardiology*, 105(3), pp. 365-377.

HEEMSKERK, H.A., DE WINTER, C.L., DE KIMPE, S.J., VAN KUIK-ROMEIJN, P., HEUVELMANS, N., PLATENBURG, G.J., VAN OMMEN, G.J., VAN DEUTEKOM, J.C. and AARTSMA-RUS, A. (2009). In vivo comparison of 2'-O-methyl phosphorothioate and morpholino antisense oligonucleotides for Duchenne muscular dystrophy exon skipping. *The journal of gene medicine*, 11(3), pp. 257-266.

HELBLING-LECLERC, A., ZHANG, X., TOPALOGLU, H., CRUAUD, C., TESSON, F., WEISSENBACH, J., TOME, F.M., SCHWARTZ, K., FARDEAU, M. and TRYGGVASON, K. (1995). Mutations in the laminin alpha 2-chain gene (LAMA2) cause merosin-deficient congenital muscular dystrophy. *Nature genetics*, 11(2), pp. 216-218.

HILL, J.J., DAVIES, M.V., PEARSON, A.A., WANG, J.H., HEWICK, R.M., WOLFMAN, N.M. and QIU, Y. (2002). The myostatin propeptide and the follistatin-related gene are inhibitory binding proteins of myostatin in normal serum. *The Journal of biological chemistry*, 277(43), pp. 40735-40741.

KANG, J.K., MALERBA, A., POPPLEWELL, L., FOSTER, K. and DICKSON, G. (2011). Antisense-induced myostatin exon skipping leads to muscle hypertrophy in mice following octa-guanidine morpholino oligomer treatment. *Molecular therapy* 19(1), pp. 159-164.

KINALI, M., ARECHAVALA-GOMEZA, V., FENG, L., CIRAK, S., HUNT, D., ADKIN, C., GUGLIERI, M., ASHTON, E., ABBS, S., NIHOYANNOPOULOS, P., GARRALDA, M.E., RUTHERFORD, M., MCCULLEY, C., POPPLEWELL, L., GRAHAM, I.R., DICKSON, G., WOOD, M.J., WELLS, D.J., WILTON, S.D., KOLE, R., STRAUB, V., BUSHBY, K., SEWRY, C., MORGAN, J.E. and MUNTONI, F. (2009). Local restoration of dystrophin expression with the morpholino oligomer AVI-4658 in Duchenne muscular dystrophy: a single-blind, placebo-controlled, dose-escalation, proof-of-concept study. *Lancet neurology*, 8(10), pp. 918-928.

KOO, T., MALERBA, A., ATHANASOPOULOS, T., TROLLET, C., BOLDRIN, L., FERRY, A., POPPLEWELL, L., FOSTER, H., FOSTER, K. and DICKSON, G. (2011). Delivery of AAV2/9-microdystrophin genes incorporating helix 1 of the coiled-coil motif in the C-terminal domain of dystrophin improves muscle pathology and restores the level of alpha1-syntrophin and alpha-dystrobrevin in skeletal muscles of mdx mice. *Human Gene Therapy*, 22(11), pp. 1379-1388.

KOO, T., OKADA, T., ATHANASOPOULOS, T., FOSTER, H., TAKEDA, S. and DICKSON, G. (2011). Long-term functional adeno-associated virus-microdystrophin expression in the dystrophic CXMDj dog. *The journal of gene medicine*, 13(9), pp. 497-506.

KORNEGAY, J.N., TULER, S.M., MILLER, D.M. and LEVESQUE, D.C. (1988). Muscular dystrophy in a litter of golden retriever dogs. *Muscle & nerve*, 11(10), pp. 1056-1064.

KUMAMOTO, T., FUJIMOTO, S., ITO, T., HORINOUCHI, H., UEYAMA, H. and TSUDA, T. (2000). Proteasome expression in the skeletal muscles of patients with muscular dystrophy. *Acta Neuropathologica*, 100(6), pp. 595-602.

LONGMAN, C., BROCKINGTON, M., TORELLI, S., JIMENEZ-MALLEBRERA, C., KENNEDY, C., KHALIL, N., FENG, L., SARAN, R.K., VOIT, T., MERLINI, L.,

SEWRY, C.A., BROWN, S.C. and MUNTONI, F. (2003). Mutations in the human LARGE gene cause MDC1D, a novel form of congenital muscular dystrophy with severe mental retardation and abnormal glycosylation of alpha-dystroglycan. *Human molecular genetics*, 12(21), pp. 2853-2861.

LOVERING, R.M., PORTER, N.C. and BLOCH, R.J. (2005). The muscular dystrophies: from genes to therapies. *Physical Therapy*, 85(12), pp. 1372-1388.

MALERBA, A., SHARP, P.S., GRAHAM, I.R., ARECHAVALA-GOMEZA, V., FOSTER, K., MUNTONI, F., WELLS, D.J. and DICKSON, G. (2011). Chronic systemic therapy with low-dose morpholino oligomers ameliorates the pathology and normalizes locomotor behavior in mdx mice. *Molecular therapy : the journal of the American Society of Gene Therapy*, 19(2), pp. 345-354.

MATSAKAS, A., FOSTER, K., OTTO, A., MACHARIA, R., ELASHRY, M.I., FEIST, S., GRAHAM, I., FOSTER, H., YAWORSKY, P., WALSH, F., DICKSON, G. and PATEL, K. (2009). Molecular, cellular and physiological investigation of myostatin propeptide-mediated muscle growth in adult mice. *Neuromuscular disorders : NMD*, 19(7), pp. 489-499.

MCCARTY, D.M. (2008). Self-complementary AAV vectors; advances and applications. *Molecular therapy : the journal of the American Society of Gene Therapy*, 16(10), pp. 1648-1656.

MCPHERRON, A.C., LAWLER, A.M. and LEE, S.J. (1997). Regulation of skeletal muscle mass in mice by a new TGF-beta superfamily member. *Nature*, 387(6628), pp. 83-90.

MCPHERRON, A.C. and LEE, S.J. (1997). Double muscling in cattle due to mutations in the myostatin gene. *Proceedings of the National Academy of Sciences of the United States of America*, 94(23), pp. 12457-12461.

MENDELL, J.R., CAMPBELL, K., RODINO-KLAPAC, L., SAHENK, Z., SHILLING, C., LEWIS, S., BOWLES, D., GRAY, S., LI, C., GALLOWAY, G., MALIK, V., COLEY, B., CLARK, K.R., LI, J., XIAO, X., SAMULSKI, J., MCPHEE, S.W., SAMULSKI, R.J. and WALKER, C.M. (2010). Dystrophin immunity in Duchenne's muscular dystrophy. *The New England journal of medicine*, 363(15), pp. 1429-1437.

MOSHER, D.S., QUIGNON, P., BUSTAMANTE, C.D., SUTTER, N.B., MELLERSH, C.S., PARKER, H.G. and OSTRANDER, E.A. (2007). A mutation in the myostatin gene increases muscle mass and enhances racing performance in heterozygote dogs. *PLoS genetics*, 3(5), pp. e79.

MOULTON, H.M., FLETCHER, S., NEUMAN, B.W., MCCLOREY, G., STEIN, D.A., ABES, S., WILTON, S.D., BUCHMEIER, M.J., LEBLEU, B. and IVERSEN, P.L. (2007). Cell-penetrating peptide-morpholino conjugates alter pre-mRNA splicing of DMD (Duchenne muscular dystrophy) and inhibit murine coronavirus replication in vivo. *Biochemical Society transactions*, 35(Pt 4), pp. 826-828.

MUCHIR, A., BONNE, G., VAN DER KOOI, A.J., VAN MEEGEN, M., BAAS, F., BOLHUIS, P.A., DE VISSER, M. and SCHWARTZ, K. (2000). Identification of mutations in the gene encoding lamins A/C in autosomal dominant limb girdle muscular dystrophy with atrioventricular conduction disturbances (LGMD1B). *Human molecular genetics*, 9(9), pp. 1453-1459.

MUELLER, C. and FLOTTE, T.R. (2008). Clinical gene therapy using recombinant adeno-associated virus vectors. *Gene therapy*, 15(11), pp. 858-863.

NERI, M., TORELLI, S., BROWN, S., UGO, I., SABATELLI, P., MERLINI, L., SPITALI, P., RIMESSI, P., GUALANDI, F., SEWRY, C., FERLINI, A. and MUNTONI, F. (2007). Dystrophin levels as low as 30% are sufficient to avoid muscular dystrophy in the human. *Neuromuscular disorders : NMD*, 17(11-12), pp. 913-918.

PEAULT, B., RUDNICKI, M., TORRENTE, Y., COSSU, G., TREMBLAY, J.P., PARTRIDGE, T., GUSSONI, E., KUNKEL, L.M. and HUARD, J. (2007). Stem and progenitor cells in skeletal muscle development, maintenance, and therapy. *Molecular therapy : the journal of the American Society of Gene Therapy*, 15(5), pp. 867-877.

PISTILLI, E.E., BOGDANOVICH, S., GONCALVES, M.D., AHIMA, R.S., LACHEY, J., SEEHRA, J. and KHURANA, T. (2011). Targeting the activin type IIB receptor to improve muscle mass and function in the mdx mouse model of Duchenne muscular dystrophy. *The American journal of pathology*, 178(3), pp. 1287-1297.

POPPLEWELL, L.J., ADKIN, C., ARECHAVALA-GOMEZA, V., AARTSMA-RUS, A., DE WINTER, C.L., WILTON, S.D., MORGAN, J.E., MUNTONI, F., GRAHAM, I.R. and DICKSON, G. (2010). Comparative analysis of antisense oligonucleotide sequences targeting exon 53 of the human DMD gene: Implications for future clinical trials. *Neuromuscular disorders : NMD*, 20(2), pp. 102-110.

RODINO-KLAPAC, L.R., HAIDET, A.M., KOTA, J., HANDY, C., KASPAR, B.K. and MENDELL, J.R. (2009). Inhibition of myostatin with emphasis on follistatin as a therapy for muscle disease. *Muscle & nerve*, 39(3), pp. 283-296.

RUEGG, U.T., NICOLAS-METRAL, V., CHALLET, C., BERNARD-HELARY, K., DORCHIES, O.M., WAGNER, S. and BUETLER, T.M. (2002). Pharmacological control of cellular calcium handling in dystrophic skeletal muscle. *Neuromuscular disorders : NMD*, 12 Suppl 1, pp. S155-61.

SAMPAOLESI, M., BLOT, S., D'ANTONA, G., GRANGER, N., TONLORENZI, R., INNOCENZI, A., MOGNOL, P., THIBAUD, J.L., GALVEZ, B.G., BARTHELEMY, I., PERANI, L., MANTERO, S., GUTTINGER, M., PANSARASA, O., RINALDI, C., CUSELLA DE ANGELIS, M.G., TORRENTE, Y., BORDIGNON, C., BOTTINELLI, R. and COSSU, G. (2006). Mesoangioblast stem cells ameliorate muscle function in dystrophic dogs. *Nature*, .

SHARMA, M., KAMBADUR, R., MATTHEWS, K.G., SOMERS, W.G., DEVLIN, G.P., CONAGLEN, J.V., FOWKE, P.J. and BASS, J.J. (1999). Myostatin, a transforming growth factor-beta superfamily member, is expressed in heart muscle and is upregulated in cardiomyocytes after infarct. *Journal of cellular physiology*, 180(1), pp. 1-9.

SHIMATSU, Y., KATAGIRI, K., FURUTA, T., NAKURA, M., TANIOKA, Y., YUASA, K., TOMOHIRO, M., KORNEGAY, J.N., NONAKA, I. and TAKEDA, S. (2003). Canine X-linked muscular dystrophy in Japan (CXMDJ). *Experimental animals / Japanese Association for Laboratory Animal Science*, 52(2), pp. 93-97.

SICINSKI, P., GENG, Y., RYDER-COOK, A.S., BARNARD, E.A., DARLISON, M.G. and BARNARD, P.J. (1989). The molecular basis of muscular dystrophy in the mdx mouse: a point mutation. *Science (New York, N.Y.)*, 244(4912), pp. 1578-1580.

SKUK, D., GOULET, M., ROY, B., PIETTE, V., COTE, C.H., CHAPDELAINE, P., HOGREL, J.Y., PARADIS, M., BOUCHARD, J.P., SYLVAIN, M., LACHANCE, J.G. and TREMBLAY, J.P. (2007). First test of a "high-density injection" protocol for myogenic cell transplantation throughout large volumes of muscles in a Duchenne muscular dystrophy patient: eighteen months follow-up. *Neuromuscular disorders : NMD*, 17(1), pp. 38-46.

TANABE, Y., ESAKI, K. and NOMURA, T. (1986). Skeletal muscle pathology in X chromosome-linked muscular dystrophy (mdx) mouse. *Acta Neuropathologica*, 69(1-2), pp. 91-95.

THIES, R.S., CHEN, T., DAVIES, M.V., TOMKINSON, K.N., PEARSON, A.A., SHAKEY, Q.A. and WOLFMAN, N.M. (2001). GDF-8 propeptide binds to GDF-8 and antagonizes biological activity by inhibiting GDF-8 receptor binding. *Growth factors (Chur, Switzerland)*, 18(4), pp. 251-259.

TOBIN, J.F. and CELESTE, A.J. (2005). Myostatin, a negative regulator of muscle mass: implications for muscle degenerative diseases. *Current opinion in pharmacology*, 5(3), pp. 328-332.

TORRENTE, Y., BELICCHI, M., MARCHESI, C., DANTONA, G., COGIAMANIAN, F., PISATI, F., GAVINA, M., GIORDANO, R., TONLORENZI, R., FAGIOLARI, G., LAMPERTI, C., PORRETTI, L., LOPA, R., SAMPAOLESI, M., VICENTINI, L., GRIMOLDI, N., TIBERIO, F., SONGA, V., BARATTA, P., PRELLE, A., FORZENIGO, L., GUGLIERI, M., PANSARASA, O., RINALDI, C., MOULY, V., BUTLER-BROWNE, G.S., COMI, G.P., BIONDETTI, P., MOGGIO, M., GAINI, S.M., STOCCHETTI, N., PRIORI, A., D'ANGELO, M.G., TURCONI, A., BOTTINELLI, R., COSSU, G., REBULLA, P. and BRESOLIN, N. (2007). Autologous transplantation of muscle-derived CD133+ stem cells in Duchenne muscle patients. *Cell transplantation*, 16(6), pp. 563-577.

TURK, R., STERRENBURG, E., DE MEIJER, E.J., VAN OMMEN, G.J., DEN DUNNEN, J.T. and 'T HOEN, P.A. (2005). Muscle regeneration in dystrophin-deficient mdx mice studied by gene expression profiling. *BMC genomics*, 6, pp. 98.

VALENTINE, B.A., COOPER, B.J., DE LAHUNTA, A., O'QUINN, R. and BLUE, J.T. (1988). Canine X-linked muscular dystrophy. An animal model of Duchenne muscular dystrophy: clinical studies. *Journal of the neurological sciences*, 88(1-3), pp. 69-81.

VALENTINE, B.A., WINAND, N.J., PRADHAN, D., MOISE, N.S., DE LAHUNTA, A., KORNEGAY, J.N. and COOPER, B.J. (1992). Canine X-linked muscular dystrophy as an animal model of Duchenne muscular dystrophy: a review. *American Journal of Medical Genetics*, 42(3), pp. 352-356.

VAN DEUTEKOM, J.C., BREMMER-BOUT, M., JANSON, A.A., GINJAAR, I.B., BAAS, F., DEN DUNNEN, J.T. and VAN OMMEN, G.J. (2001). Antisense-induced exon skipping restores dystrophin expression in DMD patient derived muscle cells. *Human molecular genetics*, 10(15), pp. 1547-1554.

VAN DEUTEKOM, J.C., JANSON, A.A., GINJAAR, I.B., FRANKHUIZEN, W.S., AARTSMA-RUS, A., BREMMER-BOUT, M., DEN DUNNEN, J.T., KOOP, K., VAN DER KOOI, A.J., GOEMANS, N.M., DE KIMPE, S.J., EKHART, P.F., VENNEKER, E.H., PLATENBURG, G.J., VERSCHUUREN, J.J. and VAN OMMEN, G.J. (2007). Local dystrophin restoration with antisense oligonucleotide PRO051. *The New England journal of medicine*, 357(26), pp. 2677-2686.

WELCH, E.M., BARTON, E.R., ZHUO, J., TOMIZAWA, Y., FRIESEN, W.J., TRIFILLIS, P., PAUSHKIN, S., PATEL, M., TROTTA, C.R., HWANG, S., WILDE, R.G., KARP, G., TAKASUGI, J., CHEN, G., JONES, S., REN, H., MOON, Y.C., CORSON, D., TURPOFF, A.A., CAMPBELL, J.A., CONN, M.M., KHAN, A., ALMSTEAD, N.G.,

HEDRICK, J., MOLLIN, A., RISHER, N., WEETALL, M., YEH, S., BRANSTROM, A.A., COLACINO, J.M., BABIAK, J., JU, W.D., HIRAWAT, S., NORTHCUTT, V.J., MILLER, L.L., SPATRICK, P., HE, F., KAWANA, M., FENG, H., JACOBSON, A., PELTZ, S.W. and SWEENEY, H.L. (2007). PTC124 targets genetic disorders caused by nonsense mutations. *Nature,* 447(7140), pp. 87-91.

WHITEHEAD, N.P., YEUNG, E.W. and ALLEN, D.G. (2006). Muscle damage in mdx (dystrophic) mice: role of calcium and reactive oxygen species. *Clinical and experimental pharmacology & physiology,* 33(7), pp. 657-662.

WILLIAMSON, R.A., HENRY, M.D., DANIELS, K.J., HRSTKA, R.F., LEE, J.C., SUNADA, Y., IBRAGHIMOV-BESKROVNAYA, O. and CAMPBELL, K.P. (1997). Dystroglycan is essential for early embryonic development: disruption of Reichert's membrane in Dag1-null mice. *Human molecular genetics,* 6(6), pp. 831-841.

WILLMANN, R., POSSEKEL, S., DUBACH-POWELL, J., MEIER, T. and RUEGG, M.A. (2009). Mammalian animal models for Duchenne muscular dystrophy. *Neuromuscular disorders : NMD,* 19(4), pp. 241-249.

WORMAN, H.J. and COURVALIN, J.C. (2000). The inner nuclear membrane. *The Journal of membrane biology,* 177(1), pp. 1-11.

XIONG, F., ZHANG, C., XIAO, S.B., LI, M.S., WANG, S.H., YU, M.J. and SHANG, Y.C. (2007). Construction of recombinant adenovirus including microdystrophin and expression in the mesenchymal cells of mdx mice. *Sheng wu gong cheng xue bao = Chinese journal of biotechnology,* 23(1), pp. 27-32.

YIN, H., MOULTON, H.M., BETTS, C., MERRITT, T., SEOW, Y., ASHRAF, S., WANG, Q., BOUTILIER, J. and WOOD, M.J. (2010). Functional rescue of dystrophin-deficient mdx mice by a chimeric peptide-PMO. *Molecular therapy : the journal of the American Society of Gene Therapy,* 18(10), pp. 1822-1829.

YOKOTA, T., LU, Q.L., PARTRIDGE, T., KOBAYASHI, M., NAKAMURA, A., TAKEDA, S. and HOFFMAN, E. (2009). Efficacy of systemic morpholino exon-skipping in Duchenne dystrophy dogs. *Annals of Neurology,* 65(6), pp. 667-676.

YUGETA, N., URASAWA, N., FUJII, Y., YOSHIMURA, M., YUASA, K., WADA, M.R., NAKURA, M., SHIMATSU, Y., TOMOHIRO, M., TAKAHASHI, A., MACHIDA, N., WAKAO, Y., NAKAMURA, A. and TAKEDA, S. (2006). Cardiac involvement in Beagle-based canine X-linked muscular dystrophy in Japan (CXMDJ): electrocardiographic, echocardiographic, and morphologic studies. *BMC cardiovascular disorders,* 6, pp. 47.

Section 2

Current Advances and Future Promises

6

From Basic Research to Clinical Trials: Preclinical Trial Evaluation in Mouse Models

Sasha Bogdanovich[1,3] and Emidio E. Pistilli[2]
[1]University of Pennsylvania School of Medicine and Pennsylvania Muscle Institute,
Department of Physiology, Philadelphia, Pennsylvania
[2]West Virginia University School of Medicine,
Division of Exercise Physiology, Morgantown, West Virginia
[3]Current address: University of Kentucky College of Medicine,
Department of Ophthalmology and Visual Sciences, Lexington, Kentucky
USA

1. Introduction

Duchenne Muscular Dystrophy (DMD) is a fatal, X chromosome-inherited disease which affects the whole world population equally and has an incidence of 1 in 3500 boys. The disease is progressive in nature with the first signs of muscle wasting appearing as early as age 3 (Dubowitz 1975; Jennekens et al. 1991). The disease slowly weakens the skeletal muscles of the arms and legs (mostly muscles of shoulder and pelvic girdles) and abdomen. By the early teens, heart and respiratory muscles may also become affected. Nearly all children with DMD lose the ability to walk between the age of 7 and the early teen years, with activities involving the arms, legs or trunk requiring assistance or mechanical support. Patients are typically confined to a wheelchair and they rarely survive the fourth decade of their life. Most DMD patients die due to respiratory or cardiac failure because of the progressive damage to the diaphragm or cardiac myopathy. A milder form of muscular dystrophy, termed Becker Muscular Dystrophy (BMD), has been characterized with a milder clinical presentation (Becker 1955). Children with this variation remain physically active and independent later in life compared to DMD patients. Symptoms begin to appear after 20 years of age and patients live longer compared to DMD patients.

Histologically, muscles from DMD patients are characterized by increased variation in muscle fiber size, necrosis of individual muscle fibers and replacement of necrotic fibers by fibrofatty tissue (Emery 1995; Engel 1994). In addition, an increase in serum Creatine Kinase (CK), derived from degenerating muscle fibers, has been recognized as one of the main diagnostic characteristics of the disease (Engel 1994; Guyton 1995). In 1983, Kay Davies of London, England found linkage between a DNA marker and the DMD gene located on the short arm of the X chromosome (Xp21) (Davies et al. 1983). This discovery finally confirmed the long time theory that DMD inheritance is through the X chromosome and explained Duchenne's notes of affected boys while girls remained without symptoms.

The culmination of DMD research occurred in 1986 when Louis Kunkel of Boston, United States of America (USA) isolated and cloned the gene which caused DMD / BMD (Kunkel et al. 1986). One year later (1987) Eric Hoffman from the same laboratory identified the protein product of the DMD / BMD gene (Hoffman et al. 1987). This protein was called dystrophin. The discovery of the dystrophin gene mutation as the cause of DMD opened the door for diagnostic development and therapeutic strategies for this disease (Bogdanovich et al. 2004).

1.1 Dystrophin

Disease symptoms are progressive and characterized by quantitative and qualitative changes in dystrophin protein (Brown 1997; Khurana et al. 1990). The dystrophin gene is located on the short arm of chromosome Xp21 and is a large gene comprised of 79 exons. With a total size of 3Mb, the gene represents about 0.1% of the entire human genome. The dystrophin protein consists of 3645 amino acids (AA) and has a molecular mass of 426 kDa (Coffey et al. 1992; Monaco et al. 1986). The molecule can be divided into 4 parts: an N-terminal actin binding domain, a central rod, a cysteine rich segment and a C-terminal end (Einbond & Sudol 1996; Koenig et al. 1988; Ponting et al. 1996; Roberts et al. 1996;). Dystrophin forms a link between the extra and intra-cellular cytoskeleton, and it is hypothesized that dystrophin acts to neutralize stressful events that come from outside the cell toward the intracellular matrix, although the full function of dystrophin is still unknown. With a lack of dystrophin protein, the sarcolemma is susceptible to contraction-induced ruptures and permanent cell damage is inevitable (Wrogemann & Pena 1976). Previous experiments have demonstrated an influx of extracellular Ca^{2+} or sarcoplasmatic reticulum leakage due to membrane disruption, which can result in proteolitic activities by Ca^{2+} dependent proteases. This cycle leads to necrosis, inflammatory cell infiltration, and phagocytosis. Additionally, the presence of mast cells can stimulate the release of basic fibroblast growth factor (bFGF) which contributes to fibrotic changes in dystrophic muscle.

The clinical presentation of DMD depends on the nature of the *dystrophin* gene mutation mutation. Nonsense mutations in the *DMD* gene lead to a premature stop codon that blocks dystrophin translation (Hoffman et al. 1987). In the case of a frame shift mutation, there is an exchange of one nucleotide base with another, resulting in the synthesis of shorter or longer dystrophin variants. These mutations result in a milder clinical presentation, namely BMD, where expression of dystrophin protein is present but reduced (Monaco et al. 1988). Dystrophin mutations can be localized in any of its 4 parts and the mutation localization is in direct correlation with the severity of clinical disease presentation. The most severe cases of DMD are described with mutations in the cystein rich component because of its multiple functions (Beggs et al. 1991; Koenig et al. 1989), while mutations in the other 3 parts result in milder clinical presentation.

Disease diagnosis starts with taking a careful history of the disease as well as laboratory testing. The level of CK in the blood is significantly higher in DMD patients, especially at the beginning of the disease, where it can often be 10 times higher compared to normal (Engel 1994). Many advantages are achieved by genetic analysis of DMD mutations. It is possible to discover mutations in the DMD gene using polymerase chain reaction (Flanigan et al. 2003; White et al. 2002). These methods are used routinely in prenatal diagnosis of male fetuses. Typically, DMD patients become wheelchair bound before 13 years of age, while BMD patients can remain physically active after 16 years of age. More invasive methods such as electrodiagnostics and muscle biopsy are used in cases of negative genetic analysis, for the differential diagnosis between DMD and BMD, and especially in autosomal disorders such as Limb-Girdle Muscular Dystrophy, where big differences between clinical presentations and laboratory testing do not exist (Laval & Bushby 2004). In such cases, muscle biopsy samples are used for histopathology and immunohistochemistry examination.

2. Mouse models of DMD

The identification and utilization of animal models in biomedical research is a necessary step in evaluating disease pathology and designing effective therapies for that disease (Table 1). In 1984, a mouse model of DMD was identified and has been termed the *mdx* mouse (*mdx* = muscular disease x-chromosome). The identification of a mouse model for DMD proved to be useful for further understanding of both the normal function of dystrophin and the pathology of the disease (Petrof et al. 1993; Stedman et al. 1991), and the *mdx* mouse currently remains the most widely used mouse model of DMD (Brockdorff et al. 1987; Cavanna et al. 1988). *Mdx* mice have a natural mutation in the dystrophin gene, caused by a point mutation. Compared to human DMD patients, *mdx* mice have a relatively mild disease presentation, characterized by periods of muscle fiber degeneration and regeneration starting approximately 2 weeks after birth although not all muscles are similarly affected. Despite the milder disease phenotype in these mice, the characteristic cycles of muscle fiber degeneration and regeneration provide a variable to evaluate therapies in this mouse model. In addition, biochemical analyses have demonstrated that there is a consistent increase in serum CK in the *mdx* mouse, mirroring an important biomarker in human patients (Bulfield et al. 1984; Moens et al. 1993). Inasmuch as there are recognized limitations of this mouse model, the *mdx* mouse remains a widely used animal in biomedical research.

The *mdx* mouse is very suitable for experiments designed to elucidate function and causality of the disease, as well as for gene and pharmaceutical therapy. It is in fact proving to be useful for furthering our understanding on both the normal function of dystrophin and the pathology of the disease. Experiments using *mdx* mice have provided us with invaluable information regarding the function of the gene product involved in DMD as well as the dystrophin-associated proteins (DAP) and the dystroglycan/sarcoglycan complex (DGC/SGC).

Additional allelic variants of the original *mdx* mouse mutation were created by treating mice with the mutagen, N-ethylnitrosourea (Rafael et al. 2000). This resulted in the formation of 4 new mouse models with specific mutations in the dystrophin gene and relevant increases in circulating CK levels in the blood. These mouse models have been described previously (Chapman et al. 1989; Cox et al. 1993; Im et al. 1996). Briefly, the *mdx*[2cv] mouse has a mutation in intro 42; the *mdx*[3cv] mouse has a mutant splice acceptor site in nintron 65; the *mdx*[4cv] mouse has a "C" to "T" substitution in exon 53; and *mdx*[5cv] has an "A" to "T" transition in exon 10. Due to the different sites of these point mutations, different dystrophin isoforms can be expressed in the form of revertant fibers. It has been proposed that these strains of *mdx* mice may be usefule to elucidate the role of these various dystrophin isoforms, although the original *mdx* variant remains the mouse model most utilized (Banks & Chamberlain 2008).

The mild phenotype of *mdx* mice is a recognized limitation of this mouse model. For example, *mdx* mice maintain cage activity and do not have significant exercise limitations (De Luca et al. 2003). Indeed, forced treadmill exercise has been used as a way to increase the degree of muscle pathology present in these mice (Fraysse et al. 2004). Also, there is only approximately a 20% difference in the lifespan of the *mdx* mouse compared to wild-type, thus limiting the ability to detect a therapy-based improvement on lifespan (Chamberlain et al. 2007). For these reasons, a more severe mouse model was developed that introduced the knockout of the utrophin gene into the *mdx* mouse; thus creating the dystrophin:utrophin double knockout mouse (DKO) (Deconinck et al. 1997, 1998; Grady et al. 1997; Huang et al. 2011). These mice have a severely limited lifespan coupled with severe impairments in muscle function (Chamberlain et al. 2007).

Most commonly used mouse models in muscular dystrophies		
Muscular Dystrophy	**Gene product**	**Mouse model**
Duchenne/Becker MD	Dystrophin	*mdx, mdx²-⁵ᶜᵛ, mdx:utr⁻ᐟ*
Limb-Girdle MD		
Type 1C	Caveolin 3	*cav3⁻ᐟ*
Type 2A	Calpain 3	*capn3⁻ᐟ*
Type 2B (Miyoshi myopathy)	Dysferlin	SJL, A/J
Type 2C	γ-Sarcoglycan	*Sgcg⁻ᐟ*
Type 2D	a-Sarcoglycan (Adhalin)	*sgca⁻ᐟ*
Type 2E	β-Sarcoglycan	*sgcb⁻ᐟ*
Type 2F	δ-Sarcoglycan	*sgcd⁻ᐟ*
Congenital MD (CMD)		*dy, dy²ᴶ, dy³ᵏ, dyʷ, dyᴾᴬˢ*

Table 1. Mouse models in MDs

3. Current progress and evaluation

It has recently been proposed that a set of standard operating procedures be established for evaluating pre-clinical testing data in *mdx* mice (Grounds et al. 2008; Nagaraju & Willmann 2009; Spurney et al. 2009; Willmann et al. 2011). Through the universal adoption of standardized laboratory assays, the results of multiple pre-clinical trials performed in independent laboratories could be evaulated. The laboratory assays that we have employed in designing our new scaling system have been identified as robust tests for evaluating endpoints in the *mdx* mouse (Spurney et al. 2009). Before introducing the new scaling methodology, we will review the results of a number of preclinical trials performed in the *mdx* mouse. The data from these trials will then be utilized in presenting and evaulating the new scaling system, we call the Multiparametric Muscle Improvement Score (MMIS). These preclinical trials use a variety of parameters to establish the beneficial effect of the administered compound, and can be catogorized as either functional, morphological, or biochemical. Functional evaluation was done using a specially designed system to quantify *ex vivo* isometric and eccentric contractions (ECC) in freshly dissected muscle. Morphologic measures were quantified from hematoxylin and eosin (H&E) or immuno-stained muscle sections, and included counting of total muscle fibers, single fiber cross-sectional area, and the percentage of centrally nucleated fibers. Determination of serum creatine kinase and up-regulation of utrophin constituted the biochemical evaluation. Improvement in any of these individual parameters would suggest a therapy-based improvement in the dystrophic phenotype in *mdx* mice. However, some parameters are suggestive of more significant clinical improvement (i.e. greater muscle force, lower serum CK) and are therefore given more weight in our scaling system.

Preclinical trials were performed to determine the extent that small molecule therapies could up-regulate utrophin, and therefore functionally compensate for the loss of dystrophin in the muscles of *mdx* mice. These small moleculaes included heregulin (Krag et al. 2004) and biglycan (Amenta et al. 2011). In general, these utrophin-based up-regulation strategies resulted in very similar benefits in the *mdx* mouse. Parameters that were improved included isometric force following ECC, increased regenerative capacities of *mdx* muscle (i.e. greater number of regenerative fibers), and less necrotic areas in the diaphragm muscle. However, these strategies did not show improvements isometric force producing capacity of limb muscles or the levels of serum creatine kinase. The improvements in the ECC force coupled with the up-regulation of utrophin demonstrate that utrophin can functionally substitute for the loss of dystrophin. However, the incomplete amelioration of the dystrophic phenotype suggests that these therapies have limitations when administered individually.

A number of preclinical studies were performed to analyze the effects of blocking the activity of myostatin, a negative regulator of muscle growth and member of the TGF-β family (McPherron et al. 1997; McPherron & Lee 1997). Strategies included using antibodies directed against myostatin and administration of the myostatin propeptide, to sequester circulating myostatin and neutralize its activity. Administration of these compounds to *mdx* mice resulted in significant improvements in overall body and skeletal muscle mass. Muscle mass increases were greater in response to the myostatin propeptide, and may be due to a higher binding affinity for myostatin compared to the myostatin antibody (Bogdanovich et al. 2002, 2005). In addition, muscle function was improved as evidenced by greater absolute forces in muscles from treated mice in both trials. However, the propeptide-based strategy also resulted in improvements in specific force (i.e. force normalized to muscle cross-sectional area). Both strategies demonstrated improvements in overall muscle histopathology and the levels of serum creatine kinase, suggesting an improvement in the sarcolemma by a utrophin independent mechanism. Collectively, these myostatin blockade strategies were effective in stimulating increases in muscle mass and muscle function, along with measures of muscle histopathology and serum CK. However, complete amelioration of the dystrophic phenotype was not accomplished due to the fact that no improvements were noted in the force loss following eccentric lengthening contractions.

Furthermore, we wanted to determine whether myostatin blockade would be beneficial to additional mouse models of muscular dystrophy. We utilized the myostatin-antibody strategy in gamma sarcoglycan (*Sgcg-/-*) knockout mice, a model of Limb-Girdle 2C muscular dystrophy (LGMD 2C) (Bogdanovich et al. 2008). Interestingly, myostatin antibody blockade did not show desired improvement in this mouse model. Improvement was minimal and evident in body and muscle weight increases. Physiological improvement was notable only in one parameter, absolute force improvement. Histopathological and biochemical parameters were unchaged when compared to control mice. Therefore, unique disease charactersitics of LGMD 2C compared to DMD in mouse models may have led to these differing results and a preferential benefit in the *mdx* mouse.

Recently, we tested the efficacy of a novel myostatin blockade strategy using a soluble form of the activin type IIB receptor (ActRIIB) (Pistilli et al. 2011). The ActRIIB is the receptor for myostain as well as other member of the TGF-β superfamily. The solubilized form of the receptor (sActRIIB) would be able to bind to and sequester multiple TGF-β superfamily members, thereby potentially providing a greater therapeutic effect. In this preclinical trial, two doses of sActRIIB were utilized, a low dose of 1,0 mg/kg bodyweight and a high dose 10,0 mg/kg bodyweight. Notable differences were observed when comparing these two dosing strategies. The high dose of sActRIIB resulted in dramatic increases in body weight and lean muscle mass, while minimal changes in overall body mass were noted in the response to the low dose. Both doses of sActRIIB improved absolute forces produced by limb muscles. However, the low dose significantly improved specific force, indicating an improvement in force producing capacity independent of muscle size. Serum CK levels were also lower in sActRIB treated mice. Unfortunately, force loss follwing eccentric lengthening contractions and muscle histopathology were not significantly improved in these trials. Therefore, as with the myostatin antibody and the myostatin propeptide, complete amelioration of the dystrophic phenotype was not observed with sActRIIB therapy.

The results of these trials demonstrate that small molecule-based therapies have the potential to improve a number of paremeters related to the dystrophic phenotype in *mdx* mice. However, as noted, no therapy has been able to completely ameliorate the phenotype and rescue the *mdx* mouse. Also, evaluating the therapeutic efficacy of drugs identified through preclinical trials is inefficient, due to the large number of preclinical trials published

Multiparametric Muscle Improvement Score -MMIS	
Bogdanovich / Khurana points	
Body weight (g)	1
Muscle weights (mg)	2
Absolute force, twitch (mN)	1
Specific force, twitch (mN/mm^2)	3
Absolute force, tetanus (mN)	4
Specific force, tetanus (mN/mm^2)	5
Eccentric contractions improvement	5
Centrally nucleated fibers	5
Loss of fibrotic changes	3
Decreased CK value	5
Total score	**34**

Total umeric score: 34
01-08 no improvement
09-22 intermediate
23-34 optimal

Table 2. Multiparametric Muscle Improvement Score

in animal models, and the differential methodology used to evaluate the data. Therefore, a scaling system that can evaluate the therapeutic efficacy of independent preclinical trials would be useful to identify those compounds with the most therapeutic promise. The purpose of this research was to formulate a single, objective scoring system to evaluate preclinical trial data arising from multiple laboratories. More detailed and precise quantification of different therapies can be obtained by utilizing the Multiparametric Muscle Improvement Score (MMIS) system (Bogdanovich 2009).

4. Methods

The authors have complied preclinical trial data acquired during the last 10 years, and evaluated the data using the MMIS scoring system (Bogdanovich 2009). This system consists of ten of the most important anatomical, physiological and biochemical elements directly related to improvement of the dystrophic phenotype in mouse models of muscular dystrophy. These include: body and muscle weight changes, muscle force production during isometric and lengthening contractions, evidence of histological improvement, and reductions in circulating creatine kinase (see Table 2). These elements are weighted with one single numerical value from 1 (least important) to 5 (most important). Only statistically significant improvements in measured parameters can be scored. Scoring is done in such a way that every parameter receives maximal value if there is improvement. Scored elements are summarized at the end and the final number is the improvement score.

Comparison of possible therapeutic strategies for muscular dystrophies (before MMIS system)						
Mice	*mdx*	*mdx*	*Sgcg[−/−]*	*mdx*	*mdx*	*mdx*
	Myostatin blockade or inhibition				**Utrophin upregulation**	
	Antibody	Propeptide	Antibody	sActRIIB 1mg/kg 10mg/kg	Heregulin	Biglycan
Treatment	Bogdanovich et al. 2002 (Nature)	Bogdanovich et al. 2005 (FASEB J)	Bogdanovich et al. 2007 (Muscle&Nerve)	Pistilli et al. 2011 (Am. J. Pathol.)	Krag et al. 2004 (PNAS)	Amenta et al. 2010 (PNAS)
Body weight (g)	+	+	+	− +	−	−
Muscle weights (mg)	+	+	+	+	−	−
Absolute force, twitch (mN)	+	+	+	+	−	−
Specific force, twitch (mN/mm²)	−	−	−	+	−	−
Absolute force, tetanus (mN)	+	+	+	+	−	−
Specific force, tetanus (mN/mm²)	−	+	−	+	−	−
Eccentric contractions	−	−	−	−	+	+
Centrally nucleated fibers	+	−	−	−	+	+
Loss of fibrotic changes	+	+	−	−	+	+
Decreased CK value	+	+	−	+	−	−

Legend: *Sgcg[−/−]*, gamma sarcoglycan (LGMD 2C mouse model); −, no improvement; +, positive improvement

Table 3. Evaluation of possible therapeutic stratagies for muscular dystrophy (before MMIS system)

5. Results

The scoring system is objective and excludes human error. It is possible to review and rank therapies based on a final single numeric score using the MMIS scale. With the MMIS scale, we have objectively assessed the therapeutic efficacy of multiple drug therapies in mouse models of muscular dystrophy (*mdx* mouse, *Sgcg-/-* mouse) (Table 3, 4). However, the limitations of these promising methods were identified objectively using the MMIS scale. Despite significant effects on muscle mass and muscle force production, neither strategy completely ameliorated the dystrophic phenotype with regards to eccentric lenghtening contractions or histological improvement as identified using the MMIS scale.

Comparison of possible therapeutic strategies for muscular dystrophies (MMIS system)							
Mice	*mdx*	*mdx*	*Sgcg-/-*	*mdx*		*mdx*	*mdx*
	Myostatin blockade or inhibition					Utrophin upregulation	
	Antibody	Propeptide	Antibody	sActRIIB 1mg/kg 10mg/kg		Heregulin	Biglycan
Treatment	Bogdanovich *et al.* 2002 (Nature)	Bogdanovich *et al.* 2005 (FASEB J)	Bogdanovich *et al.* 2007 (Muscle&Nerve)	Pistilli *et al.* 2011 (Am. J. Pathol.)		Krag *et al.* 2004 (PNAS)	Amenta *et al.* 2010 (PNAS)
Body weight (g)	1	1	1	0	1	0	0
Muscle weights (mg)	2	2	2	2	2	0	0
Absolute force, twitch (mN)	1	1	1	1	1	0	0
Specific force, twitch (mN/mm²)	0	0	0	3	0	0	0
Absolute force, tetanus (mN)	4	4	4	4	4	0	0
Specific force, tetanus (mN/mm²)	0	5	0	5	0	0	0
Eccentric contractions	0	0	0	0	0	5	5
Centrally nucleated fibers	5	0	0	0	0	5	5
Loss of fibrotic changes	3	3	0	0	0	3	3
Decreased CK value	5	5	0	5	5	0	0
Total score	21	21	8	20	13	13	13

Legend: *Sgcg-/-*, gamma sarcoglycan (LGMD 2C mouse model) ; Total numeric score: 34; 01-08 no improvement; 09-22 intermediate; 23-34 optimal

Table 4. Possible therapeutic stratagies for muscular dystrophy (MMIS system)

6. Conclusion

Currently, there is a need for standardization of measurement and objective evaluation of different preclinical studies of the muscular dystrophies, which would allow for a better understanding of the disease and its response to potential therapies. We suggest that the MMIS provides a single numeric value useful for cross-comparing different preclinical studies and prioritizing drug development for muscular dystrophy therapy. We suggest that the use of the MMIS scale will allow for precise and rigorous evaluation of functional improvements of therapeutic interventions performed in preclinical trials.

7. Acknowledgment

We would like to thank to Dr. T. S. Khurana (University of Pennsylvania, USA) for helpful discussion on this topic.

8. References

Amenta, A. R.; Yilmaz, A., et al. (2011). Biglycan recruits utrophin to the sarcolemma and counters dystrophic pathology in mdx mice. *Proc Natl Acad Sci U S A*, Vol.108, No.2, (Jan 11 2011), pp. 762-767, ISSN 1091-6490 (Electronic); 0027-8424 (Linking)

Banks, G. B. & Chamberlain, J. S. (2008). The value of mammalian models for duchenne muscular dystrophy in developing therapeutic strategies. *Curr Top Dev Biol*, Vol.84, 2008), pp. 431-453, ISSN 0070-2153 (Print); 0070-2153 (Linking)

Becker, P. E., Kiener, F (1955). [A new x-chromosomal muscular dystrophy]. *Arch. Psychiatr. Nervenkr Z Gesamte Neurol Psychiatr.*, Vol.193 (n.d.) No.4, pp. 427-448, PMID 13249581

Beggs, A. H.; Hoffman, E. P., et al. (1991). Exploring the molecular basis for variability among patients with Becker muscular dystrophy: dystrophin gene and protein studies. *Am J Hum Genet*, Vol.49, No.1, (Jul 1991), pp. 54-67, ISSN 0002-9297 (Print) 0002-9297 (Linking)

Bogdanovich, S. (2009). *Myostatin blockade for functional improvement of Duchenne's dystrophic phenotype.* Doctoral dissertation. University of Novi Sad Faculty of Medicine. UCK 616.8-009.5-08:612.085, Novi Sad, Serbia.

Bogdanovich, S.; Krag, T. O., et al. (2002). Functional improvement of dystrophic muscle by myostatin blockade. *Nature*, Vol.420, No.6914, (Nov 28 2002), pp. 418-421, ISSN 0028-0836 (Print); 0028-0836 (Linking)

Bogdanovich, S.; McNally, E. M., et al. (2008). Myostatin blockade improves function but not histopathology in a murine model of limb-girdle muscular dystrophy 2C. *Muscle Nerve*, Vol.37, No.3, (Mar 2008), pp. 308-316, ISSN 0148-639X (Print); 0148-639X (Linking)

Bogdanovich, S.; Perkins, K. J., et al. (2004). Therapeutics for Duchenne muscular dystrophy: current approaches and future directions. *J Mol Med (Berl)*, Vol.82, No.2, (Feb 2004), pp. 102-115, ISSN 0946-2716 (Print); 0946-2716 (Linking)

Bogdanovich, S.; Perkins, K. J., et al. (2005). Myostatin propeptide-mediated amelioration of dystrophic pathophysiology. *FASEB J*, Vol.19, No.6, (Apr 2005), pp. 543-549, ISSN 1530-6860 (Electronic); 0892-6638 (Linking)

Brockdorff, N.; Cross, G. S., et al. (1987). The mapping of a cDNA from the human X-linked Duchenne muscular dystrophy gene to the mouse X chromosome. *Nature*, Vol.328, No.6126, (Jul 9-15 1987), pp. 166-168, ISSN 0028-0836 (Print); 0028-0836 (Linking)

Brown, S. C. & Lucy, J. A. (Ed.) (1997) *Dystrophin Gene, Protein and Cell Biology.* Cambridge University Press, ISBN 0-521-55033-5, Cambridge, United Kingdom

Bulfield, G.; Siller, W. G., et al. (1984). X chromosome-linked muscular dystrophy (mdx) in the mouse. *Proc Natl Acad Sci U S A*, Vol.81, No.4, (Feb 1984), pp. 1189-1192, ISSN 0027-8424 (Print); 0027-8424 (Linking)

Cavanna, J. S.; Coulton, G., et al. (1988). Molecular and genetic mapping of the mouse mdx locus. *Genomics*, Vol.3, No.4, (Nov 1988), pp. 337-341, ISSN 0888-7543 (Print); 0888-7543 (Linking)

Chamberlain, J. S.; Metzger, J., et al. (2007). Dystrophin-deficient mdx mice display a reduced life span and are susceptible to spontaneous rhabdomyosarcoma. *FASEB J*, Vol.21, No.9, (Jul 2007), pp. 2195-2204, ISSN 1530-6860 (Electronic); 0892-6638 (Linking)

Chapman, V. M.; Miller, D. R., et al. (1989). Recovery of induced mutations for X chromosome-linked muscular dystrophy in mice. *Proc Natl Acad Sci U S A*, Vol.86, No.4, (Feb 1989), pp. 1292-1296, ISSN 0027-8424 (Print); 0027-8424 (Linking)

Coffey, A. J.; Roberts, R. G., et al. (1992). Construction of a 2.6-Mb contig in yeast artificial chromosomes spanning the human dystrophin gene using an STS-based approach. *Genomics*, Vol.12, No.3, (Mar 1992), pp. 474-484, ISSN 0888-7543 (Print); 0888-7543 (Linking)

Cox, G. A.; Phelps, S. F., et al. (1993). New mdx mutation disrupts expression of muscle and nonmuscle isoforms of dystrophin. *Nat Genet*, Vol.4, No.1, (May 1993), pp. 87-93, ISSN 1061-4036 (Print); 1061-4036 (Linking)

Davies, K. E.; Jackson, J., et al. (1983). Linkage analysis of myotonic dystrophy and sequences on chromosome 19 using a cloned complement 3 gene probe. *J Med Genet*, Vol.20, No.4, (Aug 1983), pp. 259-263, ISSN 0022-2593 (Print); 0022-2593 (Linking)

De Luca, A.; Pierno, S., et al. (2003). Enhanced dystrophic progression in mdx mice by exercise and beneficial effects of taurine and insulin-like growth factor-1. *J Pharmacol Exp Ther*, Vol.304, No.1, (Jan 2003), pp. 453-463, ISSN 0022-3565 (Print); 0022-3565 (Linking)

Deconinck, A. E.; Rafael, J. A., et al. (1997). Utrophin-dystrophin-deficient mice as a model for Duchenne muscular dystrophy. *Cell*, Vol.90, No.4, (Aug 22 1997), pp. 717-727, ISSN 0092-8674 (Print); 0092-8674 (Linking)

Deconinck, N.; Rafael, J. A., et al. (1998). Consequences of the combined deficiency in dystrophin and utrophin on the mechanical properties and myosin composition of some limb and respiratory muscles of the mouse. *Neuromuscul Disord*, Vol.8, No.6, (Aug 1998), pp. 362-370, ISSN 0960-8966 (Print); 0960-8966 (Linking)

Dubowitz, V. (1975). Neuromuscular disorders in childhood. Old dogmas, new concepts. *Arch Dis Child*, Vol.50, No.5, (May 1975), pp. 335-346, ISSN 1468-2044 (Electronic); 0003-9888 (Linking)

Einbond, A. & Sudol, M. (1996). Towards prediction of cognate complexes between the WW domain and proline-rich ligands. *FEBS Lett*, Vol.384, No.1, (Apr 8 1996), pp. 1-8, ISSN 0014-5793 (Print); 0014-5793 (Linking)

Emery, A. H. E., Emery, M.L.H (1995) *The History of a Gentic Disease*. Royal Society of Medicine Press, ISBN 978-0-19-959147-3, London, United Kingdom

Engel, A. G., Franzini-Armstrong, C (2004) *Myology*. McGraw-Hill, ISBN 0-07-137180-X, New York, USA

Flanigan, K. M.; von Niederhausern, A., et al. (2003). Rapid direct sequence analysis of the dystrophin gene. *Am J Hum Genet*, Vol.72, No.4, (Apr 2003), pp. 931-939, ISSN 0002-9297 (Print); 002-9297 (Linking)

Fraysse, B.; Liantonio, A., et al. (2004). The alteration of calcium homeostasis in adult dystrophic mdx muscle fibers is worsened by a chronic exercise in vivo. *Neurobiol Dis*, Vol.17, No.2, (Nov 2004), pp. 144-154, ISSN 0969-9961 (Print); 0969-9961 (Linking)

Grady, R. M.; Teng, H., et al. (1997). Skeletal and cardiac myopathies in mice lacking utrophin and dystrophin: a model for Duchenne muscular dystrophy. *Cell*, Vol.90, No.4, (Aug 22 1997), pp. 729-738, ISSN 0092-8674 (Print); 0092-8674 (Linking)

Grounds, M. D.; Radley, H. G., et al. (2008). Towards developing standard operating procedures for pre-clinical testing in the mdx mouse model of Duchenne muscular dystrophy. *Neurobiol Dis*, Vol.31, No.1, (Jul 2008), pp. 1-19, ISSN 1095-953X (Electronic); 0969-9961 (Linking)

Guyton, A. (2011) *Textbook of Medical Physiology*. Saunders ISBN 978-1-4160-4574-8, New York, USA

Hoffman, E. P.; Brown, R. H., Jr., et al. (1987). Dystrophin: the protein product of the Duchenne muscular dystrophy locus. *Cell*, Vol.51, No.6, (Dec 24 1987), pp. 919-928, ISSN 0092-8674 (Print); 0092-8674 (Linking)

Huang, P.; Cheng, G., et al. (2011). Impaired respiratory function in mdx and mdx/utrn(+/-) mice. *Muscle Nerve*, Vol.43, No.2, (Feb 2011), pp. 263-267, ISSN 1097-4598 (Electronic); 0148-639X (Linking)

Im, W. B.; Phelps, S. F., et al. (1996). Differential expression of dystrophin isoforms in strains of mdx mice with different mutations. *Hum Mol Genet*, Vol.5, No.8, (Aug 1996), pp. 1149-1153, ISSN 0964-6906 (Print); 0964-6906 (Linking)

Jennekens, F. G.; ten Kate, L. P., et al. (1991). Diagnostic criteria for Duchenne and Becker muscular dystrophy and myotonic dystrophy. *Neuromuscul Disord*, Vol.1, No.6, 1991), pp. 389-391, ISSN 0960-8966 (Print); 0960-8966 (Linking)

Khurana, T. S.; Hoffman, E. P., et al. (1990). Identification of a chromosome 6-encoded dystrophin-related protein. *J Biol Chem*, Vol.265, No.28, (Oct 5 1990), pp. 16717-16720, ISSN 0021-9258 (Print); 0021-9258 (Linking)

Koenig, M.; Beggs, A. H., et al. (1989). The molecular basis for Duchenne versus Becker muscular dystrophy: correlation of severity with type of deletion. *Am J Hum Genet*, Vol.45, No.4, (Oct 1989), pp. 498-506, ISSN 0002-9297 (Print); 0002-9297 (Linking)

Koenig, M.; Monaco, A. P., et al. (1988). The complete sequence of dystrophin predicts a rod-shaped cytoskeletal protein. *Cell*, Vol.53, No.2, (Apr 22 1988), pp. 219-228, ISSN 0092-8674 (Print); 0092-8674 (Linking)

Krag, T. O.; Bogdanovich, S., et al. (2004). Heregulin ameliorates the dystrophic phenotype in mdx mice. *Proc Natl Acad Sci U S A*, Vol.101, No.38, (Sep 21 2004), pp. 13856-13860, ISSN 0027-8424 (Print); 0027-8424 (Linking)

Kunkel, L. M.; Monaco, A. P., et al. (1986). Molecular genetics of Duchenne muscular dystrophy. *Cold Spring Harb Symp Quant Biol*, Vol.51 Pt 1, 1986), pp. 349-351, ISSN 0091-7451 (Print); 0091-7451 (Linking)

Laval, S. H. & Bushby, K. M. (2004). Limb-girdle muscular dystrophies--from genetics to molecular pathology. *Neuropathol Appl Neurobiol*, Vol.30, No.2, (Apr 2004), pp. 91-105, ISSN 0305-1846 (Print); 0305-1846 (Linking)

McPherron, A. C.; Lawler, A. M., et al. (1997). Regulation of skeletal muscle mass in mice by a new TGF-beta superfamily member. *Nature*, Vol.387, No.6628, (May 1 1997), pp. 83-90, ISSN 0028-0836 (Print); 0028-0836 (Linking)

McPherron, A. C. & Lee, S. J. (1997). Double muscling in cattle due to mutations in the myostatin gene. *Proc Natl Acad Sci U S A*, Vol.94, No.23, (Nov 11 1997), pp. 12457-12461, ISSN 0027-8424 (Print); 0027-8424 (Linking)

Moens, P.; Baatsen, P. H., et al. (1993). Increased susceptibility of EDL muscles from mdx mice to damage induced by contractions with stretch. *J Muscle Res Cell Motil*, Vol.14, No.4, (Aug 1993), pp. 446-451, ISSN 0142-4319 (Print); 0142-4319 (Linking)

Monaco, A. P.; Bertelson, C. J., et al. (1988). An explanation for the phenotypic differences between patients bearing partial deletions of the DMD locus. *Genomics*, Vol.2, No.1, (Jan 1988), pp. 90-95, ISSN 0888-7543 (Print); 0888-7543 (Linking)

Monaco, A. P.; Neve, R. L., et al. (1986). Isolation of candidate cDNAs for portions of the Duchenne muscular dystrophy gene. *Nature*, Vol.323, No.6089, (Oct 16-22 1986), pp. 646-650, ISSN 0028-0836 (Print); 0028-0836 (Linking)

Nagaraju, K. & Willmann, R. (2009). Developing standard procedures for murine and canine efficacy studies of DMD therapeutics: report of two expert workshops on "Preclinical testing for Duchenne dystrophy": Washington DC, October 27th-28th 2007 and Zurich, June 30th-July 1st 2008. *Neuromuscul Disord*, Vol.19, No.7, (Jul 2009), pp. 502-506, ISSN 1873-2364 (Electronic); 0960-8966 (Linking)

Petrof, B. J.; Shrager, J. B., et al. (1993). Dystrophin protects the sarcolemma from stresses developed during muscle contraction. *Proc Natl Acad Sci U S A*, Vol.90, No.8, (Apr 15 1993), pp. 3710-3714, ISSN 0027-8424 (Print); 0027-8424 (Linking)

Pistilli, E. E.; Bogdanovich, S., et al. (2011). Targeting the activin type IIB receptor to improve muscle mass and function in the mdx mouse model of Duchenne muscular dystrophy. *Am J Pathol*, Vol.178, No.3, (Mar 2011), pp. 1287-1297, ISSN 1525-2191 (Electronic); 0002-9440 (Linking)

Ponting, C. P.; Blake, D. J., et al. (1996). ZZ and TAZ: new putative zinc fingers in dystrophin and other proteins. *Trends Biochem Sci*, Vol.21, No.1, (Jan 1996), pp. 11-13, ISSN 0968-0004 (Print); 0968-0004 (Linking)

Rafael, J. A.; Nitta, Y., et al. (2000). Testing of SHIRPA, a mouse phenotypic assessment protocol, on Dmd(mdx) and Dmd(mdx3cv) dystrophin-deficient mice. *Mamm Genome*, Vol.11, No.9, (Sep 2000), pp. 725-728, ISSN 0938-8990 (Print); 0938-8990 (Linking)

Roberts, R. G.; Freeman, T. C., et al. (1996). Characterization of DRP2, a novel human dystrophin homologue. *Nat Genet*, Vol.13, No.2, (Jun 1996), pp. 223-226, ISSN 1061-4036 (Print); 1061-4036 (Linking)

Spurney, C. F.; Gordish-Dressman, H., et al. (2009). Preclinical drug trials in the mdx mouse: assessment of reliable and sensitive outcome measures. *Muscle Nerve*, Vol.39, No.5, (May 2009), pp. 591-602, ISSN 0148-639X (Print); 0148-639X (Linking)

Stedman, H. H.; Sweeney, H. L., et al. (1991). The mdx mouse diaphragm reproduces the degenerative changes of Duchenne muscular dystrophy. *Nature*, Vol.352, No.6335, (Aug 8 1991), pp. 536-539, ISSN 0028-0836 (Print); 0028-0836 (Linking)

White, S.; Kalf, M., et al. (2002). Comprehensive detection of genomic duplications and deletions in the DMD gene, by use of multiplex amplifiable probe hybridization. *Am J Hum Genet*, Vol.71, No.2, (Aug 2002), pp. 365-374, ISSN 0002-9297 (Print); 0002-9297 (Linking)

Willmann, R.; De Luca, A., et al. (2011). Enhancing translation: Guidelines for standard preclinical experiments in mdx mice. *Neuromuscul Disord*, Vol.(Jul 5 2011), pp. 1873-2364 ISSN 0960-8966 (Linking)

Wrogemann, K. & Pena, S. D. (1976). Mitochondrial calcium overload: A general mechanism for cell-necrosis in muscle diseases. *Lancet*, Vol.1, No.7961, (Mar 27 1976), pp. 672-674, ISSN 0140-6736 (Print); 0140-6736 (Linking)

7

Myotonic Dystrophy Type 1:
Focus on the RNA Pathology and Therapy

Nikolaos P. Mastroyiannopoulos,
Andrie Koutsoulidou and Leonidas A. Phylactou*
Department of Molecular Genetics, Function & Therapy,
The Cyprus Institute of Neurology & Genetics,
Cyprus

1. Introduction

Almost 100 years ago, Steinert (1909), Batten and Gibb (1909), independently described Myotonic Dystrophy type 1 (DM1) that is now recognized as the most common form of muscular dystrophies in adults and the second most common type of muscular dystrophy after Duchenne Muscular Dystrophy, affecting 1 in 8000 individuals globally (Harper, 1989). DM1 is a genetic disorder, which is inherited in an autosomal dominant fashion (the mutation in one copy of the affected allele is enough to cause the disease). Although the disease affects mainly the skeletal muscle, it is considered a multi-systemic disorder with variable clinical symptoms affecting skeletal muscle, heart, and the central nervous system (CNS) (Larkin & Fardaei, 2001). Individual patients with DM1 are often identified as having congenital, juvenile or adult-onset disease based on the age of symptom onset. Congenital cases display the most severe phenotype and face a neonatal mortality rate of 25% (Harper, 1989).

The involvement of skeletal muscle in DM1 is highly characteristic and largely unwavering. Skeletal muscle in DM1 displays progressive weakness and wasting, myotonia and pain. Moreover, at the early stages of the disease, DM1 patients exhibit facial and neck flexion muscle weaknesses. Also, ptosis and weakness of eye and mouth closure are classical facial changes observed in DM1 patients. Weakness of neck flexion is an early sign, and patients may notice difficulty in lifting their heads from the pillow or experience tendency for the head to fall backwards during acceleration of the vehicle in which they are traveling (Machuca-Tzili et al., 2005). At a later stage in the course of the disease, distal weakness in the limbs, affecting particularly the finger flexors causes substantial disability. Less marked but often occurring, the weakness of ankle dorsiflexion causes foot drop. The combination of facial muscle weakness (with ptosis) and distal muscle weakness in DM1, even in the absence of myotonia, does not occur in any other disease (Ranum & Day, 2002). Respiratory failure due to the weakness of the respiratory muscles can also occur. This may be lethal in some cases, and is presented mainly in DM1 patients that experienced anesthesia or suffered from various chest infections (Machuca-Tzili et al., 2005). Myotonia is demonstrable in most

* Corresponding Author

symptomatic adults, whatever their symptoms. The commonest symptom of myotonia is difficulty in relaxing the grip. Myotonia can also affect the facial muscles, tongue, and other bulbar muscles, causing problems when talking, chewing and swallowing. Muscle pain is clearly independent to myotonia and more common in the lower limbs, where myotonia is usually not observed (Machuca-Tzili et al., 2005; Ranum & Day, 2002). Biopsies of DM1 muscle show a markedly increased variation in fibre diameter that ranges from 10μm to greater than 100μm. Severely atrophic fibres have pygnotic nuclei with minimal remaining contractile elements. DM1 muscle observations also showed ring fibre and central nuclear chains. Moreover, ATPase staining of the affected muscle sections showed atrophy of type 1 fibres. Finally, basophilic regenerating fibres, splitting fibres, fibrosis and adipose deposition are common muscle abnormalities of DM1, always depending on the extent of muscle involvement (Vihola et al., 2003).

Antrioventricular and intraventricular conduction abnormalities are very common in DM1 and require regular monitoring. DM1 patients were shown to be more vulnerable to cardiac conduction abnormalities than impaired myocardial function. Atrial fibrillation, ventricular arrhythmias and cardiomyopathy are also very common abnormalities in DM1 affected individuals (Phillips & Harper, 1997). Sudden death, due to heart block, is not common in DM1, but does occur in severe DM1 patients, as a result of extreme sinus bradycardia or tachyarrhythmia, necessitating the use of pacemakers and implantable defibrillators by these patients (Colleran et al., 1997). There is extensive evidence for CNS involvement in DM1. Cognitive impairment / mental retardation, specific patterns of psychological dysfunction and personality traits, are widely recognized features of congenital and juvenile DM1 affected patients. In addition to the above, DM1 patients develop CNS white matter and cerebral blood flow abnormalities (Ogata et al., 1998). Central hypersomnia, another recognized CNS effect of DM1, appears to occur in adulthood. Excessive daytime sleepiness is very common and in some cases very disabling. Apathy, epilepsy, stroke and parkinsonism are rarely observed in adult DM1 patients, but are fairly common in congenitally affected patients (Rubinsztein et al., 1997). Posterior capsular, iridescent, multicoloured opacities are regularly seen in DM1 patients. Cataracts can be detected in DM1 patients at a very early stage in the course of the disease by slit-lamp examination. When vision is significantly impaired, surgical intervention is required (Klesert et al., 2000). Irritable bowel-like symptoms such as constipation, diarrhea, colicky abdominal pain and pseudo-obstruction are extremely common in DM1. The upper gastrointestinal tract is affected in later stages of the disease and can cause dysphagia and aspiration resulting in serious chest infections that can cause morbidity and mortality of DM1 patients. DM1 patients display a large variety of endocrine abnormalities. Testicular failure, hypotestosteronism and oligospermia are associated with the reduced fertility of these patients. Laboratory observations have also shown a reduction in the serum levels of IgG and IgM and as a result, hypogammaglobulinemia can affect these patients. Insulin resistance is also seen in DM1 patients, but even in severe cases, type 2 diabetes clinical symptoms are not linked with the disease, whilst recent evidence supports that there is alteration in the normal functioning of the insulin receptor (Moxley et al., 1984).

DM1 is caused by an unstable expansion of CTG repeats in the 3'-untranslated region (3' UTR) of the *dystrophia myotonica protein kinase (DMPK)* gene on chromosome 19q13.3 (Aslanidis et al., 1992; Brook et al., 1992; Davies et al., 1983). The number of CTG repeats is in the range of 5-35 in the normal population and increases to between 50 and several thousand in DM1 patients. The variation in the number of CTG repeats is closely related to the phenomenon of 'anticipation': The number of CTG repeats can increase through successive generations, due to mitotic and meiotic instabilities (Martorell et al., 1999; Monckton et al., 1995). Interesting is also the fact that DM1 patients might show difference in the number of CTG repeats from one cell to another (genetic heterogeneity). 3'UTR is a region that is transcribed into RNA but not translated into protein therefore the CTG expansion at the DM1 locus does not alter the protein sequence encoded by DMPK. The mechanism of pathogenesis in DM1 is different from other genetic disorders. Three different mechanisms of pathogenesis have been proposed to explain how repeat expansions in the DMPK gene result in DM1 (Tapscott & Thornton, 2001):

i.   The mutant RNA accumulates in discrete foci in the cell nucleus rather than being transported to the cytoplasm (Davis et al., 1997; Taneja et al., 1995), where translation of mRNA into protein normally takes place. According to experimental evidence this causes deficiency in the production of DMPK (DMPK Haploinsufficiency) (Jansen et al., 1996; Reddy et al., 1996).

ii. The second mechanism of pathogenesis, involves the disruption of the expression and function of DMPK neighboring genes. Scientific evidence showed that the expanded CTG repeats interfere with the nucleosome assembly and therefore on the total chromatin structure. This process disrupts and prevents the binding of necessary factors for the expression of neighboring genes (Klesert et al., 1997; Wang & Griffith, 1995; Westerlaken et al., 2003).

iii. Lastly, evidence suggests that the molecular pathogenesis of DM1 is to a great extent due to the downstream effects of the retention of the mutant DMPK transcripts in the nucleus. Some of these include the inhibition of myogenesis and the defective splicing of cellular RNA molecules (Mankodi et al., 2000; Miller et al., 2000; Timchenko et al., 1996).

This book chapter will focus mainly on the pathology which arises from nuclear RNA retention and the therapeutic approaches against it. The correlation between the CTG repeat size and the severity of the disease, suggests that the repeats represent the major cause of DM1 pathogenesis. After investigations of the mutant DMPK transcripts, it was found that these form nuclear foci that are enclosed within the nucleus of the affected cells (Amack & Mahadevan, 2001; Taneja et al., 1995). Moreover, it was postulated that these nuclear foci might contribute to DM1 pathogenesis, perhaps by disrupting the transport of mRNA from DMPK and/or other genes to the cytoplasm (Alwazzan et al., 1999; Klesert et al., 1997; Otten & Tapscott, 1995; Taneja et al., 1995). Further on, cell models expressing the CTG repeat expansion, showed also nuclear localization of mutant RNA foci and extended myogenic defects (Amack & Mahadevan, 2004). These nuclear RNA foci were also shown to interact with nuclear RNA binding proteins and subsequently alter the regulation or localization (Fardaei et al., 2002; Philips et al., 1998). Mutant DMPK RNA foci were found to interact with the CUG-binding protein (Timchenko et al., 1996) and three different forms of the muscleblind binding protein (MBNL) (Ho et al., 2005). Scientific evidence, using knockout MBNL or CUGBP animal models revealed similarities to the DM1 pathophysiology, including cardiac, endocrine system and muscle abnormalities (Kanadia et al., 2003; Kanadia et al., 2003; Roberts et al., 1997).

2. RNA pathogenesis

2.1 RNA nuclear retention

Mutant DMPK alleles are transcribed in the nucleus to produce RNA molecules containing expanded CUG repeats. The expanded CUG transcript folds back on itself to form stable duplex hairpin structures. Napierala and Kryzosiak provided evidence that hairpins indeed exist in the DMPK RNA fragments containing 11–49 CUG repeats and that the stability of these structures increases with the repeat length (Napierala & Krzyzosiak, 1997). Koch and Leffert, generated secondary structures of partial and full-length DMPK mRNAs carrying variable numbers of CUG triplet repeats (up to 500) (Koch & Leffert, 1998). They suggested that CUG hairpins are the most stable structures formed and also that the DMPK mRNAs are sterically impeded from transport through nuclear pores, by giant hairpins or hairpin clusters formed by CUG repeats above a limit size (44 or less) (Koch & Leffert, 1998). Further thermal melting and nuclease mapping studies indicated that CUG repeats form highly stable hairpins (Tian et al., 2000). Michalowski et al., used electron microscopy to provide the first visual evidence that the DMPK mRNA expansion forms an RNA hairpin structure (Michalowski et al., 1999). Visualization of large RNAs containing up to 130 CUG repeats revealed perfect double-stranded RNA segments whose lengths were that expected for duplex RNA (Michalowski et al., 1999). The duplex segments were highly stable, since the hairpin structures reformed rapidly during the electron microscopy mounting procedures when the RNAs were boiled and quickly cooled, even under low salt conditions (Michalowski et al., 1999).

RNA harboring CUG repeat expansion impose dominant-negative effects by aberrantly interacting and recruiting RNA-binding proteins thus leading to nuclear retention of the mutant transcript and the formation of ribonuclear inclusions known as RNA foci. Taneja et al., used fluorochrome-conjugated and digoxigenin-conjugated oligonucleotide probes to analyze the intracellular localization of DMPK transcripts in fibroblasts derived from DM patients and normal individuals and showed a striking difference in the nuclear distribution of the DMPK transcripts, a difference that was verified in a muscle biopsy from an affected individual (Taneja et al., 1995). Davis et al., generated "myoblasts" by *MyoD* retroviral infection of DM1 fibroblast lines and showed that mutant *DMPK* transcripts were abundant in myoblasts, but could not contribute to kinase production, as the transcripts were quantitatively retained within myoblast nuclei (Davis et al., 1997). Terminally differentiated myoblasts contained no cytoplasmic mutant transcripts; instead, they formed stable, long-lived clusters that were tightly linked to the nuclear matrix (Davis et al., 1997). Myoblasts and myotubes isolated from patients with congenital myotonic dystrophy (CDM1) also showed abnormal retention of mutant RNA in nuclear foci (Furling et al., 2001).

2.2 CUG binding protein 1 (CUGBP1)

Proteins of the CELF family are a group of proteins extensively studied for their implication in DM1 pathogenesis. CELF (CUGBP and ETR-3-like factors) proteins are a family of structurally related RNA-binding proteins involved in various aspects of RNA processing including alternative splicing, translation and mRNA stability. The first member of the CELF family, CELF1/CUGBP1, was identified in investigating the molecular mechanisms of DM1 (Gallo & Spickett, 2010). Timchenko et al. reported that CUG binding protein 1

(CUGBP1) binds specifically to CUG triplet repeated sequences (Timchenko et al., 1996; Timchenko et al., 1996). Electron microscopy studies showed that CUGBP1 is primarily a single-stranded RNA-binding protein that has a binding preference for CUG-rich RNA elements but not double-stranded CUG hairpins (Michalowski et al., 1999). Moreover, CUGBP1 was visualized to localize to the base of the RNA hairpin and not along the stem (Michalowski et al., 1999). In a yeast three-hybrid system CUGBP1 was found to associate with long CUG trinucleotide repeats $((CUG)_{(11)}(CUG)_{(12)})$, but not with short repeats $((CUG)_{(12)})$ (Takahashi et al., 2000). However, using a combination of indirect immunofluorescence to detect endogenous proteins and overexpression of proteins with green fluorescent protein (GFP) tags it has been shown that CUGBP1 does not co-localise with triplet repeat foci in DM1 fibroblast cell lines (Fardaei et al., 2001).

Experiments in tissue culture and analysis of DM1 patients demonstrated that RNA CUG repeats directly affect expression and activity of CUGBP1 in DM1 myoblasts, heart, and skeletal muscle tissues (Timchenko et al., 2001). Specifically, the formation of CUGBP1 · CUG RNA complexes is accompanied by increased CUGBP1 protein stability and subsequent elevation of CUGBP1 (Timchenko et al., 2001). Furthermore, nuclear CUGBP1 levels have been found increased in DM1 patients, compared to normal subjects (Timchenko et al., 2001). These observations suggest that abnormal activation of CUGBP1 is related to DM1 pathogenesis. Furthermore, in a transgenic mice model, overexpression of CUGBP1 in heart and skeletal muscle, produced DM1-like symptoms such as central nuclei, chains of nuclei, centralized nicotinamide adenine dinucleotide (NADH) reactivity and mis-splicing (Ho et al., 2005). De Haro et al., generated a *Drosophila* model of DM1 that showed degenerative phenotypes in muscle and eye tissue and key histopathological features of the DM1, including accumulation of the expanded transcripts in nuclear foci (de Haro et al., 2006). Using this model they showed that by increasing the levels of CUGBP1 degeneration is deteriorated even though CUGBP1 distribution is not altered by the expression of the expanded triplet repeat (de Haro et al., 2006). Wang et al., generated an inducible and heart-specific DM1 mouse model expressing expanded CUG RNA in the context of DMPK 3' UTR that recapitulated pathological and molecular features of DM1 including dilated cardiomyopathy, arrhythmias, systolic and diastolic dysfunction, and mis-regulated alternative splicing (Wang et al., 2007). Combined *in situ* hybridization and immunofluorescent staining for CUGBP1 protein expressed in heart, showed increased protein levels specifically in nuclei containing foci of CUG repeat RNA (Wang et al., 2007).

Although the molecular mechanisms for increased CUGBP1 is not completely understood, Kuyumcu-Martinez et al. reported that the expression of mutant DMPK-CUG-repeat RNA results in hyperphosphorylation and stabilization of CUGBP1 through the inappropriate activation of the protein kinase C (PKC) pathway, in DM1 tissues, cells, and a DM1 mouse model (Kuyumcu-Martinez et al., 2007). Experiments performed in C2C12 mouse cell line showed that expression of a mutant DMPK 3'-UTR containing 960 CUG repeats is sufficient to increase expression and stability of an mRNA encoding the potent proinflammatory cytokine, tumor necrosis factor (TNF), which was found elevated in DM1 patients serum (Mammarella et al., 2002; Zhang et al., 2008). Moreover, activation of the protein kinase C (PKC) pathway also stabilized the TNF transcript. These results suggest that the elevated serum TNF seen in DM1 patients may be derived from muscle where it is induced by expression of toxic DMPK RNA (Zhang et al., 2008). In a more recent study, Koshelev et al.

used tetracycline-inducible CUGBP1 and heart-specific reverse tetracycline trans-activator transgenes in order to express human CUGBP1 in adult mouse heart (Koshelev et al., 2010). Up-regulation of CUGBP1 was sufficient to reproduce molecular, histopathological and functional changes observed in DM1 patients and in a DM1 mouse model thus supporting a role for CUGBP1 up-regulation in DM1 pathogenesis (Koshelev et al., 2010). In another mouse model, Ward et al. overexpressed CUGBP1 and showed that mice reproduced molecular and physiological defects of DM1 tissue, suggesting that CUGBP1 has a major role in DM1 skeletal muscle pathogenesis (Ward et al., 2010).

2.3 Muscleblind (MBNL) family proteins

Muscleblind (MBNL) family proteins, initially identified by Miller et al. were selectively associated with CUG repeat expansions and named as triplet repeat expansion (EXP) double-stranded (ds) RNA-binding proteins (Miller et al., 2000). Human EXP proteins are found to be orthologous to the *Drosophila* MBNL proteins, which are required for terminal differentiation of photoreceptors and muscle cells (Artero et al., 1998; Begemann et al., 1997). The alternative splicing factor MBNL1 binds to pyrimidine-rich pre-mRNAs containing YGCY motifs and promotes either the inclusion or the exclusion of alternative exons depending on the 5' or 3' localization of *cis*-regulatory elements (Goers et al., 2010). All three isoforms of MBNL family proteins (MBNL/MBNL1, MBLL/MBNL2 and MBXL/MBNL3) co-localize with the nuclear mutant RNA foci in DM1 cells, presumably diverting them from their normal cellular functions (Wojciechowska & Krzyzosiak, 2011). The biological significance of the interaction between mutant RNA and MBNL-family proteins has been manifested through the disruption of alternative splicing which is a characteristic feature of DM1 pathogenesis (Wojciechowska & Krzyzosiak, 2011). Fardaei et al. investigated for the first time the localization of MBNL (EXP) protein with mutant DMPK transcripts (Fardaei et al., 2001). Using indirect immunofluorescence to detect endogenous proteins and overexpression of GFP-tagged MBNL, they showed that MBNL forms foci in DM1 fibroblast cell lines and co-localises with the foci of expanded repeat transcripts in the nuclei of DM1 cells (Fardaei et al., 2001). The binding of MBNL1 with expanded CUG repeats was further verified in DM1 muscle biopsy tissues (Mankodi et al., 2003) and in a yeast three-hybrid system (Kino et al., 2004). Overexpression of MBNL1 *in vivo* using a recombinant adeno-associated viral vector rescued disease-associated muscle myotonia and aberrant splicing of specific gene transcripts, characteristic of DM1 skeletal muscle supporting the hypothesis that loss of MBNL1 activity is a primary pathogenic event in the development of the disease (Kanadia et al., 2006).

Analysis of the expression pattern of the mouse *Mbnl1*, *Mbnl2*, *Mbnl3* and *Dmpk* genes during embryonic development revealed a striking overlap between the expression of *Dmpk* and the *Mbnl* genes during development of the limbs, nervous system and various muscles, including the diaphragm and tongue (Kanadia et al., 2003). In 2003, Kanadia et al. generated the first MBNL knockout mouse model for DM1 (Kanadia et al., 2003). The disruption of the mouse *Mbnl1* gene led to muscle, eye and RNA splicing abnormalities which are characteristics of DM1 disease (Kanadia et al., 2003). Examination of DM1 post-mortem brain tissue by FISH indicated that the mutant DMPK mRNA is widely expressed in cortical and subcortical neurons and accumulated in discrete foci within neuronal nuclei (Jiang et al., 2004). Moreover, MBNL family proteins were recruited into the RNA foci and a subset of neuronal pre-mRNAs showed abnormal regulation of alternative splicing suggesting that central nervous system impairment in DM1 may result from a deleterious gain-of-function by mutant DMPK mRNA (Jiang et al., 2004). In 2005, Mankodi et al. provided evidence that accumulation of expanded CUG repeats in nuclear foci was associated with sequestration of MBNL proteins and abnormal regulation of alternative splicing in cardiac muscle tissue from DM1 patients (Mankodi et al., 2005).

In a *Drosophila* model of DM1 expressing CTG repeats in the 3'-UTR of a marker gene CUG repeats form discrete ribonuclear foci in muscle cells that co-localize with MBNL (Houseley et al., 2005). Moreover, MBNL was also revealed as having a previously unrecognized role in stabilizing CUG transcripts (Houseley et al., 2005). In another *Drosophila* model of DM1 that shows degenerative phenotypes in muscle and eye tissue as well as key histopathological features of the DM1, including accumulation of the expanded transcripts in nuclear foci and their co-localization with MBNL1 protein, reduced levels of MBNL1 aggravate the muscle and eye phenotypes of DM1 flies whereas MBNL1 overexpression suppresses the degenerative phenotypes (de Haro et al., 2006). *Mbnl2*-deficient mice developed myotonia, skeletal muscle pathology consistent with human DM1 and defective CLCN1 mRNA splicing in skeletal muscle, supporting the hypothesis that MBNL proteins and specifically MBNL2 contribute to the pathogenesis of human DM1 (Hao et al., 2008). These results are consistent with the notion that *Mbnl1* deficiency alone is not sufficient to fully replicate the human DM1 phenotype (Kanadia et al., 2003). An additional mouse DM1 model with inducible and skeletal muscle-specific expression of 960 CTG repeats in the context of DMPK exon 15 recapitulated many findings associated with DM1 skeletal muscle, such as nuclear foci with MBNL1 protein co-localization, mis-splicing, myotonia, characteristic histological abnormalities, and increased CUGBP1 protein levels (Orengo et al., 2008). Importantly, this DM1 mouse model exhibited severe muscle wasting, which has not been reported previously in models in which MBNL1 depletion was the main feature (Orengo et al., 2008). More recently, Machuca-Tzili et al. generated an *mbnl2* knockdown zebrafish model, which exhibits features of DM (Machuca-Tzili et al., 2011). They showed that loss of zebrafish mbnl2 function causes muscle defects and splicing abnormalities of clcn1 and tnnt2 transcripts, similar to those observed in DM1 patients (Machuca-Tzili et al., 2011).

Wheeler et al., showed that CUG expanded RNA is also expressed in subsynaptic nuclei of muscle fibers and in motor neurons in DM1 patients, causing sequestration of MBNL1 protein in both locations (Wheeler et al., 2007). Additionally, in a transgenic mouse model, expression of CUG expanded RNA at high levels in extrajunctional nuclei replicates many features of DM1, including myotonia, spliceopathy, internal nuclei, ring fibers, and sarcoplasmic masses, but the toxic RNA is poorly expressed in subsynaptic nuclei and mice fail to develop denervation-like features of DM1 myopathology (Wheeler et al., 2007). These findings suggest that subsynaptic nuclei and motor neurons are at risk for DM1-induced mis-splicing, which may affect function or stability of the neuromuscular junction (Wheeler et al., 2007). MBNL1 protein was also found in the human brain, and consists of several isoforms, as shown by RT-PCR and sequencing. In the brain tissue of DM1 patients, a fetal isoform of MBNL1 was found overexpressed (Dhaenens et al., 2008). The expression of this fetal isoform can also be reproduced by the ectopic expression of long CUG repeats *in vitro* (Dhaenens et al., 2008).

2.4 Mis-regulation of alternative splicing

At the molecular level, one of the best-characterized trans-dominant effects induced by the mutant *DMPK* RNAs in DM1 is the mis-regulation of alternative splicing of a subset of pre-mRNAs. Alternative splicing is a process by which the exons of the transcribed pre-mRNA are reconnected in multiple ways to give rise to different mRNAs which are in turn translated into different protein isoforms. To date, more than twenty transcripts have been found to be mis-spliced in different tissues of DM1 patients (Klein et al., 2011).

2.4.1 CUGBP1 and MBNL1 significance in alternative splicing mis-regulation

Mis-splicing events observed in DM1 result from an inappropriate regulation of alternative splicing due to altered activities of splicing regulators such as CUGBP1 and MBNL1. The biological significance of CUGBP1 overexpression and MBNL family proteins sequestration to nuclear RNA foci has been manifested through the disruption of alternative splicing, which is a characteristic feature of DM1 pathogenesis. Muscle wasting and weakness, heart problems and insulin resistance are associated with aberrant alternative splicing of a range of pre-mRNAs.

2.4.1.1 Cardiac troponin T (cTNT)

The first mis-regulation of alternative splicing described in DM1 was the abnormal inclusion of exon 5 in cardiac troponin T (cTNT) in cardiac muscle (Philips et al., 1998). CUGBP1 was found to bind to the human cTNT pre–mRNA and regulate its alternative splicing. Splicing of cTNT was disrupted in DM1 striated muscle and in normal cells expressing CUG expanded RNAs (Philips et al., 1998). Transgenic mice with a targeted deletion of *Mbnl1* exon 3 (E3) (*Mbnl1$^{\Delta E3/\Delta E3}$*) in adult heart showed abnormal retention of the *cTNT* "fetal" exon 5, as was observed in DM1 (Kanadia et al., 2003; Philips et al., 1998). Ho et al., involved for the first time all three MBNL family members with mis-regulation of alternative splicing in DM1 (Ho et al., 2004). MBNL proteins were found to act antagonistically to CELF proteins on the human and chicken cTNT pre-mRNAs (Ho et al., 2004). MBNL1 binds a common motif near the human and chicken cTNT alternative exons within intronic regions, which appear to be single stranded (Ho et al., 2004). Furthermore, CELF and MBNL proteins bind to distinct *cis*-elements and minigenes containing CELF- or MBNL-binding site mutations thus showing that regulation by one family does not require responsiveness to the other (Ho et al., 2004). However, modified cTNT minigenes made nonresponsive to the *trans*-dominant effects of CUG repeat RNA still respond to MBNL depletion, suggesting that CUG repeat RNA affects splicing by a mechanism more complex than MBNL depletion alone (Ho et al., 2004).

2.4.1.2 Insulin receptor (IR)

Three years after the discovery of the first pre-mRNA that is mis-spliced in DM1, Savkur et al., described the second pre-mRNA that undergoes mis-regulation of alternative splicing in DM1 skeletal tissue (Savkur et al., 2001). Alternative splicing of the insulin receptor (IR) pre-mRNA was aberrantly regulated in DM1, resulting in predominant expression of the lower-signaling non-muscle isoform (IR-A) of the receptor (Savkur et al., 2001). IR-A also predominates in DM1 skeletal muscle cultures, which exhibit a reduced responsiveness to the metabolic effects of insulin (Savkur et al., 2001). Furthermore, the aberrant regulation of

IR alternative splicing was reproduced in normal cells by the expression of CUG-repeat RNA (Savkur et al., 2001). Additionally, overexpression of CUGBP1 also induced a switch to IR-A in normal cells (Savkur et al., 2001). The CUGBP1 protein mediates this switch through an intronic element located upstream of the alternatively spliced exon 11, and specifically binds within this element *in vitro* (Savkur et al., 2001). The research group suggested a model in which increased expression CUGBP1 splicing regulator contributes to insulin resistance observed in DM1 by affecting IR alternative splicing (Savkur et al., 2001).

In addition to CUGBP1, IR alternative splicing was found to be regulated by MBNL1 (Ho et al., 2004). Down-regulation of MBNL1 and MBNL2 in normal myoblasts resulted in abnormal splice pattern observed in DM1 (Dansithong et al., 2005). Moreover, CUGBP1 was found to regulate the equilibrium of splice site selection by antagonizing the facilitatory activity of MBNL1 and MBNL2 on IR exon 11 splicing in a dose-dependent manner (Dansithong et al., 2005). Rescued experiments in DM1 myoblasts demonstrated that loss of MBNL1 function is the critical event, whereas CUGBP1 overexpression plays a secondary role in the aberrant alternative splicing of IR RNA in DM1 (Dansithong et al., 2005). Therefore, these experiments demonstrated that MBNL1 sequestration is the primary determinant of the IR pre-mRNA abnormal splicing in DM1 myoblasts (Dansithong et al., 2005).

2.4.1.3 Chloride channel - 1 (ClC-1)

In a transgenic mouse model of DM1, the expression of expanded CUG repeats reduced the transmembrane chloride conductance to an extent sufficient to account for myotonia (Mankodi et al., 2002). These mice showed abnormal splicing of pre-mRNA encoding chloride channel – 1 (ClC-1), the main chloride channel in skeletal muscle, resulting in loss of ClC-1 protein from the surface membrane (Mankodi et al., 2002). Furthermore, the induction of abnormal ClC-1 splicing, the corresponding loss of ClC-1 protein from the muscle membrane, and the development of myotonia were tightly correlated with the level of expanded CUG repeats in different transgenic lines (Mankodi et al., 2002). Additional to the mice models, similar effects on CLC-1 splicing and protein accumulation in muscle tissue from patients with DM1 (Mankodi et al., 2002). These findings suggest that mis-regulation of ClC-1 pre-mRNA alternative splicing is an important factor that leads to myotonia observed in DM1 patients. In an additional study, loss of ClC-1 mRNA and protein due to aberrant splicing of the ClC-1 pre-mRNA was detected in DM1 skeletal muscle tissue (Charlet et al., 2002). Specifically, the majority of ClC-1 mRNAs contained premature termination codons due to retention of intron 2 or inclusion of two novel exons between exons 6 and 7 (Charlet et al., 2002). CUGBP1, which is found elevated in DM1 striated muscle, bound to the ClC-1 pre-mRNA, and overexpression of CUGBP1 in normal cells reproduced the aberrant pattern of ClC-1 splicing observed in DM1 skeletal muscle (Charlet et al., 2002). In particular, CUGBP1 induced retention of intron 2 by binding to a U/G-rich motif common to other pre-mRNA targets of CUGBP1 thus suggesting that increased CUGBP1 activity in DM1 causes aberrant regulation of ClC-1 alternative splicing (Charlet et al., 2002).

2.4.1.4 Tau

Tau protein belongs to the family of microtubule-associated proteins whose transcript undergoes complex regulated splicing in the mammalian nervous system. They are essentially expressed in neurons where their essential function is to regulate the microtubule network. In the adult human central nervous system, alternative splicing of exons 2, 3 and 10 of the single *tau* gene transcript gives six tau isoforms (Sergeant et al., 2001). The tau isoforms aggregated in DM1 brain lesions consists mainly of the shortest human tau isoform suggesting that the $(CTG)_n$ expansion is altering the processing of tau pre-mRNA splicing and gives rise to symptoms such as dementia (Sergeant et al., 2001).

2.4.1.5 Myotubularin-related 1 (MTMR1)

The *myotubularin-related 1 (MTMR1)* gene belongs to a highly conserved family of phosphatases with at least 11 isoforms in humans (Buj-Bello et al., 2002). One of the transcripts resulting from MTMR1 alternative slicing is muscle-specific and is induced during myogenesis both *in vitro* and *in vivo*, and represents the major isoform in adult skeletal muscle (Buj-Bello et al., 2002). MTMR1 splicing pattern was found strikingly altered in cultured muscle cells, in skeletal muscle from patients with congenital myotonic dystrophy (CDM1) and in DM1 muscle biopsies (Buj-Bello et al., 2002; Santoro et al., 2010).

2.4.1.6 Ryanodine receptor 1 (RyR1) and sarcoplasmic/endoplasmic reticulum Ca2+-ATPase (SERCA) 1 or 2

Ryanodine receptor 1 (RyR1) and sarcoplasmic/endoplasmic reticulum Ca2+-ATPase (SERCA) 1 or 2 which are the main sarcoplasmic reticulum regulators of intracellular Ca^{2+} homeostasis in skeletal muscle cells (Kimura et al., 2005). The fetal variants, ASI(-) of RyR1 which lacks residue 3481-3485, and SERCA1b which differs at the C-terminal were found significantly increased in skeletal muscles from DM1 patients and a transgenic mouse model of DM1 thus suggesting that aberrant splicing of RyR1 and SERCA1 mRNAs might contribute to impaired Ca^{2+} homeostasis in DM1 muscle (Kimura et al., 2005).

2.4.1.7 Myocyte enhancer factor 2 (Mef2)

MBNL3 regulates the splicing pattern of the muscle transcription factor myocyte enhancer factor 2 (Mef2) (Lee et al., 2010). MBNL3 antagonizes muscle differentiation by disrupting the expression of (+)β isoform of Mef2D which is transcriptionally more active (Lee et al., 2010). Using a DM1 cell culture model and DM1 patient tissue, they provided evidence that expression of CUG expanded RNAs can lead to an increase in MBNL3 expression accompanied by a decrease in Mef2D β-exon splicing (Lee et al., 2010). These studies suggest that an increase in MBNL3 activity may play a role in the skeletal muscle degeneration experienced by DM1 patients (Lee et al., 2010).

2.4.1.8 Bridging integrator-1 (BIN1)

Bridging integrator-1 (BIN1) is a myc box-dependent-interacting protein involved in tubular invaginations of membranes and is required for the biogenesis of muscle T tubules, which are specialized skeletal muscle membrane structures essential for excitation-contraction coupling (Fugier et al., 2011). Mutations in the *BIN1* gene cause centronuclear myopathy, which shares some histopathological features with myotonic dystrophy (Jungbluth et al., 2008). BIN1's function is regulated by alternative splicing which was found altered in skeletal muscle samples of people with CDM1 and DM1 (Fugier et al., 2011). Particularly, MBNL1 was detected to bind the BIN1 pre-mRNA and regulate the alternative splicing of the exon 11 (Fugier et al., 2011). Sequestration of MBNL1 by expanded CUG repeats in DM1 patients resulted in expression of an inactive form of BIN1 lacking phosphatidylinositol 5-

phosphate-binding and membrane-tubulating activities (Fugier et al., 2011). Consistent with a defect of BIN1, muscle T tubules found altered in DM1 patients, and membrane structures were restored upon expression of the normal splicing form of BIN1 in muscle cells of such individuals (Fugier et al., 2011). Finally, reproducing BIN1 splicing alteration in mice was sufficient to promote T tubule alterations and muscle weakness, a predominant feature of DM1 (Fugier et al., 2011).

2.4.1.9 Myomesin 1 (MYOM1)

Myomesin 1 (MYOM1) is a constituent of the M band of the sacromere which is the basic unit of a muscle (Lange et al., 2005). The fact that MYOM1 is a structural constituent of muscle suggests that it could be involved in muscle impairment in patients with DM1. Koebis et al. used exon array and identified aberrant inclusion of *MYOM1* exon 17a as a novel splicing abnormality in DM1 muscle (Koebis et al., 2011). A cellular splicing assay using a *MYOM1* minigene revealed that MBNL and CELF family proteins function as *trans*-acting factors in the alternative splicing of *MYOM1* exon 17a (Koebis et al., 2011). Expression of expanded CUG repeat impeded MBNL1 activity but did not affect CUGBP1 activity on the splicing of *MYOM1* minigene (Koebis et al., 2011). These results suggested that the downregulation of MBNL proteins should lead to the abnormal splicing of *MYOM1* exon 17a in DM1 muscle (Koebis et al., 2011).

2.5 Myogenic defects

DM1-associated molecular events, such as abberant recruitment of RNA-binding proteins into ribonuclear foci and mis-splicing, could eventually provoke alterations in global cell function. Notably, a critical disorder of DM1 that distinguishes it from other muscular dystrophies is the defects observed in muscle differentiation. Fetal muscle development is affected in fetuses with congenital myotonic dystrophy whereas muscle regeneration is compromised in adult patients (Amack & Mahadevan, 2004).

Initial experiments performed in the mouse myoblast cell line C2C12 showed that overexpression of the mouse *dmpk* gene leads to markedly inhibition of both fusion and terminal differentiation of the cell line (Okoli et al., 1998). Further experiments performed on C2C12 cell line showed that overexpression of human DMPK mRNA caused a marked inhibition of terminal differentiation accompanied by a reduction of myogenin mRNA levels (Sabourin et al., 1997). These results suggest that overexpression of the DMPK 3'-UTR may interfere with the expression of muscle-specific mRNAs leading to a delay in muscle terminal differentiation (Sabourin et al., 1997). Amack et al. used reporter assays to provide unambiguous evidence that the expression of the mutant *DMPK* 3'-UTR mRNA with $(CUG)_{200}$ selectively inhibited myogenic differentiation of C2C12 myoblasts (Amack et al., 1999). In agreement, overexpression of DMPK 3'-UTR including either wild-type or expanded CTG repeats resulted in aberrant and delayed muscle development in fetal transgenic mice and displayed muscle atrophy at 3 months of age. Moreover, primary myoblast cultures from both wild-type and expanded CTG repeat mice showed reduced fusion potential with greater reduction observed in the expanded repeat cultures (Storbeck et al., 2004). Interestingly, the differentiation defect was confirmed in muscle cell cultures derived from DM1 fetuses and patients (Furling et al., 2001; Timchenko et al., 2001).

Molecular studies have begun to uncover the effect of the mutant DMPK mRNA on myogenesis inhibition. Various studies implicate CUGBP1 protein with myogenic impairment in DM1, since it is a key regulator of translation of proteins that are involved in muscle development and differentiation. Timchenko et al. reported that cultured myoblasts isolated from DM1 patients failed to permanently withdraw from the cell cycle when stimulated to differentiate (Timchenko et al., 2001). Skeletal muscle cells from DM1 patients failed to induce cytoplasmic levels of CUGBP1, while normal differentiated cells accumulate CUGBP1 in the cytoplasm (Timchenko et al., 2001). In normal cells, CUGBP1 up-regulates p21 translation during differentiation by binding to a GC-rich sequence located within the 5' region of p21 mRNA (Timchenko et al., 2001). DM1 cultured cells failed to accumulate CUGBP1 in the cytoplasm thus leading to a significant reduction of p21 and to alterations of other proteins responsible for the cell cycle withdrawal (Timchenko et al., 2001). In normal cells, activity of cdk4 declines during differentiation, whereas in DM1 cells cdk4 is highly active during all stages of differentiation (Timchenko et al., 2001). Furthermore, DM1 cells do not form Rb/E2F repressor complexes that are abundant in differentiated cells from normal individuals (Timchenko et al., 2001). These data provide evidence for an impaired cell cycle withdrawal in DM1 muscle cells and suggest that alterations in the CUGBP1 activity causes disruption of p21-dependent control of cell cycle arrest (Timchenko et al., 2001). Another study showed that CUGBP1 is phosphorylated by different kinases during myoblast proliferation and differentiation and that phosphorylation of CUGBP1 at different sites directs CUGBP1 to different mRNA targets (Salisbury et al., 2008). Specifically, Akt kinase and cyclinD3-cdk4/6 phosphorylate CUGBP1 during proliferation and differentiation, respectively (Salisbury et al., 2008). Cyclin D3-cdk4-mediated phosphorylation of CUGBP1 increases the interactions of CUGBP1 with eIF2 during normal myogenesis, a pathway found to be reduced in DM1 cells (Salisbury et al., 2008). Moreover, ectopic expression of cyclin D3 in DM1 cells enhances fusion of DM1 myoblasts and leads to the correction of differentiation (Salisbury et al., 2008). A more recent study, showed that human skeletal muscle satellite cells isolated from fetal congenital DM1 patients bearing large CTG expansions (>3000) secrete prostaglandin E2 (PGE(2)) that inhibits the fusion of normal myoblasts in culture by decreasing the intracellular levels of calcium (Beaulieu et al., 2011). Authors suggest that the delay in muscle maturation observed in congenital DM1 patients may result, at least in part, from an altered autocrine mechanism (Beaulieu et al., 2011).

3. Therapeutic approaches for DM1

3.1 Restoring MBNL1 and CUGBP1 protein activity

It is widely accepted that MBNL and CUGBP play a major role in the pathogenesis of DM1 and are therefore targets for the reversal of the defective splicing and subsequent alleviation of symptoms in the disease. MBNL activity is compromised due to its sequestration in RNA foci. Therefore an approach to increase its expression levels and hence its activity could serve as a potential route for restoring alternative splicing. Kanadia et al. used intramuscular injection with an AAV (adeno-associated virus) expressing MBNL1 protein in a transgenic mouse model of DM1. This transgenic mouse model carries the human skeletal *a-actin (HSA)* gene modified by insertion of 250 CTG repeats within the 3' untranslated region. These mice develop severe myotonia and dystrophic muscle features characteristic of DM1 disease. Overexpression of MBNL1 saturated the expanded CUG binding sites of the mutant DMPK transcripts and free MBNL1 was able to cause the reversal of muscle hyperexcitability, myotonia and spliceopathy (Kanadia et al., 2006). These results, demonstrated that the elevated expression of MBNL1 alone was sufficient to rescue myotonia, a key pathological feature of DM1, and aberrant splicing of specific gene transcripts, characteristic of the DM1 skeletal muscle. In a parallel study, de Haro et al. used a *Drosophila* model of DM1 expressing mRNA transcripts containing 480 CUG repeats, which accumulate in nuclear foci and show degenerative phenotypes in muscle (muscle wasting) and eye tissue (disorganization and fusion of the ommatidia as well as loss and duplication of inter-ommatidial bristles) as well as other key histopathological features of DM1. Furthermore, this DM1 model shows altered levels of MBNL1 and CUGBP1, as observed in DM1 pathogenesis. Overexpression of MBNl1 in this DM1 model showed to suppress the muscle and eye phenotypes of DM1. Interestingly, expanded RNA transcripts that accumulated in nuclear foci within muscle cells were decreased in flies expressing the mutant RNA transcripts that also overexpress MBNL1 (de Haro et al., 2006).

CUGBP1 has been shown to be up-regulated in DM1 as a result of PKC activation and subsequent CUGBP1 protein hyperphosphorylation and stabilization (Kuyumcu-Martinez et al., 2007). Wang et al. created a heart specific Tamoxifen-inducible mouse model containing 960 CTG repeats within the last exon of the DMPK. These mice exhibited high mortality, conduction abnormalities, and systolic and diastolic dysfunction as well as molecular changes seen in DM1 patients, such as increased levels of CUGBP1, colocalization of MBNL1 with RNA foci and reversion of splicing to embryonic patterns. Blocking of PKC activity, using a specific PKC inhibitor (Ro-31-8220), in this heart-specific DM1 mouse model ameliorated several DM1 symptoms, including cardiac conduction defects and contraction abnormalities (Wang et al., 2009). The inhibitor also reduced the splicing defects regulated by CUGBP1, but not those regulated by MBNL1, suggesting distinct roles for these proteins in DM1 cardiac pathogenesis (Wang et al., 2009). As previously described, DM1 mouse models showed elevated levels of CUGBP1 that leads to a delay of muscle development and differentiation. Salisbury et al. presented evidence that two signal transduction pathways regulate CUGBP1 activity in normal muscle and that these pathways are altered in DM1 cells. CUGBP1 was found to be phosphorylated by different kinases, during myoblast proliferation and differentiation and that phosphorylation of CUGBP1 at different sites directs CUGBP1 to different mRNA targets. Moreover, cyclin D3-cdk4-mediated phosphorylation of CUGBP1 increases the interactions of CUGBP1 with eIF2 during normal myogenesis. Furthermore, it was found that cyclin D3-cdk4 pathway is reduced in DM1 cells and that the normalization of cyclin D3 expression in DM1 cells leads to the correction of differentiation (Salisbury et al., 2008).

Overexpression of MBNL1 and downregulation of CUGBP1 or modulation of their counterparts showed encouraging results towards the development of rational therapies for DM1. These two key proteins play a major role in the pathogenesis of the disease and any attempt to normalize their function will be beneficial.

3.2 Targeting the mutant DMPK transcripts

A promising gene therapy approach is to target the mutant DMPK transcripts. Most of the attempts to eliminate toxic *DMPK* transcripts in DM1 cells and animal models used catalytic

RNA (ribozymes) (Langlois et al., 2003; Phylactou et al., 1998), chemically modified antisense oligonucleotides (Furling et al., 2003; Mulders et al., 2009) and siRNA duplexes (Langlois et al., 2005).

Ribozymes are RNA molecules that adopt a tertiary structure and function as catalysts. The hammerhead, hairpin and hepatitis delta virus (HDV) ribozyme motifs can be characterized by their ability for self-cleavage of a particular phosphodiester bond. Hammerhead ribozymes have the ability to suppress gene expression through specific cleavage of RNA molecules (Phylactou et al., 1998; Tedeschi et al., 2009). Langlois et al. designed a hammerhead ribozyme with significant accessibility to a specific target site within the 3' UTR of the DMPK mRNA. Utilizing this system, a significant reduction of mutant and normal DMPK 3' UTR transcripts was observed. Furthermore, these human DM1 myoblasts showed a significant reduction of nuclear RNA foci and a partial restoration of insulin receptor isoform B expression. This study demonstrated for the first time intracellular ribozyme-mediated cleavage of nuclear-retained mutant DMPK mRNAs, providing a potential gene therapy agent for the treatment of myotonic dystrophy (Langlois et al., 2003). Beside degradation of their targets, ribozymes can lead to splicing events that replace target RNA with embedded sequences. Group I Intron ribozymes can be characterized by their capacity for self-splicing by cleavage and ligation of phosphodiester bonds (Cech, 1990; Fiskaa & Birgisdottir, 2010). Group I intron ribozymes can be designed to act in *trans* by recognition and separation of RNA molecules in a sequence specific manner, and ligation of a new RNA sequence to the separated RNA molecules. In their 1998 study, Phylactou et al. created a group I intron ribozyme to cleave, *in vitro*, a DMPK RNA containing 12 repeats and replace them with 5 repeats. Furthermore, it was shown that similar splicing was able to be achieved in human cultured fibroblasts (Phylactou et al., 1998). Another promising approach is to target the mutant DMPK transcripts with antisense oligonucleotides. In 2003, Furling et al. showed that by infecting DM1 cells in culture with an adenoviral vector expressing an antisense RNA to the CUG repeat sequence, the mutant DMPK mRNA was significantly reduced. In addition, effective restoration of human DM1 myoblast functions such as myoblast fusion and the uptake of glucose was achieved (Furling et al., 2003). Furthermore, DM1 cells expressing the antisense RNA indicated a correction of CUGBP1 expression in infected DM1 cells. Muscle differentiation and insulin resistance in DM1 were found to be in close proximity with the misregulation of CUGBP1 protein levels.

Alternative approaches towards targeting the mutant DMPK transcripts in DM1, include the use of chemically modified antisense oligonucleotides. A recent report showed convincingly the therapeutic effect of 2-O-methyl phosphorothioate modified $(CAG)_7$ oligonucleotides in DM1 mouse models and in patient myoblast cultures (Mulders et al., 2009). The addition of 2-O-methyl groups to a phosphorothioate-modified oligonucleotide confirms increased stability of binding and reduced nonspecific effects. Local administration of the modified oligonucleotide in skeletal muscle resulted in approximately 50% reduction of expanded *DMPK* RNA. As a result, RNA foci were also reduced and defective splicing corrected. Such findings demonstrate that a low (CUG) n RNA dosage can still be beneficial to patients and be an attractive therapeutic approach. Myotonia is one of the key features of DM1 and is associated with abnormal alternative splicing of the muscle-specific chloride channel (ClC-1) and reduced conductance of chloride ions in the sarcolemma. Wheeler et al. developed a morpholino antisense oligonucleotide targeting the 3' splice site of ClC-1 exon 7a and reversed the defect of ClC-1 alternative splicing in two mouse models of

DM1. The levels of ClC-1 mRNA and eventually protein were found to be upregulated. Moreover, treated mice had a fully functional chloride channel and lack myotonia (Wheeler et al., 2007).

In one approach to inhibit the sequestration of MBNL1 with the expanded CUG repeats, Wheeler et al. used a (CAG) $_{25}$ antisense oligonucleotide morpholino. Antisense morpholinos are unable to cause the cleavage of their target RNAs. *In vitro*, these morpholinos were able to bind to the expanded CUG repeats forming a stable RNA-morpholino heteroduplex that was able to block the formation of MBNL1-RNA complexes and disrupt complexes that had already formed. *In vivo*, intramuscular injection and electroporation of the (CAG) $_{25}$ antisense oligonucleotide morpholino in a transgenic mouse model that accumulate expanded CUG RNA and MBNL1 protein in nuclear foci in skeletal muscle, caused the reduction of nuclear foci and redistribution of MBNL1 protein. 14 weeks after treatment, myotonia was significantly reduced and ClC-1 function restored. The same approach was used to test the effect of this morpholino in an mbnl-1 deficient mouse, which mimics most of the splicing abnormalities of DM1. The morpholino had no effect, confirming that the morpholino specifically acts on the expanded repeats, which are not present in the mbnl1 knockout model (Wheeler et al., 2009).

RNAi has also been used successfully to degrade mutant *DMPK* transcripts. SiRNA duplexes induce the specific cleavage of target RNAs in mammalian cells. Although most of the RNAi applications rely on the cytoplasmic effect of these molecules, it has been shown that RNAi phenomena can occur in the nucleus of primary DM1 cells by targeting nuclear retained *DMPK* mRNAs (Langlois et al., 2005). Krol et al. attempted to target particularly long hairpin structures formed from the interactions of CUG repeats rather than the targeting of nascent RNA in general. In this study it was demonstrated that these long CUG repeat hairpins are under the control of a ribonuclease Dicer, involved in the RNA interference pathway whose main function is to induce the fragmentation of double-stranded RNA duplexes into shorter duplexes, which then act as endogenous siRNAs and trigger the downstream silencing effect. Furthermore, it was shown that the transduction of synthetic (CAG) $_7$ siRNAs into DM1 patient fibroblasts, leads towards a selective reduction of mutant transcripts containing long CUG repeats (Krol et al., 2007).

An alternative approach to confront the toxicity of nuclear RNA retention is to block the binding of RNA-binding proteins to mutant *DMPK* transcripts using small chemical molecules with high affinity towards the mutant *DMPK* transcripts. The binding of these molecules on the mutant *DMPK* transcripts should prevent the binding and therefore the sequestration of RNA-binding proteins, such as MBNL1, and restore aberrant splicing (Mastroyiannopoulos et al., 2010). Several approaches have been performed with the most promising of these being the use of pentamidine, a small molecule that binds to the expanded CUG RNA sequence with high affinity and specificity causing reduction of CUG repeat foci formation and relieves MBNL1 sequestration (Warf et al., 2009). Moreover, pentamidine reversed the mis-splicing of 4 different pre-mRNAs affected in DM1 (Warf et al., 2009). Gareiss et al. used resin-bound dynamic combinatorial chemistry in order to identify the compounds that are able to inhibit MBNL1 binding to expanded CUG RNA. Screening of 11,325 members yielded several molecules with significant selectivity for binding to CUG repeat RNA. These compounds were also able to inhibit the interaction of expanded CUG with MBNL1 *in vitro* (Gareiss et al., 2008). In another report, the design of high affinity ligands that bind to expanded CUG and CAG repeats and inhibit the formation of RNA-protein complexes that are implicated in DM1 was described (Pushechnikov et al., 2009). Similarly, Garcia-Lopez et al. identified molecules that aim to target toxic CUG RNA transcripts when applied on a *Drosophila* model of DM1. By performing a positional scanning combinatorial peptide library screen, a D-amino acid hexapeptide (ABP1) that reduced CUG-induced toxicity in fly eyes and muscles was identified. Furthermore, ABP1 reversed muscle histopathology and splicing misregulation of MBNL1 targets in DM1 model mice. *In vitro*, ABP1 was found bound to CUG hairpins and induced a switch to a single-stranded conformation (Garcia-Lopez et al., 2011). In another study, Arambula et al. created a ligand with high nanomolar affinity to CUG RNA or CTG DNA repeats. This ligand is a triaminotriazine-acridine conjugate designed to hydrogen bond to both U's or T's in the U-U or T-T mismatch, interactions observed between binding of multi CUG and CTG repeats. This ligand was found to destabilize the interactions of MBNL1 with multi CUG repeats (Arambula et al., 2009).

3.3 Induction of mutant DMPK transcripts nuclear export

Few studies have attempted to determine whether the export of mutant DMPK transcripts is beneficial for the disease. The export of mutant DMPK RNA transcripts from the nucleus to the cytoplasm will have as a result the recovery of these cells from DM1 pathogenic events. The export of mRNA from the nucleus is a highly ordered and complicated procedure that implicates several molecules. As previously described, mutant DMPK RNA carrying long CUG repeats form haipin structures which then interact with proteins such as MBNL1 and CUGBP1. These interactions most possibly prohibit the export of these transcripts to the cytoplasm and cause nuclear retention in the form of foci.

Mastroyiannopoulos et al. have demonstrated nuclear export of mutant DMPK 3'-UTR transcripts by introducing a viral post-transcriptional regulatory element. The WPRE (Woodchuck post-transcriptional regulatory element) has been widely used as an enhancer during transgene expression (Lee et al., 2005). It is also known to enhance gene expression through stimulation of nuclear RNA export (Donello et al., 1998). WPRE was inserted downstream of the 3'-end of a mutant DMPK 3'-UTR sequence and was shown to bypass nuclear entrapment. With the use of fluorescence *in situ* hybridization it was shown that the mutant DMPK transcripts that carried the WPRE sequence were localized mainly in the cytoplasm of C2C12 cells in the form of foci. WPRE mediated nuclear export enhanced muscle cell differentiation (Mastroyiannopoulos et al., 2005) and more specifically initial fusion of myoblasts (Mastroyiannopoulos et al., 2008). In another study, cardiac cells, identified from a transgenic mouse in which 400 CTG repeats were positioned downstream of the reporter *LacZ* gene and upstream of the bovine growth hormone polyadenylation signal, localized CUG aggregates exclusively in the cytoplasm of cells (Dansithong et al., 2005). Aggregation of CUG RNAs within the cytoplasm resulted both in MBNL1 sequestration and in approximately 2-fold increase in both nuclear and cytoplasmic CUGBP1 levels. Significantly, and despite these changes, RNA splice defects were not observed, and functional analysis revealed only subtle cardiac dysfunction. These results demonstrate that the presence of mutant DMPK transcripts in the cytoplasm in the form of foci is insufficient to elicit DM1 defects. Interestingly, Garcia-Lopez et al. described a transgenic *Drosophila* model expressing expanded CTG repeats which exhibit an extended

DM1 phenotype. Such as, muscle degeneration, ribonuclear formation, interactions with muscleblinds including misregulated alternative splicing of muscle genes and CUG depended central nervous system alterations. Genetic screens and functional assays on this *Drosophila* model identified the RNA export factor Aly as one of the causes of the phenotype. It has been shown that the Aly phenotype has a close relationship to mRNA export factors and EJC (exon junction complex) components. Mutations in Aly were shown to be associated with nuclear accumulation of CUG repeats. It is therefore important to study further the mRNA export pathway implicated in DM1 and identify candidate targets for repairing nuclear retention of the DMPK transcripts (Garcia-Lopez et al., 2008). Finally, a report proved in a very convincing way the benefit of exporting mutant DMPK transcripts to the cytoplasm. Wheeler et al. attempted to reverse the myotonic dystrophy symptoms in a well-studied animal model by interfering with the MBNL1 and CUG RNA hairpins interaction. The authors used a 25-nt antisense molecule, composed of CAG repeats, in order to prevent the interaction between MBNL1 and expanded CUG repeats by forming a heteroduplex with the hairpins. The oligonucleotide caused elimination of foci and released the trapped transcripts to the cytoplasm. Moreover, the antisense oligonucleotide repaired the defect of mis-splicing and restored the CLCN1 function and myotonia. This paper provided proof-of concept about the therapeutic potential of molecules that prevent the deleterious interactions between proteins and RNA in diseases.

4. Discussion / conclusions

In conclusion, almost 20 years after the discovery of DM1 mutation there is a very good understanding of the pathogenic mechanisms involved in DM1. As previously stated, the mutant DM1 RNA transcripts generate most of the pathological aspects of DM1. The retention of DMPK transcripts as ribonuclear inclusions in the nucleus of DM1 cells is considered to be an important pathogenic mechanism of the disease (Mankodi et al., 2000). A growing body of evidence showed that pleiotropic effects of aberrant interactions between mutant DMPK 3' UTR transcripts and RNA-binding proteins alter the metabolism of 'target' messenger RNAs (Ho et al., 2005; Jiang et al., 2004; Timchenko et al., 1996; Timchenko et al., 2001; Timchenko et al., 2004). Members of the muscleblind family (MBNL, MBXL and MBLL), which usually regulate mRNA splicing, have been shown to colocalize with the ribonuclear inclusions. The nuclear interactions of the MBNL proteins with the mutant DMPK 3' UTR transcripts, have shown to affect the splicing of various mRNAs, such as the insulin receptor (IR), troponin T (cTNT) and the muscle-specific chloride channel (ClC-1). Another RNA-binding protein, implicated in DM1 mechanism of pathogenesis, is CUGBP1. Extensive investigations have shown that CUGBP1 activity is increased in DM cells, and results in a trans-dominant effect on gene splicing.

Although there is very good understanding of the consequences of the genetic mutation that causes DM1, the exact mechanisms responsible for the DM1 phenotype is not completely understood. DM1 pathogenesis is very complex and therefore, different potential approaches and multiple targets can be used for the development of DM1 therapies. To date, several attempts have been described as potential approaches for the therapy of the disease, either by restoring the levels of CUGBP1 and MBNL proteins, by targeting the mutant DMPK 3' UTR transcripts or by the export of this toxic RNA from the nucleus to the cytoplasm of DM1 cells. All of the above approaches hold a great promise for the future treatment of myotonic dystrophy, nevertheless it is also certain that more therapeutic approaches will be unveiled in the near future, which may be variations of the existing methods or novel ways to tackle the pathogenesis of the disease. Further research in DM1 needs to be done in order to move these therapies forward into clinical trials for the cure of DM1 disease.

5. Acknowledgements

Work carried out in the authors' laboratory and described in this chapter was supported by a grant to L.A.P. by A.G. Leventis Foundation.

6. References

Alwazzan, M., E. Newman, M. G. Hamshere & J. D. Brook (1999). "Myotonic dystrophy is associated with a reduced level of RNA from the DMWD allele adjacent to the expanded repeat." *Hum Mol Genet* 8(8): 1491-1497.

Amack, J. D. & M. S. Mahadevan (2001). "The myotonic dystrophy expanded CUG repeat tract is necessary but not sufficient to disrupt C2C12 myoblast differentiation." *Hum Mol Genet* 10(18): 1879-1887.

Amack, J. D. & M. S. Mahadevan (2004). "Myogenic defects in myotonic dystrophy." *Dev Biol* 265(2): 294-301.

Amack, J. D., A. P. Paguio & M. S. Mahadevan (1999). "Cis and trans effects of the myotonic dystrophy (DM) mutation in a cell culture model." *Hum Mol Genet* 8(11): 1975-1984.

Arambula, J. F., S. R. Ramisetty, A. M. Baranger & S. C. Zimmerman (2009). "A simple ligand that selectively targets CUG trinucleotide repeats and inhibits MBNL protein binding." *Proc Natl Acad Sci U S A* 106(38): 16068-16073.

Artero, R., A. Prokop, N. Paricio, G. Begemann, I. Pueyo, M. Mlodzik, M. Perez-Alonso & M. K. Baylies (1998). "The muscleblind gene participates in the organization of Z-bands and epidermal attachments of Drosophila muscles and is regulated by Dmef2." *Dev Biol* 195(2): 131-143.

Aslanidis, C., G. Jansen, C. Amemiya, G. Shutler, M. Mahadevan, C. Tsilfidis, C. Chen, J. Alleman, N. G. Wormskamp, M. Vooijs, J. Buxton, K. Johnson, H. J. M. Smeets, G. G. Lennon, A. V. Carrano, R. G. Korneluk, B. Wieringa & P. J. de Jong (1992). "Cloning of the essential myotonic dystrophy region and mapping of the putative defect." *Nature* 355(6360): 548-551.

Beaulieu, D., P. Thebault, R. Pelletier, P. Chapdelaine, M. Tarnopolsky, D. Furling & J. Puymirat (2011). "Abnormal prostaglandin E2 production blocks myogenic differentiation in myotonic dystrophy." *Neurobiol Dis.*

Begemann, G., N. Paricio, R. Artero, I. Kiss, M. Perez-Alonso & M. Mlodzik (1997). "muscleblind, a gene required for photoreceptor differentiation in Drosophila, encodes novel nuclear Cys3His-type zinc-finger-containing proteins." *Development* 124(21): 4321-4331.

Brook, J. D., M. E. McCurrach, H. G. Harley, A. J. Buckler, D. Church, H. Aburatani, K. Hunter, V. P. Stanton, J. P. Thirion, T. Hudson, R. Sohn, B. Zemelman, R. G. Snell, S. A. Rundle, S. Crow, J. Davies, P. Shelbourne, J. Buxton, C. Jones, V. Juvonen, K. Johnson, P. S. Harper, D. J. Shaw & D. E. Housman (1992). "Molecular basis of myotonic dystrophy: expansion of a trinucleotide (CTG) repeat at the 3' end of a transcript encoding a protein kinase family member." *Cell* 68(4): 799-808.

Buj-Bello, A., D. Furling, H. Tronchere, J. Laporte, T. Lerouge, G. S. Butler-Browne & J. L. Mandel (2002). "Muscle-specific alternative splicing of myotubularin-related 1 gene is impaired in DM1 muscle cells." *Hum Mol Genet* 11(19): 2297-2307.

Cech, T. R. (1990). "Self-splicing of group I introns." *Annu Rev Biochem* 59: 543-568.

Charlet, B. N., R. S. Savkur, G. Singh, A. V. Philips, E. A. Grice & T. A. Cooper (2002). "Loss of the muscle-specific chloride channel in type 1 myotonic dystrophy due to misregulated alternative splicing." *Mol Cell* 10(1): 45-53.

Colleran, J. A., R. J. Hawley, E. E. Pinnow, P. F. Kokkinos & R. D. Fletcher (1997). "Value of the electrocardiogram in determining cardiac events and mortality in myotonic dystrophy." *Am J Cardiol* 80(11): 1494-1497.

Dansithong, W., S. Paul, L. Comai & S. Reddy (2005). "MBNL1 is the primary determinant of focus formation and aberrant insulin receptor splicing in DM1." *J Biol Chem* 280(7): 5773-5780.

Davies, K. E., J. Jackson, R. Williamson, P. S. Harper, S. Ball, M. Sarfarazi, L. Meredith & G. Fey (1983). "Linkage analysis of myotonic dystrophy and sequences on chromosome 19 using a cloned complement 3 gene probe." *J Med Genet* 20(4): 259-263.

Davis, B. M., M. E. McCurrach, K. L. Taneja, R. H. Singer & D. E. Housman (1997). "Expansion of a CUG trinucleotide repeat in the 3' untranslated region of myotonic dystrophy protein kinase transcripts results in nuclear retention of transcripts." *Proc Natl Acad Sci U S A* 94(14): 7388-7393.

de Haro, M., I. Al-Ramahi, B. De Gouyon, L. Ukani, A. Rosa, N. A. Faustino, T. Ashizawa, T. A. Cooper & J. Botas (2006). "MBNL1 and CUGBP1 modify expanded CUG-induced toxicity in a Drosophila model of myotonic dystrophy type 1." *Hum Mol Genet* 15(13): 2138-2145.

Dhaenens, C. M., S. Schraen-Maschke, H. Tran, V. Vingtdeux, D. Ghanem, O. Leroy, J. Delplanque, E. Vanbrussel, A. Delacourte, P. Vermersch, C. A. Maurage, H. Gruffat, A. Sergeant, M. S. Mahadevan, S. Ishiura, L. Buee, T. A. Cooper, M. L. Caillet-Boudin, N. Charlet-Berguerand, B. Sablonniere & N. Sergeant (2008). "Overexpression of MBNL1 fetal isoforms and modified splicing of Tau in the DM1 brain: two individual consequences of CUG trinucleotide repeats." *Exp Neurol* 210(2): 467-478.

Donello, J. E., J. E. Loeb & T. J. Hope (1998). "Woodchuck hepatitis virus contains a tripartite posttranscriptional regulatory element." *J Virol* 72(6): 5085-5092.

Fardaei, M., K. Larkin, J. D. Brook & M. G. Hamshere (2001). "In vivo co-localisation of MBNL protein with DMPK expanded-repeat transcripts." *Nucleic Acids Res* 29(13): 2766-2771.

Fardaei, M., M. T. Rogers, H. M. Thorpe, K. Larkin, M. G. Hamshere, P. S. Harper & J. D. Brook (2002). "Three proteins, MBNL, MBLL and MBXL, co-localize in vivo with nuclear foci of expanded-repeat transcripts in DM1 and DM2 cells." *Hum Mol Genet* 11(7): 805-814.

Fiskaa, T. & A. B. Birgisdottir (2010). "RNA reprogramming and repair based on trans-splicing group I ribozymes." *N Biotechnol* 27(3): 194-203.

Fugier, C., A. F. Klein, C. Hammer, S. Vassilopoulos, Y. Ivarsson, A. Toussaint, V. Tosch, A. Vignaud, A. Ferry, N. Messaddeq, Y. Kokunai, R. Tsuburaya, P. de la Grange, D. Dembele, V. Francois, G. Precigout, C. Boulade-Ladame, M. C. Hummel, A. L. de Munain, N. Sergeant, A. Laquerriere, C. Thibault, F. Deryckere, D. Auboeuf, L. Garcia, P. Zimmermann, B. Udd, B. Schoser, M. P. Takahashi, I. Nishino, G. Bassez, J. Laporte, D. Furling & N. Charlet-Berguerand (2011). "Misregulated alternative splicing of BIN1 is associated with T tubule alterations and muscle weakness in myotonic dystrophy." *Nat Med* 17(6): 720-725.

Furling, D., L. Coiffier, V. Mouly, J. P. Barbet, J. L. St Guily, K. Taneja, G. Gourdon, C. Junien & G. S. Butler-Browne (2001). "Defective satellite cells in congenital myotonic dystrophy." *Hum Mol Genet* 10(19): 2079-2087.

Furling, D., G. Doucet, M. A. Langlois, L. Timchenko, E. Belanger, L. Cossette & J. Puymirat (2003). "Viral vector producing antisense RNA restores myotonic dystrophy myoblast functions." *Gene Ther* 10(9): 795-802.

Furling, D., D. Lemieux, K. Taneja & J. Puymirat (2001). "Decreased levels of myotonic dystrophy protein kinase (DMPK) and delayed differentiation in human myotonic dystrophy myoblasts." *Neuromuscul Disord* 11(8): 728-735.

Gallo, J. M. & C. Spickett (2010). "The role of CELF proteins in neurological disorders." *RNA Biol* 7(4): 474-479.

Garcia-Lopez, A., B. Llamusi, M. Orzaez, E. Perez-Paya & R. D. Artero (2011). "In vivo discovery of a peptide that prevents CUG-RNA hairpin formation and reverses RNA toxicity in myotonic dystrophy models." *Proc Natl Acad Sci U S A* 108(29): 11866-11871.

Garcia-Lopez, A., L. Monferrer, I. Garcia-Alcover, M. Vicente-Crespo, M. C. Alvarez-Abril & R. D. Artero (2008). "Genetic and chemical modifiers of a CUG toxicity model in Drosophila." *PLoS One* 3(2): e1595.

Gareiss, P. C., K. Sobczak, B. R. McNaughton, P. B. Palde, C. A. Thornton & B. L. Miller (2008). "Dynamic combinatorial selection of molecules capable of inhibiting the (CUG) repeat RNA-MBNL1 interaction in vitro: discovery of lead compounds targeting myotonic dystrophy (DM1)." *J Am Chem Soc* 130(48): 16254-16261.

Goers, E. S., J. Purcell, R. B. Voelker, D. P. Gates & J. A. Berglund (2010). "MBNL1 binds GC motifs embedded in pyrimidines to regulate alternative splicing." *Nucleic Acids Res* 38(7): 2467-2484.

Hao, M., K. Akrami, K. Wei, C. De Diego, N. Che, J. H. Ku, J. Tidball, M. C. Graves, P. B. Shieh & F. Chen (2008). "Muscleblind-like 2 (Mbnl2) -deficient mice as a model for myotonic dystrophy." *Dev Dyn* 237(2): 403-410.

Harper, P. S. (1989). "Gene mapping and the muscular dystrophies." *Prog Clin Biol Res* 306: 29-49.

Ho, T. H., D. Bundman, D. L. Armstrong & T. A. Cooper (2005). "Transgenic mice expressing CUG-BP1 reproduce splicing mis-regulation observed in myotonic dystrophy." *Hum Mol Genet* 14(11): 1539-1547.

Ho, T. H., B. N. Charlet, M. G. Poulos, G. Singh, M. S. Swanson & T. A. Cooper (2004). "Muscleblind proteins regulate alternative splicing." *EMBO J* 23(15): 3103-3112.

Ho, T. H., R. S. Savkur, M. G. Poulos, M. A. Mancini, M. S. Swanson & T. A. Cooper (2005). "Colocalization of muscleblind with RNA foci is separable from mis-regulation of alternative splicing in myotonic dystrophy." *J Cell Sci* 118(Pt 13): 2923-2933.

Houseley, J. M., Z. Wang, G. J. Brock, J. Soloway, R. Artero, M. Perez-Alonso, K. M. O'Dell & D. G. Monckton (2005). "Myotonic dystrophy associated expanded CUG repeat muscleblind positive ribonuclear foci are not toxic to Drosophila." *Hum Mol Genet* 14(6): 873-883.

Jansen, G., P. J. Groenen, D. Bachner, P. H. Jap, M. Coerwinkel, F. Oerlemans, W. van den Broek, B. Gohlsch, D. Pette, J. J. Plomp, P. C. Molenaar, M. G. Nederhoff, C. J. van Echteld, M. Dekker, A. Berns, H. Hameister & B. Wieringa (1996). "Abnormal myotonic dystrophy protein kinase levels produce only mild myopathy in mice." *Nat Genet* 13(3): 316-324.

Jiang, H., A. Mankodi, M. S. Swanson, R. T. Moxley & C. A. Thornton (2004). "Myotonic dystrophy type 1 is associated with nuclear foci of mutant RNA, sequestration of muscleblind proteins and deregulated alternative splicing in neurons." *Hum Mol Genet* 13(24): 3079-3088.

Jungbluth, H., C. Wallgren-Pettersson & J. Laporte (2008). "Centronuclear (myotubular) myopathy." *Orphanet J Rare Dis* 3: 26.

Kanadia, R. N., K. A. Johnstone, A. Mankodi, C. Lungu, C. A. Thornton, D. Esson, A. M. Timmers, W. W. Hauswirth & M. S. Swanson (2003). "A muscleblind knockout model for myotonic dystrophy." *Science* 302(5652): 1978-1980.

Kanadia, R. N., J. Shin, Y. Yuan, S. G. Beattie, T. M. Wheeler, C. A. Thornton & M. S. Swanson (2006). "Reversal of RNA missplicing and myotonia after muscleblind overexpression in a mouse poly(CUG) model for myotonic dystrophy." *Proc Natl Acad Sci U S A* 103(31): 11748-11753.

Kanadia, R. N., C. R. Urbinati, V. J. Crusselle, D. Luo, Y. J. Lee, J. K. Harrison, S. P. Oh & M. S. Swanson (2003). "Developmental expression of mouse muscleblind genes Mbnl1, Mbnl2 and Mbnl3." *Gene Expr Patterns* 3(4): 459-462.

Kimura, T., M. Nakamori, J. D. Lueck, P. Pouliquin, F. Aoike, H. Fujimura, R. T. Dirksen, M. P. Takahashi, A. F. Dulhunty & S. Sakoda (2005). "Altered mRNA splicing of the skeletal muscle ryanodine receptor and sarcoplasmic/endoplasmic reticulum Ca2+-ATPase in myotonic dystrophy type 1." *Hum Mol Genet* 14(15): 2189-2200.

Kino, Y., D. Mori, Y. Oma, Y. Takeshita, N. Sasagawa & S. Ishiura (2004). "Muscleblind protein, MBNL1/EXP, binds specifically to CHHG repeats." *Hum Mol Genet* 13(5): 495-507.

Klein, A. F., E. Gasnier & D. Furling (2011). "Gain of RNA function in pathological cases: Focus on myotonic dystrophy." *Biochimie*.

Klesert, T. R., D. H. Cho, J. I. Clark, J. Maylie, J. Adelman, L. Snider, E. C. Yuen, P. Soriano & S. J. Tapscott (2000). "Mice deficient in Six5 develop cataracts: implications for myotonic dystrophy." *Nat Genet* 25(1): 105-109.

Klesert, T. R., A. D. Otten, T. D. Bird & S. J. Tapscott (1997). "Trinucleotide repeat expansion at the myotonic dystrophy locus reduces expression of DMAHP." *Nat Genet* 16(4): 402-406.

Koch, K. S. & H. L. Leffert (1998). "Giant hairpins formed by CUG repeats in myotonic dystrophy messenger RNAs might sterically block RNA export through nuclear pores." *J Theor Biol* 192(4): 505-514.

Koebis, M., N. Ohsawa, Y. Kino, N. Sasagawa, I. Nishino & S. Ishiura (2011). "Alternative splicing of myomesin 1 gene is aberrantly regulated in myotonic dystrophy type 1." *Genes Cells*.

Koshelev, M., S. Sarma, R. E. Price, X. H. Wehrens & T. A. Cooper (2010). "Heart-specific overexpression of CUGBP1 reproduces functional and molecular abnormalities of myotonic dystrophy type 1." *Hum Mol Genet* 19(6): 1066-1075.

Krol, J., A. Fiszer, A. Mykowska, K. Sobczak, M. de Mezer & W. J. Krzyzosiak (2007). "Ribonuclease dicer cleaves triplet repeat hairpins into shorter repeats that silence specific targets." *Mol Cell* 25(4): 575-586.

Kuyumcu-Martinez, N. M., G. S. Wang & T. A. Cooper (2007). "Increased steady-state levels of CUGBP1 in myotonic dystrophy 1 are due to PKC-mediated hyperphosphorylation." *Mol Cell* 28(1): 68-78.

Lange, S., I. Agarkova, J. C. Perriard & E. Ehler (2005). "The sarcomeric M-band during development and in disease." *J Muscle Res Cell Motil* 26(6-8): 375-379.

Langlois, M. A., C. Boniface, G. Wang, J. Alluin, P. M. Salvaterra, J. Puymirat, J. J. Rossi & N. S. Lee (2005). "Cytoplasmic and nuclear retained DMPK mRNAs are targets for RNA interference in myotonic dystrophy cells." *J Biol Chem* 280(17): 16949-16954.

Langlois, M. A., N. S. Lee, J. J. Rossi & J. Puymirat (2003). "Hammerhead ribozyme-mediated destruction of nuclear foci in myotonic dystrophy myoblasts." *Mol Ther* 7(5 Pt 1): 670-680.

Larkin, K. & M. Fardaei (2001). "Myotonic dystrophy--a multigene disorder." *Brain Res Bull* 56(3-4): 389-395.

Lee, K. S., Y. Cao, H. E. Witwicka, S. Tom, S. J. Tapscott & E. H. Wang (2010). "RNA-binding protein Muscleblind-like 3 (MBNL3) disrupts myocyte enhancer factor 2 (Mef2) {beta}-exon splicing." *J Biol Chem* 285(44): 33779-33787.

Lee, Y. B., C. P. Glover, A. S. Cosgrave, A. Bienemann & J. B. Uney (2005). "Optimizing regulatable gene expression using adenoviral vectors." *Exp Physiol* 90(1): 33-37.

Machuca-Tzili, L., D. Brook & D. Hilton-Jones (2005). "Clinical and molecular aspects of the myotonic dystrophies: a review." *Muscle Nerve* 32(1): 1-18.

Machuca-Tzili, L. E., S. Buxton, A. Thorpe, C. M. Timson, P. Wigmore, P. K. Luther & J. D. Brook (2011). "Zebrafish deficient for Muscleblind-like 2 exhibit features of myotonic dystrophy." *Dis Model Mech* 4(3): 381-392.

Mammarella, A., P. Ferroni, M. Paradiso, F. Martini, V. Paoletti, S. Morino, G. Antonini, P. P. Gazzaniga, A. Musca & S. Basili (2002). "Tumor necrosis factor-alpha and myocardial function in patients with myotonic dystrophy type 1." *J Neurol Sci* 201(1-2): 59-64.

Mankodi, A., X. Lin, B. C. Blaxall, M. S. Swanson & C. A. Thornton (2005). "Nuclear RNA foci in the heart in myotonic dystrophy." *Circ Res* 97(11): 1152-1155.

Mankodi, A., E. Logigian, L. Callahan, C. McClain, R. White, D. Henderson, M. Krym & C. A. Thornton (2000). "Myotonic dystrophy in transgenic mice expressing an expanded CUG repeat." *Science* 289(5485): 1769-1773.

Mankodi, A., M. P. Takahashi, H. Jiang, C. L. Beck, W. J. Bowers, R. T. Moxley, S. C. Cannon & C. A. Thornton (2002). "Expanded CUG repeats trigger aberrant splicing of ClC-1 chloride channel pre-mRNA and hyperexcitability of skeletal muscle in myotonic dystrophy." *Mol Cell* 10(1): 35-44.

Mankodi, A., P. Teng-Umnuay, M. Krym, D. Henderson, M. Swanson & C. A. Thornton (2003). "Ribonuclear inclusions in skeletal muscle in myotonic dystrophy types 1 and 2." *Ann Neurol* 54(6): 760-768.

Martorell, L., M. A. Pujana, J. Valero, J. Joven, V. Volpini, A. Labad, X. Estivill & E. Vilella (1999). "Anticipation is not associated with CAG repeat expansion in parent-offspring pairs of patients affected with schizophrenia." *Am J Med Genet* 88(1): 50-56.

Mastroyiannopoulos, N. P., E. Chrysanthou, T. C. Kyriakides, J. B. Uney, M. S. Mahadevan & L. A. Phylactou (2008). "The effect of myotonic dystrophy transcript levels and location on muscle differentiation." *Biochem Biophys Res Commun* 377(2): 526-531.

Mastroyiannopoulos, N. P., M. L. Feldman, J. B. Uney, M. S. Mahadevan & L. A. Phylactou (2005). "Woodchuck post-transcriptional element induces nuclear export of myotonic dystrophy 3' untranslated region transcripts." *EMBO Rep* 6(5): 458-463.

Mastroyiannopoulos, N. P., C. Shammas & L. A. Phylactou (2010). "Tackling the pathogenesis of RNA nuclear retention in myotonic dystrophy." *Biol Cell* 102(9): 515-523.

Michalowski, S., J. W. Miller, C. R. Urbinati, M. Paliouras, M. S. Swanson & J. Griffith (1999). "Visualization of double-stranded RNAs from the myotonic dystrophy protein kinase gene and interactions with CUG-binding protein." *Nucleic Acids Res* 27(17): 3534-3542.

Miller, J. W., C. R. Urbinati, P. Teng-Umnuay, M. G. Stenberg, B. J. Byrne, C. A. Thornton & M. S. Swanson (2000). "Recruitment of human muscleblind proteins to (CUG)(n) expansions associated with myotonic dystrophy." *EMBO J* 19(17): 4439-4448.

Monckton, D. G., L. J. Wong, T. Ashizawa & C. T. Caskey (1995). "Somatic mosaicism, germline expansions, germline reversions and intergenerational reductions in myotonic dystrophy males: small pool PCR analyses." *Hum Mol Genet* 4(1): 1-8.

Moxley, R. T., A. J. Corbett, K. L. Minaker & J. W. Rowe (1984). "Whole body insulin resistance in myotonic dystrophy." *Ann Neurol* 15(2): 157-162.

Mulders, S. A., W. J. van den Broek, T. M. Wheeler, H. J. Croes, P. van Kuik-Romeijn, S. J. de Kimpe, D. Furling, G. J. Platenburg, G. Gourdon, C. A. Thornton, B. Wieringa & D. G. Wansink (2009). "Triplet-repeat oligonucleotide-mediated reversal of RNA toxicity in myotonic dystrophy." *Proc Natl Acad Sci U S A* 106(33): 13915-13920.

Napierala, M. & W. J. Krzyzosiak (1997). "CUG repeats present in myotonin kinase RNA form metastable "slippery" hairpins." *J Biol Chem* 272(49): 31079-31085.

Ogata, A., S. Terae, M. Fujita & K. Tashiro (1998). "Anterior temporal white matter lesions in myotonic dystrophy with intellectual impairment: an MRI and neuropathological study." *Neuroradiology* 40(7): 411-415.

Okoli, G., N. Carey, K. J. Johnson & D. J. Watt (1998). "Over expression of the murine myotonic dystrophy protein kinase in the mouse myogenic C2C12 cell line leads to inhibition of terminal differentiation." *Biochem Biophys Res Commun* 246(3): 905-911.

Orengo, J. P., P. Chambon, D. Metzger, D. R. Mosier, G. J. Snipes & T. A. Cooper (2008). "Expanded CTG repeats within the DMPK 3' UTR causes severe skeletal muscle wasting in an inducible mouse model for myotonic dystrophy." *Proc Natl Acad Sci U S A* 105(7): 2646-2651.

Otten, A. D. & S. J. Tapscott (1995). "Triplet repeat expansion in myotonic dystrophy alters the adjacent chromatin structure." *Proc Natl Acad Sci U S A* 92(12): 5465-5469.

Philips, A. V., L. T. Timchenko & T. A. Cooper (1998). "Disruption of splicing regulated by a CUG-binding protein in myotonic dystrophy." *Science* 280(5364): 737-741.

Phillips, M. F. & P. S. Harper (1997). "Cardiac disease in myotonic dystrophy." *Cardiovasc Res* 33(1): 13-22.

Phylactou, L. A., C. Darrah & M. J. Wood (1998). "Ribozyme-mediated trans-splicing of a trinucleotide repeat." *Nat Genet* 18(4): 378-381.

Phylactou, L. A., M. W. Kilpatrick & M. J. Wood (1998). "Ribozymes as therapeutic tools for genetic disease." *Hum Mol Genet* 7(10): 1649-1653.

Pushechnikov, A., M. M. Lee, J. L. Childs-Disney, K. Sobczak, J. M. French, C. A. Thornton & M. D. Disney (2009). "Rational design of ligands targeting triplet repeating transcripts that cause RNA dominant disease: application to myotonic muscular dystrophy type 1 and spinocerebellar ataxia type 3." *J Am Chem Soc* 131(28): 9767-9779.

Ranum, L. P. & J. W. Day (2002). "Myotonic dystrophy: clinical and molecular parallels between myotonic dystrophy type 1 and type 2." *Curr Neurol Neurosci Rep* 2(5): 465-470.

Reddy, S., D. B. Smith, M. M. Rich, J. M. Leferovich, P. Reilly, B. M. Davis, K. Tran, H. Rayburn, R. Bronson, D. Cros, R. J. Balice-Gordon & D. Housman (1996). "Mice lacking the myotonic dystrophy protein kinase develop a late onset progressive myopathy." *Nat Genet* 13(3): 325-335.

Roberts, R., N. A. Timchenko, J. W. Miller, S. Reddy, C. T. Caskey, M. S. Swanson & L. T. Timchenko (1997). "Altered phosphorylation and intracellular distribution of a (CUG)n triplet repeat RNA-binding protein in patients with myotonic dystrophy and in myotonin protein kinase knockout mice." *Proc Natl Acad Sci U S A* 94(24): 13221-13226.

Rubinsztein, J. S., D. C. Rubinsztein, P. J. McKenna, S. Goodburn & A. J. Holland (1997). "Mild myotonic dystrophy is associated with memory impairment in the context of normal general intelligence." *J Med Genet* 34(3): 229-233.

Sabourin, L. A., K. Tamai, M. A. Narang & R. G. Korneluk (1997). "Overexpression of 3'-untranslated region of the myotonic dystrophy kinase cDNA inhibits myoblast differentiation in vitro." *J Biol Chem* 272(47): 29626-29635.

Salisbury, E., K. Sakai, B. Schoser, C. Huichalaf, C. Schneider-Gold, H. Nguyen, G. L. Wang, J. H. Albrecht & L. T. Timchenko (2008). "Ectopic expression of cyclin D3 corrects differentiation of DM1 myoblasts through activation of RNA CUG-binding protein, CUGBP1." *Exp Cell Res* 314(11-12): 2266-2278.

Santoro, M., A. Modoni, M. Masciullo, T. Gidaro, A. Broccolini, E. Ricci, P. A. Tonali & G. Silvestri (2010). "Analysis of MTMR1 expression and correlation with muscle pathological features in juvenile/adult onset myotonic dystrophy type 1 (DM1) and in myotonic dystrophy type 2 (DM2)." *Exp Mol Pathol* 89(2): 158-168.

Savkur, R. S., A. V. Philips & T. A. Cooper (2001). "Aberrant regulation of insulin receptor alternative splicing is associated with insulin resistance in myotonic dystrophy." *Nat Genet* 29(1): 40-47.

Sergeant, N., B. Sablonniere, S. Schraen-Maschke, A. Ghestem, C. A. Maurage, A. Wattez, P. Vermersch & A. Delacourte (2001). "Dysregulation of human brain microtubule-associated tau mRNA maturation in myotonic dystrophy type 1." *Hum Mol Genet* 10(19): 2143-2155.

Storbeck, C. J., S. Drmanic, K. Daniel, J. D. Waring, F. R. Jirik, D. J. Parry, N. Ahmed, L. A. Sabourin, J. E. Ikeda & R. G. Korneluk (2004). "Inhibition of myogenesis in transgenic mice expressing the human DMPK 3'-UTR." *Hum Mol Genet* 13(6): 589-600.

Takahashi, N., N. Sasagawa, K. Suzuki & S. Ishiura (2000). "The CUG-binding protein binds specifically to UG dinucleotide repeats in a yeast three-hybrid system." *Biochem Biophys Res Commun* 277(2): 518-523.

Taneja, K. L., M. McCurrach, M. Schalling, D. Housman & R. H. Singer (1995). "Foci of trinucleotide repeat transcripts in nuclei of myotonic dystrophy cells and tissues." *J Cell Biol* 128(6): 995-1002.

Tapscott, S. J. & C. A. Thornton (2001). "Biomedicine. Reconstructing myotonic dystrophy." *Science* 293(5531): 816-817.

Tedeschi, L., C. Lande, A. Cecchettini & L. Citti (2009). "Hammerhead ribozymes in therapeutic target discovery and validation." *Drug Discov Today* 14(15-16): 776-783.

Tian, B., R. J. White, T. Xia, S. Welle, D. H. Turner, M. B. Mathews & C. A. Thornton (2000). "Expanded CUG repeat RNAs form hairpins that activate the double-stranded RNA-dependent protein kinase PKR." *RNA* 6(1): 79-87.

Timchenko, L. T., J. W. Miller, N. A. Timchenko, D. R. DeVore, K. V. Datar, L. Lin, R. Roberts, C. T. Caskey & M. S. Swanson (1996). "Identification of a (CUG)n triplet repeat RNA-binding protein and its expression in myotonic dystrophy." *Nucleic Acids Res* 24(22): 4407-4414.

Timchenko, L. T., N. A. Timchenko, C. T. Caskey & R. Roberts (1996). "Novel proteins with binding specificity for DNA CTG repeats and RNA CUG repeats: implications for myotonic dystrophy." *Hum Mol Genet* 5(1): 115-121.

Timchenko, N. A., Z. J. Cai, A. L. Welm, S. Reddy, T. Ashizawa & L. T. Timchenko (2001). "RNA CUG repeats sequester CUGBP1 and alter protein levels and activity of CUGBP1." *J Biol Chem* 276(11): 7820-7826.

Timchenko, N. A., P. Iakova, Z. J. Cai, J. R. Smith & L. T. Timchenko (2001). "Molecular basis for impaired muscle differentiation in myotonic dystrophy." *Mol Cell Biol* 21(20): 6927-6938.

Timchenko, N. A., R. Patel, P. Iakova, Z. J. Cai, L. Quan & L. T. Timchenko (2004). "Overexpression of CUG triplet repeat-binding protein, CUGBP1, in mice inhibits myogenesis." *J Biol Chem* 279(13): 13129-13139.

Vihola, A., G. Bassez, G. Meola, S. Zhang, H. Haapasalo, A. Paetau, E. Mancinelli, A. Rouche, J. Y. Hogrel, P. Laforet, T. Maisonobe, J. F. Pellissier, R. Krahe, B. Eymard & B. Udd (2003). "Histopathological differences of myotonic dystrophy type 1 (DM1) and PROMM/DM2." *Neurology* 60(11): 1854-1857.

Wang, G. S., D. L. Kearney, M. De Biasi, G. Taffet & T. A. Cooper (2007). "Elevation of RNA-binding protein CUGBP1 is an early event in an inducible heart-specific mouse model of myotonic dystrophy." *J Clin Invest* 117(10): 2802-2811.

Wang, G. S., M. N. Kuyumcu-Martinez, S. Sarma, N. Mathur, X. H. Wehrens & T. A. Cooper (2009). "PKC inhibition ameliorates the cardiac phenotype in a mouse model of myotonic dystrophy type 1." *J Clin Invest* 119(12): 3797-3806.

Wang, Y. H. & J. Griffith (1995). "Expanded CTG triplet blocks from the myotonic dystrophy gene create the strongest known natural nucleosome positioning elements." *Genomics* 25(2): 570-573.

Ward, A. J., M. Rimer, J. M. Killian, J. J. Dowling & T. A. Cooper (2010). "CUGBP1 overexpression in mouse skeletal muscle reproduces features of myotonic dystrophy type 1." Hum Mol Genet 19(18): 3614-3622.

Warf, M. B., M. Nakamori, C. M. Matthys, C. A. Thornton & J. A. Berglund (2009). "Pentamidine reverses the splicing defects associated with myotonic dystrophy." Proc Natl Acad Sci U S A 106(44): 18551-18556.

Westerlaken, J. H., C. E. Van der Zee, W. Peters & B. Wieringa (2003). "The DMWD protein from the myotonic dystrophy (DM1) gene region is developmentally regulated and is present most prominently in synapse-dense brain areas." Brain Res 971(1): 116-127.

Wheeler, T. M., M. C. Krym & C. A. Thornton (2007). "Ribonuclear foci at the neuromuscular junction in myotonic dystrophy type 1." Neuromuscul Disord 17(3): 242-247.

Wheeler, T. M., J. D. Lueck, M. S. Swanson, R. T. Dirksen & C. A. Thornton (2007). "Correction of ClC-1 splicing eliminates chloride channelopathy and myotonia in mouse models of myotonic dystrophy." J Clin Invest 117(12): 3952-3957.

Wheeler, T. M., K. Sobczak, J. D. Lueck, R. J. Osborne, X. Lin, R. T. Dirksen & C. A. Thornton (2009). "Reversal of RNA dominance by displacement of protein sequestered on triplet repeat RNA." Science 325(5938): 336-339.

Wojciechowska, M. & W. J. Krzyzosiak (2011). "Cellular toxicity of expanded RNA repeats: focus on RNA foci." Hum Mol Genet.

Zhang, L., J. E. Lee, J. Wilusz & C. J. Wilusz (2008). "The RNA-binding protein CUGBP1 regulates stability of tumor necrosis factor mRNA in muscle cells: implications for myotonic dystrophy." J Biol Chem 283(33): 22457-22463.

8

Duchenne Muscular Dystrophy: Experimental Models on Physical Therapy

Thais Gaiad[1], Karla Araujo[2],
Fátima Caromano[3] and Carlos Eduardo Ambrosio[4]
[1]*Department of Physical Therapy, University of
Jequitinhonha and Mucuri Valley – UFVJM,*
[2]*Department of Surgery, Sector of Anatomy, University of São Paulo – USP,*
[3]*Department of Physical Therapy, University of São Paulo – USP,*
[4]*Department of Basic Science, University of São Paulo – USP,*
Brazil

1. Introduction

Neuromuscular disorders are a heterogeneous group of genetic diseases. Nowadays, more than 30 genetically defined forms are recognized and, in the last decade, mutations in several genes have been reported to result in the deficiency or loss of function of a variety of important muscle proteins (Shelton & Engvall, 2005). Defects in components of the dystrophin-glycoprotein complex (DGC) are known to be an important cause of different forms of muscular dystrophies (Ervasti & Campbell 1993; Yoshida & Ozawa 1990). Lack of dystrophin protein in muscle cells is characteristic of Duchenne muscular dystrophy (DMD), which is a progressive and fatal X-linked genetic disorder. Many animal models have been studied to identify an efficient treatment for this disease in humans. Two mammalian models of DMD have been widely used in preclinical trials to understand the pathogenesis of the disease and development of efficient therapeutic strategies for humans. *Mdx*-mouse is the most used animal model for DMD, followed by the Golden Retriever Muscular Dystrophy (GRMD) canine model. *Mdx*-mouse morphology displays some features of muscle degeneration, but the pathogenesis of the disease is comparatively mild. This model has a slightly shorter life spam as compared to wild-type controls (Banks & Chamberlain, 2008) and muscle degeneration is different from the one seen in DMD patients. An important degeneration and regeneration of muscle fibers is observed at a young age in the *mdx*-mouse (2 to 4 weeks), which results in the muscle morphological changes of centralized nuclei and heterogeneity of fiber size. Necrosis is also observed at this early age but decreases around sixty days. Loss of muscle tissue is slow and muscle weakness is not evident until later in life. Fibrosis, a marked feature of DMD muscle, is less pronounced in *mdx*-mouse, with the exception of diaphragm muscle (Hueber et al., 2008). Dystrophin deficiency has also been reported in cats as hypertrophic feline muscular dystrophy (HFMD), in which diaphragmatic hypertrophy is often fatal (Shelton & Engvall, 2005). Similar to *mdx* pathology, the skeletal muscle of the HFMD cats undergoes repeated cycles of degeneration and regeneration but does not develop the debilitating fibrosis that is characteristic of both DMD and the canine GRMD model (Hoffman & Gorospe, 1991). The GRMD model has been widely studied (Collins & Morgan, 2003) since it presents muscle abnormalities that are closest to the ones seen in humans: increased creatine kinase (CK) activity, muscle hypotrophy associated with contractures, muscle necrosis, degeneration, endomysial and perimysial fibrosis and cardiomyopathy (Howell et al., 1997). This model also presents repeated cycles of muscular necrosis and regeneration, muscle wasting, postural abnormalities, respiratory or heart failure and premature death, as seen in DMD patients (Valentine et al., 1988). Despite the phenotype variability of this model, it has been used due to the strong similarities of body weight and pathological expression of the disease in human (Collins & Morgan, 2003). Since the coding sequence of the dystrophin gene was discovered in 1987, no treatment has been found to stop DMD progression. To improve quality of life and prevent complications of this progressive disease, patients have access to supportive therapies such as motor and respiratory physical therapy, occupational therapy, psychology, nutritional supplements and corticosteroids. Although these therapies cannot cure DMD, they should be well investigated as they intend to lead these patients to a better quality of life and to decrease the complications of their degenerative and progressive illness. Physical therapy (PT) has been used to reduce muscular, cardiac and vascular abnormalities which develop in association with muscle strength loss (Gaiad et al., 2009). The main objective of such motor physical therapy is the prevention of muscle contractures and bone deformities (Strober, 2006). However, motor PT approaches have yielded controversial recommendations (Carter et al., 2002) and there is no consensus regarding the type and intensity of PT (Cup et al., 2007). Just as other muscular dystrophies, DMD is a progressive disorder which causes death by cardiac or respiratory failure. Nevertheless, the absence of dystrophin in the sarcolema of muscle cells makes DMD a special illness regarding therapeutic exercise prescription. Research using animal models can answer questions regarding which are the best type, frequency, and intensity of therapeutic exercise, as well as highlight a beneficial approach of PT for DMD patients. This chapter aims to detail some actual studies using *mdx* and GRMD models which reported new insights in this subject contributing to future research designs of therapeutic exercise on dystrophic muscle.

2. Duchenne muscular dystrophy (DMD)

Dystrophin is located beneath the sarcolemma and is part of a large dystroglycan complex termed the dystrophin-glycoprotein complex (DGC), which includes the dystroglican complex (α and β), sarcoglycan complex (α, β, γ and δ) and syntrophin/dystrobrevin subcomplexes (Ervasti & Campbell, 1991). DGC forms a critical link for force transmission between the contractile machinery of the muscle fiber and the extracellular matrix. Where dystrophin is defective or absent, the myofiber is fragile and the sarcolemma is readily damaged in response to exercise, leading to myofiber necrosis (Hoffman et al., 1987; Sharp et al., 1989). The absence of dystrophin in dystrophic muscles leads to altered myofiber integrity, perturbed calcium homeostasis, and activation of the calcium-dependent calpain proteases and necrosis (Straub et al., 1997). The other consequence of the loss of dystrophin is the absence or great reduction of components of the DGC, as described for skeletal muscle fibers from DMD patients and the *mdx* mouse (Ervasti et al., 1990; Ohlendieck & Campbell, 1991). Loss of dystrophin leads to membrane leakiness as a result of mechanical or hypoosmotic stress. Consequently, Ca^{2+} permeability is increased and various Ca^{2+} dependent proteases such as calpain are activated under conditions of dystrophin deficiency. It has also been proposed that alteration of the expression or function of plasma membrane proteins associated with dystrophin such as neuronal nitric oxide synthase (nNOS) and various ion channels are involved in the molecular mechanisms of muscle degeneration (Straub et al., 1997). Although the defective gene of dystrophin was identified in 1987, there is still no effective treatment for DMD patients. While cell or gene therapy to replace the defective dystrophin is the ideal solution, the clinical application of such therapies has yet to become a reality (Davies & Grounds, 2006; Foster et al., 2006). The existing treatment for DMD is administration of corticosteroids, broad-based anti-inflammatory drugs that decrease inflammatory cell populations in dystrophic muscle and increase myofiber mass. However, their precise mechanism of action in DMD is not yet known and is under intense investigation (Griggs et al., 1993; Connolly et al., 2002). Disadvantages of steroid treatment include their association with severe adverse side effects such as weight gain and osteoporosis and the variable response by the individuals undergoing treatment (Muntoni et al., 2002; Moxley et al., 2005).

3. Animal models for neuromuscular diseases

Several animal models that have been identified in nature or generated in laboratory present the phenotypes observed in neuromuscular diseases. These models generally present physiological symptoms observed in human patients and can be used as important tools for genetic, clinic, and histopathological studies (Vainzof et al., 2008). Animal models are essential for elucidation of the disease pathogenicity and for assessment of efficacy and toxicity during therapy development. Two mammalian models of DMD have been widely used in preclinical trials to understand the pathogenesis of the disease and to develop efficient therapeutic strategies for humans. *Mdx*-mouse is the most used animal model for DMD, followed by the Golden Retriever Muscular Dystrophy (GRMD) canine model.

3.1 Mouse model (*mdx*-mouse)

A mouse X-chromosome mutant (*mdx*) was first discovered in 1984 due to the observations of elevated plasma levels of muscle creatine kinase and pyruvate kinase enzymes and histological lesions characteristic of muscular dystrophy. In the *mdx* model the mutations cause a premature stop codon in exon 23 due a single base substitution (Sicinski et al., 1989). *Mdx*-mouse shows a mild non-progressive phenotype associated with comparatively moderate muscle pathology and muscle degeneration followed by subsequent significant regeneration (Dangain & Vrbova, 1984). Though the mouse models have slightly shorter life spans compared to wild-type controls (Banks & Chamberlain, 2008), they are indispensable for elucidation of the pathogenic mechanism and for development of therapeutic approaches, since they can be easily and reliably reproduced (Nakamura & Takeda, 2011).

3.1.1 Pathogenesis in the *mdx* mouse

Muscle degeneration in the *mdx* mouse is different from that seen in DMD patients. The progression of pathology in the *mdx* mouse is influenced by growth (Grounds, 2008) and may be divided into three main phases: (1) the pre-weaning phase (0–3 weeks of age), which is strongly influenced by growth and corresponds roughly to the first 6 months of human patients, (2) the post-weaning phase, with an acute onset of pathology around 3 weeks, followed at about 8 weeks by (3) the adult phase with a reduced low level of chronic damage that persists throughout life (Willmann et al., 2011). An important degeneration and regeneration of muscle fibers is observed at a young age of *mdx*-mouse (2 to 4 weeks) which results in the muscle morphological changes such as centralized nuclei and heterogeneity of fiber size. In mature limb muscle, the murine model is characterized by successive degeneration/regeneration processes and does not exhibit the progressive muscle wasting and accumulation of connective tissue observed during development of the human disease (Coulton et al., 1988). Necrosis is also observed at this early age but decreases around sixty days. Loss of muscle tissue is slow and muscle weakness is not evident until later in life. Fibrosis, a marked feature of DMD muscle, is less pronounced in *mdx*-mouse, with the exception of diaphragm muscle (Hueber et al., 2008). For this reason, histological analysis of the diaphragm, one of the most severely affected muscles of the *mdx*, is often used as a marker of weakness progression, once it reproduces the degenerative changes of muscular dystrophy.

3.2 Feline muscular dystrophy

Dystrophin deficiency has also been reported in cats, called hypertrophic feline muscular dystrophy (HFMD). The HFMD cat has a large deletion of muscle and Purkinje promoters resulting in a lack of dystrophin in the skeletal and cardiac muscle. These animals have a unique phenotypic expression of hypertrophy of the tongue, neck, and shoulder muscles, lingual calcification, excessive salivation, megaesophagus, gait disturbance manifesting as bunny hopping, dilated cardiomyopathy, hepatosplenomegaly, and kidney failure (Winand et al., 1994). Diaphragmatic hypertrophy is the principal cause of death in these animals (Shelton & Engvall, 2005). Similar to *mdx* pathology, the skeletal muscle of the HFMD cat undergoes repeated cycles of degeneration and regeneration but does not develop the debilitating fibrosis that is characteristic of both DMD and GRMD (Hoffman & Gorospe, 1991). Muscular dystrophy associated with absence of Merosin (laminin α2) was described in cats that presented muscle atrophy and marked weakness or progressive spasticity and contractions, as well as the serum creatine kinase (CK) at moderate levels (O'Brien et al., 2001). Other muscular dystrophies that have been reported are α-dystroglycan deficiency in Sphynx and Devon Rex cats (Martin et al., 2008) and reduced β- sarcoglycan in a shorthair male cat (Salvadori et al., 2009).

3.3 Canine muscular dystrophy

Numerous sporadic cases of canine muscular dystrophy have been recognized in the last two decades, but the Golden Retriever Muscular Dystrophy (GRMD) has been the most extensively examined and characterized (Cooper et al., 1988). GRMD is a degenerative myopathy homologue to Duchenne muscular dystrophy (DMD) in humans. A frame-shift point mutation in the dystrophin gene is responsible for the GRMD phenotype (Sharp et al., 1992), whereas deletions are the most frequent mutations in DMD patients. Nevertheless, in both DMD and GRMD patients, dystrophin protein is lacking (Hoffman et al., 1987; Cooper et al., 1988). Canine dystrophinopathies have also been reported in many other purebred and mixed breed dogs. In addition to the Golden Retriever (Kornegay et al., 1988), genetic mutations have also been characterized in Labrador Retriever (Bergman et al., 2002; Cosford et al., 2008), Irish Terrier (Wentink et al., 1972), German shorthaired pointer (Schatzberg et al., 1999), Samoieda (Presthus & Nordstoga, 1993), Japanese Spitz (Jones et al., 2004), English Spaniel (Van Ham et al., 1995), Old English Sheepdog (Wieczorek et al., 2006), Schnauzer miniature (Paola et al.,1993), Weimaraner (Baltzer et al., 2007), and Boston Terrier (Deitz et al., 2008). GRMD dogs closely resemble DMD patients in terms of both body weight and in the pathological expression of the disease (Collins & Morgan, 2003). However, their phenotype is variable (Banks & Chamberlain, 2008), as some pups survive only for a few days, while others are ambulant for months or even years (Ambrosio et al, 2008). Animal trials employing these dogs have substantial animal welfare implications and high costs associated with both maintenance and treatment (Nakamura & Takeda, 2011).

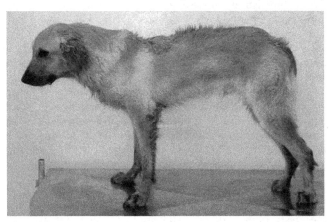

Fig. 1. Golden Retriever muscular dystrophy dog (GRMD model). (Ambrosio et al. 2009)

Researchers have developed a strain of medium sized dystrophic Beagles, designated as canine X-linked muscular dystrophy in Japan (CXMDj). They show atrophy and weakness of limb muscles which appear at 2-3 months, followed by development of macroglossia, dysphasia, gait disturbance, and joint contracture around 4 months of age. These symptoms rapidly progress until around 10 months of age, after which the progression of the disease is retarded (Shimatsu et al., 2005). The GSHPMD (German shorthaired pointer muscular dystrophy) is a spontaneous canine dystrophin 'knockout' model with complete lack of dystrophin immune reactivity. These dogs have been useful for dystrophin gene therapy trials, myoblast transfer, and in combination of the two. Any dystrophin transcripts or protein detected in GSHP skeletal muscle after therapeutic intervention could therefore only be produced by the dystrophin delivery vehicle (Schatzberg et al., 1999). Due to the common genetic basis of the disease in dog and human, the GRMD and other inbred dystrophic dog lines descended from animals with spontaneous mutations have been extensively used in preclinical settings, particularly for cell and gene therapy studies. An interesting Becker-like dystrophy with a truncated form of dystrophin was recently identified in a family of Japanese Spitz dogs (Jones et al., 2004). In these dogs, a 70–80 kDa protein on immunoblots that reacted with antibodies to the C-terminal domain of dystrophin was found, but not with antibodies to the rod domain. Canine models with deficient sarcoglycan (SG) proteins have been identified in Boston Terriers and Cocker Spaniels. The phenotype includes failure to thrive and exercise intolerance. Serum CK is highly elevated, and muscle histopathology shows a dystrophic pattern and a variable degree of loss of SG proteins staining (Shelton & Engvall 2005). A dystrophic myopathy should be considered in any young dog or cat (male or female, mixed breed or purebred) with persistent muscle weakness, muscle atrophy or hypertrophy, gait abnormality, or contractures beginning in the first few months of life

(Shelton & Engvall, 2002). The breed of an affected animal is one of the most useful distinguishing diagnostic criteria. A DNA-based test is commercially available for the dystrophin mutation in Golden Retrievers, but not yet for mutations in dystrophin or related proteins in other breeds. Diagnosis of Muscular Dystrophy (MD) in companion animals has been based on clinical presentation, markedly elevated serum creatine kinase concentration, and the presence of a dystrophic phenotype based on histopathological evaluation of muscle biopsy specimens (Shelton, 2010). Such analysis can be done by immunohistochemical localizations of dystrophin, dystrophin-associated proteins, laminin and other proteins. This is a cost-effective and sensitive method which can be performed directly on fresh-frozen biopsy specimens. Results of immunohistochemical staining using various monoclonal and polyclonal antibodies against skeletal muscle proteins involved in the muscular dystrophies can guide the direction of mutational analyses and development of diagnostic tests for specific mutations (Shelton, 2004). Serum CK activity should be part of every neuromuscular minimum database, most importantly for preneuter evaluations in young dogs because increased activity may be an early indicator of underlying muscle disease. Marked or persistent increases of CK activity may be indicative of a congenital or inherited muscle disease even if the animal is clinically asymptomatic (Shelton, 2010). The most marked increases in serum CK activity (420,000 U/L) are associated with necrotizing myopathies or MD (Kornegay et al., 1988; Bergman et al., 2002).

3.3.1 Pathogenesis in the GRMD dog

Mutations in the dystrophin protein result in membrane damage allowing massive infiltration of immune cells, chronic inflammation, necrosis, and severe muscle degeneration (Valentine et al., 1990b). The histopathological changes in the muscle are similar to the ones seen in humans and include muscle fiber degeneration and regeneration, fiber splitting, numerous fibers with centralized myonuclei, and intense connective tissue replacement. Myofiber hypertrophy and variability in myofiber size are likely to be an early change associated with dystrophin deficiency rather than a compensatory mechanism related to muscle impairment (Hoffman & Gorospe, 1991). Dystrophin deficiency in *mdx* mice and HFMD cats does not lead to significant muscle weakness (Hoffman & Gorospe, 1991). GRMD dogs, as well as DMD patients, suffer from repeated cycles of muscular necrosis and regeneration, muscle wasting and fibrosis, postural abnormalities, respiratory or heart failure, and premature death (Valentine et al, 1988). The clinical signs in GRMD dogs include the gradual loss of muscle mass and the development of contractures that often lead to skeletal deformities (Cooper et al., 1988). A prominent feature in dystrophic dogs is enlargement of the base of the tongue due to muscle fiber hypertrophy and pseudohypertrophy. Dysphagia, regurgitation and drooling associated with pharyngeal and esophageal dysfunction can be observed (Shelton and Engvall, 2005). GRMD dogs can present difficulty in opening the mouth, exercise intolerance, and atrophy of the trunk, limbs and *temporallis* muscle (Valentine et al., 1988). Elevation of serum CK is a feature of both canine and human muscular dystrophies (Cooper et al., 1998; Valentine et al., 1988). CK values were significantly elevated in GRMD dogs and increased with exercise. Serum ALT activity was also elevated, a finding which has been identified in Duchenne-like muscular dystrophy in dogs. The degree of elevation of the CK and ALT did not correlate with the severity of the clinical signs in any dog (Valentine et al, 1990a, Ambrosio et al., 2009). Gaiad et al. (2011) have found no correlation between clinical features or premature death in GRMD dogs and CK levels. Female dogs present a variety of clinical signs including generalized weakness, muscle wasting, tremors, exercise intolerance, gait abnormalities, and limb deformity. Elevation of serum creatine kinase activity may vary (Shelton et al., 2001). The gait abnormalities in GRMD dogs during growth and disease progression using an ambulatory gait analyzer (3D-accelerometers) showed that speed, stride length, total power and force had already significantly decreased (p < 0.01) at the age of 2 months. The decrease of stride frequency was a later event, secondarily contributing to the reduction of speed (Barthélémy et al., 2011).

3.3.2 Therapeutic approaches using canine model of muscular dystrophy

Papers have been recently published using the canine model of muscular dystrophy to develop various therapeutic approaches such as gene therapy, cell therapy, and pharmaceutical agents. As an animal model for DMD therapy, GRMD dogs were used in preclinical trials examining the transfer of dystrophin gene (Howell et al., 1998), utrophin gene (Cerletti et al., 2003) or oligonucleotides (Bartlett et al., 2000). These therapeutic strategies were all applied to a single muscle after local intramuscular injection. However, dystrophin deficiency appears as a generalized muscle defect, therefore achieving clinically relevant improvement may likely require intravascular delivery of genetic material. Gene therapy using viral vectors has been extensively investigated. Adeno-associated virus (AAV) vectors are the most appropriate tools for viral vector gene therapy because they are nonpathogenic due to a replication defect and have low immunogenicity as well as an effective ability to infect non dividing cells (Nakamura & Takeda, 2011). The intravenous administration of a dystrophin cDNA plasmid in the dystrophin-deficient *mdx* mouse resulted in significant dystrophin expression (Liu et al., 2001). This gene transfer was carried out on 5-week-old *mdx* mice diaphragm muscles, in which fibrosis is still minimal. It is not certain that similar gene transfer efficiency would be achieved in heavily compromised muscles, such as those occurring in GRMD and DMD. However, the treatment using myoblast or mesenchymal stem cell implantation in GRMD dogs during the early 1990s did not show improvement of muscle condition, even though other studies had demonstrated success in the mdx mouse. Similarly, hematopoietic stem cell transplantation did not restore dystrophin expression in affected dogs despite promising results in mdx mice (Dell'Agnola et al., 2004). In older GRMD dogs, fibrosis seems to be the major factor influencing microvascular architecture in skeletal muscles. Increasing extent of connective tissue correlated with lower microvessel density and longer intercapillary distance. The fibrosis might create a physical barrier between the capillary contour and the myofiber membrane. Thus, endomysial fibrosis, the hallmark of muscle pathology in DMD patients and GRMD dogs, may compromise intravascular therapeutic trials performed in the late stage of the dystrophic process. Anti-fibrotic treatment may be a necessary prerequisite to systemic genetic transfer in dystrophin-deficient canine and human muscles (Nguyen et al., 2005). Among these therapeutic strategies, exon skipping using antisense oligonucleotides (AOs) is considered to be one of the most promising therapies for the restoration of dystrophin expression at the sarcolemma in dystrophin-deficient muscle. The therapy involves a multiexon-skipping technique for targeting exons 6 and 8 to convert an out-of-frame mutation into an in-frame mutation using PMOs (Yokota et al., 2009). Kerkis et al. (2008) have reported the transplantation of human immature dental pulp stem cells from baby teeth to GRMD dogs by local and systemic via. Moreover, they have analyzed the efficiency of single and consecutive early transplantation of these cells. Their results show that Human Immature Dental Pulp Stem Cells (hIDPSC) presented significant engraftment in GRMD dog muscles, although human dystrophin expression was modest and limited to several muscle fibers. Better clinical condition was also observed in the dog which received monthly arterial injections and was still clinically stable at 25 months of age. Systemic myostatin inhibition in GRMD dogs by liver directed gene transfer of a vector designed to express a secreted negative myostatin peptide showed increase in muscle mass in these dogs assessed by MRI (Magnetic Resonance Imaging) and confirmed by muscle histology (Bish et al., 2011).

4. Pre-clinical therapeutic studies using animal models

The availability of standardized operating procedures (SOPs) to unify experimental protocols used to test the effects of new treatment in animal models is a step that will undoubtedly improve the comparability of studies from different laboratories (http://www.treat-nmd.eu/research/preclinical/dmd-sops/). To date, the main attempt to evaluate the relative translational benefit from an animal species to human subjects has focused on the minimal levels of dystrophin protein required for functional stabilization of dystrophic myofibers. Many factors need to be considered. This protective effect will depend not only on the amount of dystrophin protein within an individual myofibers, but also on the extent of distribution within all myofibers, the size of the nuclear domain (how far dystrophin protein extends along the sarcolema from the myonuclei where the mRNA is generated) and on when during development the dystrophin must be produced (Willmann et al., 2011). This situation was considered by Chamberlain (1997) who concluded from analysis of mosaic transgenic mice and viral vector delivery with suboptimal doses into *mdx* mice, that >50% of myofibers need to express dystrophin, and that these must accumulate approximately 20% of wild-type levels of dystrophin for a significant correction of the muscle pathology in mice. Factors to consider in the selection of outcome measurements (Determination and evaluation of the results of an activity, plan, process, or program and their comparison with the intended or projected results) for pre-clinical therapeutic studies using mouse model include reproducibility, objectivity, blind assessment, relevance to disease biology (e.g. muscle histology), and similarity of measures in the *mdx* mice (e.g. locomotion and in vivo muscle strength) to human clinical trials endpoints (e.g. ability to walk and muscle strength testing). Depending on the presumed mechanism of action and the intended target of the experimental agent, additional outcome measures (e.g. to assess cardiac function) may be appropriate (Willmann et al., 2011). Standardized protocols for the assessment of most of the recommended parameters have already been produced by specialized working groups of experts and are reported in brackets (PDFs available http://www.treat-nmd.eu/research/preclinical/dmd-models/). Based on the mechanism of action, different drugs may be more or less effective depending on the age at which treatment is initiated and the time period over which the drug is administered (i.e. treatment duration). Due to the ultimate translational aim of the pre-clinical experiments, it is important to consider the relationship between the age of the *mdx* mice and possible equivalence in DMD patients. A comparison of developmental stages in mice and humans is described in details elsewhere (Grounds et al., 2008). The recovery score is a tool that can be used to compare different therapies applied to mice or results obtained by different laboratories with the same therapy.

$$\text{Recovery score } (\%) \frac{[\text{treated}mdx] - [\text{untreated}mdx]}{[\text{wild type}] - [\text{untreated}mdx]} \times 100$$

A score of 100% indicates that the parameter in treated *mdx* mice is equal to that of control wild type mice, and 0% indicates that no improvement was obtained relative to untreated *mdx* mice (Gillis et al., 2002) Therefore, this calculation represents a tool to evaluate the effective recovery achieved by the treatment tested. Although this implies the need to include a wild type group of mice in any pre-clinical therapeutic study, we encourage the calculation of the recovery score in all studies where this effort is feasible (Willmann et al., 2011). Measurements of muscle strength, joint contractures, and timed function tests were made in dogs to evaluate recovery of muscular function after drugs or gene therapy. The evaluation of muscle by magnetic resonance imaging (MRI) was performed by Kornegay et al. (2010) after single intravenous injection of an AAV9 vector (1.5×1014 vector genomes/kg) carrying a human codon-optimized human mini-dystrophin gene under control of the cytomegalovirus (CMV) promoter. Earlier, the same research group performed analysis of muscle strength by measuring isometric force decrement after eccentric contraction (Childers et al., 2002) and by measuring the titanic isometric force at the tibiotarsal joint in vivo (Kornegay et al., 1994). The MRI evaluation has several strengths that include studying distribution of pathology, pathophysiology, monitoring of therapies, assessment of heart and diaphragm, and morphometry (Bish et al., 2011).

5. What's new on exercise training that can guide physical therapy for DMD related to *mdx* and GRMD models?

The coding sequence of the dystrophin gene in DMD was discovered and deciphered in 1987 (Koenig et al., 1987). Its discovery has brought hope for a cure of DMD through gene therapy, although it has not happened yet. Several therapeutic strategies are being investigated in developing a cure for this disease. Nowadays, DMD patients have access to therapeutic and supportive care aiming to prevent complications and improve their quality of life. Among them, drug therapy with corticosteroids has been widely studied in DMD and there is some controversy in its use mainly due to its multiple side effects. Nutritional supplements, psychology, occupational and physical therapy are the most used supportive therapies.

Although these therapies cannot lead to a cure of DMD, they should be well investigated because they intend to lead these patients to a better quality of life and to decrease complications of their degenerative and progressive illness. Physical therapy (PT) has been used to reduce muscular, skeletal, cardiac, and vascular abnormalities which develop in association with muscle strength loss (Gaiad et al., 2009). The main objective of such motor therapy is the prevention of muscle contractures and bone deformities (Strober, 2006). However, motor PT approaches have yielded controversial recommendations (Carter et al., 2002) and there is no consensus regarding the type and intensity of physical therapy (Cup et al., 2007). The recommendations often include exercise therapy to improve or preserve muscle strength or endurance and aerobic capacity to prevent the secondary problems of contractures, pain and fatigue. According to the review published by Grange & Call (2007) the same exercise used to increase muscle strength and endurance in normal individuals can exacerbate muscle damage in a dystrophic muscle. The authors suggested that a threshold must be defined to guide suitable exercise prescription for DMD patients (Grange & Call, 2007; Cup et al., 2007). Kimura et al. (2006) showed in a case report that immobility could reduce muscle fiber necrosis in muscular dystrophy cases. They reported a case of a three-year-old boy with a diagnosis of spina bifida and DMD. A muscle biopsy on this patient showed that necrosis and regeneration of muscle fiber was more prevalent in the biceps brachii (with normal movement) than in the gastrocnemius muscle (without movement). The authors suggest that immobility reduces muscle fiber necrosis in dystrophin-deficient muscle and attribute this characteristic to the movement restriction in the lower extremity of this patient. Reduced physical activity by *mdx* mice could theoretically be a muscle sparing strategy (Landisch et al., 2008). On the other hand, authors suggest that patients should undergo some physical activity in order to avoid muscle disuse associated with the intrinsic loss of muscle mass related to the disease progression (Ansved, 2005; Eagle, 2002, McDonald, 2002 and Caromano, 1999). Once physical therapies display an important role on DMD patients' quality of life, the prescription of its parameters must be evidence-based and well documented. In the last few years, some researchers have brought some insights into the subject of therapeutic exercise using experimental animal models for DMD. There are many publications on gene, cellular and pharmacological therapies using the DMD animal models, *mdx*-mice and GRMD dogs, but these models also have much remaining to contribute to the therapeutic exercise approach (Mercuri et al., 2008). The contribution of animal models, mainly the GRMD model, on prescription of type, frequency and modality of PT was also suggested by Grange & Call (2007).

According to Markert et al. (2011) the effect of exercise on DMD has poorly researched parameters (frequency, intensity, time and type) and until now it is unknown whether therapeutic exercise is beneficial or detrimental to dystrophic skeletal muscle. Despite the difference between *mdx*-mice and humans DMD patients in terms of regenerative ability and compensatory protein expression, this model is still the most used one to investigate exercise prescription for this population. Reasons for the wide use of *mdx*-mouse, despite its limitations, are well detailed in the first topic of this chapter.

In 2002, Eagle published a consensus about exercise recommendations for patients with neuromuscular disorders. Among them, they suggest maintenance or improvement of muscle stretch, improvement of functional ability and use of nocturnal orthesis to avoid contractures. More recently, Bushby et al. (2010) have brought some recommendations for management of rehabilitation of DMD patients. Regarding stretching, authors suggested that during ambulatory and non-ambulatory phases a regular active, active-assisted and/or passive stretching to prevent or minimize contractures should be performed a minimum of 4-6 days per week for any specific joint or muscle group. The authors agree that only limited research has been carried out on type, frequency and intensity of exercise for DMD. Although, their recommendations are in accordance with the known pathophysiology and animal studies which show contraction-induced muscle injury in dystrophinopathies. According to these authors, PT should avoid high-resistance strength training and eccentric exercise due to the knowing contraction-induced muscle fiber injury. They recommend that patients should undergo regular submaximum functional strengthening activity, including a combination of swimming-pool exercises and recreation-based exercises in the community. Based on these questions and recommendations of exercise prescription on DMD, some recent publications using animal models will be detailed in order to highlight the contribution of these models to PT prescription and recommendations.

5.1 PT exercise prescription

Kumar & Boriek (2003) studied the effects of passive mechanical stretch on the activation of nuclear factor-kappaB (NF-kB) pathways in skeletal muscles from normal and *mdx* mouse. Nuclear factor-kappaB (NF-kB) is a transcription factor which regulates genes involved in the inflammatory and acute stress response. They found that this factor in the diaphragm muscle was increased by the application of mechanical stress in a time-dependent manner. Their results show that one of the stretch exercises, mechanical stretch, activates the classical NF-kB pathway and it seems to be more active in DMD muscle than control muscle. Another study investigated the morphological effect of two different protocols of passive stretch on the immobilized soleus mucle of healthy rats (Gomes et al., 2007). They have analyzed the morphology and the proportion of fibers types (I, II and C) of four groups: control, immobilized, immobilized and stretched every 3 days, and immobilized and stretched every 7 days. The passive stretch was 40 minutes long. They found that signs of cell degeneration were more intense in the group immobilized and stretched three times a week. The authors suggest that the passive stretching applied to the soleus muscle during immobilization induce muscle fiber injury, suggesting that this therapeutic tool should be applied carefully to disused muscles, such as dystrophic ones. Even if stretch exercises are widely used in PT, its real implication on muscle structure and morphology must be better investigated, especially on dystrophic muscle. Exercise-induced muscle injury in healthy humans occurs mainly after unaccustomed exercise, particularly if the exercise involves a large amount of eccentric (muscle lengthening) contractions (Clarkson & Hubal, 2002). The exact mechanism of this injury remains unknown, but it has been ascribed to mechanical disruption of the fiber, and subsequent damage is linked to inflammatory processes and to changes in excitation-contraction coupling within the muscle. According to Childers et al. (2002) a cycle of weakness, stretch, damage, and further weakness might explain observations of selective involvement of eccentric-contraction in dystrophic muscles. This mode of exercise has not been widely recommended for DMD patients (de Araujo Leitão et al., 1995; Eagle, 2002; Ansved, 2005; Cup et al., 2007; Bushby et al., 2010). This exercise-induced dystrophic muscle damage due to eccentric contraction was also attested in the *mdx*-mouse and GRMD models (Childers et al., 2002; Tegeler et al., 2010; Mathur et al., 2010) and humans DMD patients (Marqueste et al., 2008). Childers et al. (2002) have investigated the eccentric injury in dystrophic GRMD dogs. They have found that dystrophic canine flexor muscles of hindlimbs are more susceptible than normal ones to eccentric contraction-induced injury analyzing muscle torque three days after the eccentric contraction. Clinical implications of this study show that dystrophic muscle is preferentially injured by mechanical stress. Another study by the same group of Childers and co-authors (Tegeler et al., 2010) has shown that dystrophic muscles of GRMD dogs undergo damage immediately after the eccentric contraction. Mathur et al. (2010) studied the effects of downhill and horizontal running on the magnetic resonance imaging (MRI) in *mdx*-mouse. A higher percentage of pixels with elevated T_2 were observed in *mdx*-mouse compared with controls pre-exercise, which suggest muscle damage. Moreover, downhill running which is dependent on lengthening muscle contraction induced acute changes in *mdx*-mouse muscle after exercise. Also using the MRI technique, Marqueste et al. (2008) investigated the effect of acute and successive bouts of downhill running on muscle performance of healthy rats. Their results show less muscle injury effect due to repetition of exercise bouts at a low frequency (one session per week) probably due to muscle adaptation and to the inflammatory phase occurring for a week after a single eccentric exercise bout. Another interesting result of this study is the specificity of the stimulated muscle. Soleus and gastrocnemius muscle have shown different responses to lengthening contractions on MRI analysis. The author suggested that this muscle specificity might be linked to different anatomical properties, such as fiber pennation angles, typology and/or exhausting nature of the downhill running sessions. This last result is quite interesting because in PT sessions it is more difficult to isolate a single muscle as it is possible in an experimental model. So, care must be taken when translating experimental data to human therapy. On the other hand, it is important to keep in mind that a single therapeutic exercise can influence different muscles of the same limb in different manners. In agreement with the results presented by Kimura et al. (2006) that immobility can lead to preservation of dystrophic muscle in humans DMD Mokhtarian et al. (1999) investigated whether immobilization of the hindlimbs of the *mdx*-mice would prevent the occurrence of muscle degeneration. The authors clarify that dystrophin-deficient skeletal muscle of *mdx*-mice undergo their first rounds of degeneration-regeneration at the age of 14-28 days. They have mechanically immobilized the hindlimbs of 3 week old *mdx*-mice to restrain the *Soleus* and *Extensor digitorum longus* muscles in the stretched or shortened position. The position had no influence in the final result that showed low percentage of regenerated myofibers in Soleus and Extensor digitorum longus muscles when compared to the same muscles of the contralateral limb. Regenerated myofibers was attested by the presence of central nuclei in dystrophic fibers. According to these authors (Mokhtarian et al. 1999), limb immobilization prevents the occurrence of the first round of myofibers necrosis in *mdx*-mice and reinforces the idea that muscle contractions play a role in the skeletal muscle degeneration of dystrophin-deficient muscles. Even though some authors have suggested that restriction of movement prevent cycles of degeneration and regeneration in dystrophic muscle, we should consider that restriction of movement leads to muscle disuse and has drastic consequences to the patients, e.g. contractures, bone deformities, cardiovascular disease, obesity, and osteoporosis over time. It is imperative that a balanced threshold of therapeutic exercise must be well-defined and that more research on this subject is necessary. Over the last ten years, the number of papers aiming to define the threshold of PT prescription has grown. Outcome measurements of these investigations generally use morphological features of dystrophic muscle, enzymatic, protein localization and quantification, and/or biomechanical analyses. Podhorska-Okolow et al. (1998) have studied apoptosis of myofibers and the presence of satellite cells in skeletal muscle of healthy mice after spontaneous exercise wheel running. Exercised mice have run for sixteen hours and were sacrificed after a period of 6 or 96 hours. For analysis, the authors have counted the numbers of myofibers with central nuclei, (indicative of regenerated myofibers), performed immune histochemistry, quantified by Western blot proteins related to cell death, and used electron microscopy to find satellite cells. Their results show that spontaneous running in sedentary mice increases the number of apoptotic nuclei in adult muscle fibers and in endothelial cells. These results suggested that voluntary exercise plays an important and detrimental role on disused muscle, which can be applied to dystrophic muscle. In general, any study that used voluntary wheel running detrimentaly affected the hindlimbs of *mdx* mice (Landisch et al., 2008). Studies that have investigated non-voluntary exercise have shown muscle injury in *mdx* model mainly when animals are running downhill. Landisch et al. (2008) investigated whether a voluntary endurance type of exercise could be beneficial to dystrophic muscle;

assessing cellular adaptations that typically occur in response to endurance exercise. They hypothesized that a voluntary endurance type of exercise would improve *mdx* mouse muscle to the same extent that exercise improves healthy muscle. They analyzed the histological features by counting the central nuclei, fiber types, capillarity and mitochondrial enzymes activity. In part their hypothesis was true, except that mitochondrial adaptations did not occur in *mdx* mouse muscles. They suggest that this type of exercise can improve skeletal muscle weakness and fatigue as well as prevent secondary consequences of the inactivity. In 2009, Gaiad et al. reported the effect of the free walking activity during 24weeks/3 times perweek during 45 minutes in GRMD dogs. Muscle collagen area was quantified by histomorphometry and collagen types I, III and IV were localized by immunohistochemistry. Passive joint range of motion (ROM) was measured to investigate the secondary consequences of the exercise on the muscle skeletal system. There was an improvement on tarsal ROM in dogs of the treated group. Muscle collagen area was different between the groups after treatment, and an increasing trend in these values was observed in non-treated group. This suggests a higher muscle fibrosis in dogs that have not undergone exercise. Collagen types I and III were observed in both groups. The authors suggest that the modality of free walking activity can improve ROM without increasing muscle fibrosis in dystrophic dogs. Studying markers of oxidative stress in skeletal muscle of *mdx*-mouse, Kacsor et al. (2007) applied low intensity training through treadmill running 30 minutes per day, 2 times per week during 8 weeks. They considered 9 meters perminute as a training of low intensity based on previous studies with the same animal model. This intensity of training has not been able to provoke any adaptation on healthy mice (wild type). In *mdx*-mouse, low intensity training has lead to physiologic adaptations evidenced by decrease of markers of oxidative stress. New studies should be conducted following this same intensity of training for new analyses. The investigation of creatine quinase (CK) enzyme, muscle fibrosis and morphology, as well as clinical and behavioral features of these animals can elucidate aspects of the best threshold of exercise for DMD patients. With this focus, van Putten and co-authors (2010) have investigated some functional tools on the disease progression of 4-week-old mdx mice using CK analysis and muscle morphology (measuring percentage of fibrotic/necrotic area). They suggest four functional tests (forelimb grip strength, rotarod analysis, and two and four limb hanging wire) that may be suitable for short-term functional evaluation of therapeutic approaches in the *mdx* mouse without affecting dystrophy progression. Aiming to validate parameters of functional evaluation on pre-clinical trials for DMD, Gaiad et al. (2011) investigated the use of PT assessment tools to evaluate disease progression and phenotype variability in GRMD dogs. In this study the outcome measurements were passive joint range of motion, limb and thorax circumferences, weight, CK analysis, and physical features of each of the dogs using a physical exam score previously described by Thibaud et al. (2007). The author have described the physical and behavioral features of 11 dystrophic dogs during 9 months and these PT measurements tools were considered reliable and useful to evaluate disease progression in GRMD dogs.

6. Conclusion

In the last ten years, research on exercise prescription using *mdx* mouse and GRMD dogs has increased and much of the research were discussed here. We have much to discover about the effects of type, frequency, and intensity of therapeutic exercise on DMD.

Regarding the type of exercise, it is possible to say that eccentric/lengthening contraction has no beneficial effects on dystrophic muscle, and that concentric or aerobic training should be better investigated. Free or voluntary activities seem to prevent secondary consequences of disuse while not leading to detrimental effects. The morphological and clinical effects of the intensity of exercise must be well investigated once it seems near the threshold that must still be defined. Low intensity training leads to beneficial effects though the parameters of this intensity must also be well defined and afterwards, translated to human patients. The harmonization of assessment tools for exercise research with both animal models is another important point on this subject. The definition of assessment tools to pre-clinical trials on animal models will enable the advancement of research on this subject and bring knowledge to the prescription of beneficial therapeutic exercise to DMD patients.

7. References

Ambrosio, CE; Fadel, L.; Gaiad, TP; Martins, DS; Araújo, KPC; Zucconi, E.; Brolio, MP; Giglio, RF; Morini, AC; Jazedje, T; Froes, TR; Feitosa, MLT; Valadares, MC; Beltrão-Braga, PCB; Meirelles, FV & Miglino, MA. (2009). Identification of three distinguishable phenotypes in golden retriever muscular dystrophy. *Genetics and Molecular Research*, v: 8, n: 2, pp. 389-396.

Ambrosio, CE; Valadares, MC; Zucconi, E; Cabral, R; Pearson, PL; Gaiad TP; Canovas, M; Vainzof, M; Miglino, MA & Zatz, M. (2008). Ringo, a golden retriever muscular dystrophy (grmd) dog with absent dystrophin but normal strength. *Neuromuscular Disorders*, v. 18, n. 11, pp. 892-3.

Baltzers, WI; Calise, DV; Levine, J M; Shelton, GD; Edwards, JF & Steiner, JM. (2007). Dystrophin-deficient muscular dystrophy in Weimaraner. *Journal of the American Hospital Association*, v. 43, pp. 227-232.

Banks, GB. & Chamberlain, J.S. (2008). The value of mammalian models for Duchenne Muscular Dystrophy in developing therapeutic strategies. In: *Current Topics in Developmental Biology*, Krauss, R.S. (Ed.). 431-453, Burlington: Academic Press.

Barthélémy, I; Barrey, E; Aguilar, P; Uriarte, A; Le Chevoir, M; Thibaud J; Voit, T; Blot, S & Hogrel, J. (2011). Longitudinal ambulatory measurements of gait abnormality in dystrophin-deficient dogs. *Musculoskeletal Disorders*, v.12, pp. 75 (http://www.biomedcentral.com/1471-2474/12/75).

Bartlett, RJ; Stockinger, S; Denis, MM; Bartlett, WT; Inverardi, L; Le, TT; thi Man, N; Morris, GE; Bogan, DJ; Metcalf-Bogan, J & Kornegay, JN. (2000). In vivo targeted repair of a point mutation in the canine dystrophin gene by a chimeric RNA/DNA oligonucleotide. *Nature Biotechnology*, v. 18, pp. 615–22.

Bergman, RL; Inzana, KD; Monroe, WE; Shell, LG; Liu, LA; Engvall, E & Shelton, GD. (2002). Dystrophin-deficient muscular dystrophy in Labrador retriever. *Journal of the American Animal Hospital Association*, v. 38, pp. 255-261.

Bish, TB; Sleeper, MM; Forbes, SC; Morine, KJ; Reynolds, C.; Singletary, GE; Trafny, D; Pham, J; Bogan, J; Kornegay, JN; Vandenborne, K; Walter, GA & Sweeney, HL. (2011). Long-term systemic myostatin inhibition via liver-targeted gene transfer in Golden Retriever Muscular Dystrophy. *Human gene Therapy*, [Epub ahead of print].

Carter, GT; Abresch, RT; Fowler, WM Jr. (2002). Adaptations to exercise training and contraction-induced muscle injury in animal models of muscular dystrophy. *American Journal of Physical Medicine and Rehabilitation*,v. 81, Suppl 11, pp.151-61.

Cerletti, M; Negri, T; Cozzi, F; Colpo, R; Andreetta, F; Croci, D; Davies, KE; Cornelio, F; Pozza, O; Karpati, G; Gilbert, R & Mora, M. (2003). Dystrophic phenotype of canine X-linked muscular dystrophy is mitigated by adenovirus-mediated utrophin gene transfer. *Gene Therapy*, v.10, pp. 750–7.

Chakkalakal, JV; Thompson, J; Parks, RJ &Jasmin, BJ. (2005). Molecular, cellular, and pharmacological therapies for Duchenne/Becker muscular dystrophies. *The FASEB Journal*, v. 19, pp. 880-895.

Chamberlain, JS. (1997). Dystrophin levels required for genetic correction of duchenne muscular dystrophy. *Basic and Applied Myology*, v. 7, pp. 251–5.

Childers, MK; Okamura, CS; Bogan, DJ; Bogan, JR; Petroski, GF; McDonald, K. & Kornegay, JN. Eccentric contraction injury in dystrophic canine muscle (2002). *Archives of Physical Medicine and Rehabilitation*, vol.83, pp. 1572-1578.

Clarkson, PM. & Hubal, MJ.(2002). Exercised-induced muscle damage in humans. *American Journal of Physical Medicine and Rehabilitation*, v.81(Suppl.), pp. S52-69.

Collins, CA & Morgan, JE. (2003). Duchenne's muscular dystrophy: animal models used to investigate pathogenesis and develop therapeutic strategies. *International Journal of Experimental Pathology*, v. 84, pp. 165-172.

Connolly, AM; Schierbecker, J; Renna, R & Florence, J. (2002). High dose weekly oral prednisone improves strength in boys with Duchene muscular dystrophy. *Neuromuscular Disorders*, v. 12, pp. 917-925.

Cosford, KL; Taylor, SM; Thompson, L; Shelton, GD. (2008). A possible new inherited myopathy in young Labrador retriever. *Canadian Veterinary Journal*, v. 49, p. 393-397.

Coulton, GR.; Morgan, JE.; Partridge, TA & Sloper, JC. (1988). The *mdx* mouse skeletal muscle myopathy: I. A histological, morphometric and biochemical investigation. *Neuropathology and Applied Neurobiology*, v. 14, n. 1, pp. 53–70.

Cup, EH; Pieterse, AJ; Broek-Pastoor, JM; Munneke, M; van Engelen, BG; Hendricks, HT; van der Wilt, G. & Oostendorp, RA. (2007). Exercise therapy and other types of physical therapy for patients with neuromuscular diseases: A Systematic review. *Archives of Physical Medicine and Rehabilitation*, v. 88, pp. 1452-64.

Dangain, J & Vrbova, G. (1984). Muscle development in (*mdx*) mutant mice. *Muscle & Nerve*, v. 7, pp. 700–704.

Davies, KE & Grounds, MD. (2006). Treating Muscular Dystrophy with stem cells? *Cell*, v. 127, n. 7, pp. 1304-1306.

Dell'Agnola, C; Want, Z; Storb, R; Tapscott, SJ; Kuhr, CS; Hauschka, SD; Lee, RS; Sale, GE; Zellmer, E; Gisburne, S; Bogan, J; Kornegay, JN; Cooper, BJ; Gooley, TA & Little, MT. (2004). Hematopoietic stem cell transplantation does not restore dystrophin expression in Duchenne muscular dystrophy dogs. *Blood*, v. 104, pp. 4311-4318.

Deitz, K; Morrison, JA; Kline, K; Guo, LT & Shelton, GD. (2008). Sarcoglycan-Deficient Muscular Dystrophy in a Boston Terrier. *Journal of Veterinary Intern Medicine*, v.22, pp. 476–480.

Ervasti, JM; Ohlendieck, K; Kahl, SD; Gaver, MG & Campbell, KP. (1990). Deficiency of glycoprotein component of the dystrophin complex in dystrophic muscle. *Nature*, v. 345, p. 315-319.

Ervasti, JM &Campbell, KP. (1991). Membrane organization of the dystrophin glycoprotein complex. *Cell*, v. 66, pp. 1121-1131.

Foster, K; Foster, H & Dickson, JG. (2006). Gene therapy progress and prospects: Duchenne muscular dystrophy. *Gene Therapy*, v.13, pp. 1677–1685,

Gaiad, TP; Silva, MB; Silva, GCA; Caromano, FA; Miglino, MA. & Ambrosio, CE. (2011). Physical therapy assessment tools to evaluate disease progression and phenotype variability in Golden Retriever Muscular Dystrophy. *Research in Veterinary Science*, v. 9, [Epub ahead of print].

Gaiad, TP; Miglino, MA; Zatz, M; Hamlett, WC & Ambrosio, CE. (2009). Effect of physical therapy on joint range of motion and muscle collagen deposition in the Golden Retriever Muscular Dystrophy (GRMD) model. *Brazilian Journal of Physical Therapy*, v.13, n. 3, pp. 244-51.

Gillis, JM. (2002). Multivariate evaluation of the functional recovery obtained by the overexpression of utrophin in skeletal muscles of the *mdx* mouse. *Neuromuscular Disorders*, v. 12(Suppl 1), pp. S90-94.

Griggs, RC; Mendell, JR; Fenichel, GM; Brooke, MH; Pestronk, A; Miller, JP; Cwik, VA; Pandya, S & Robison, J. (1993). Duchenne dystrophy: randomized, controlled trial of prednisone (18 months) and azathioprine (12 months). *Neurology*, v. 43, pp. 520-527.

Gomes, AR; Cornachione, A; Salvini, TF & Mattiello-Sverzuti, AC. (2007). Morphological effects of two protocols of passive stretch over the immobilized rat soleus muscle. *Journal of Anatomy*, v. 210, n. 3, p. 328-335.

Grange, RW & Call, JA. (2007). Recommendations to define exercise prescription for Duchenne Muscular Dystrophy. *Exercise and Sport Sciences Review*, v. 35, n. 1, pp. 12-7.

Grounds, M.D., Radley, H.G., Lynch, G.S., Nagaraju, K, de Luca, A. (2008). Towards developing standard operating procedures for pre-clinical testing in the mdx mouse model of Duchenne muscular dystrophy. *Neurobiology of Disease*, v. 31, pp. 1-19.

Hoffman, EP &, Gorospe, JRM. (1991). The animal-models of duchenne muscular-dystrophy - windows on the pathophysiological consequences of dystrophin deficiency. *Current Topics in Membranes*, v. 38, pp. 113-154.

Hoffman, EP; Brown Jr., RH & Kunkel, LM. (1987). Dystrophin: the protein product of the Duchenne Muscular Dystrophy locus. *Cell*, v. 51, pp. 919-928.

Howell, JM; Fletcher, S; Kakulas, BA; O'Hara, M; Lochmuller, H & Kaparti, G. (1997). Use of the dog model for Duchenne muscular dystrophy in gene therapy trials. Neuromuscular disorders, v. 7, n. 5, pp. 325-8.

Howell, JM; Lochmuller, H; O'Hara, A; Fletcher, S; Kakulas, BA; Massie, B; Nalbantoglu, J & Karpati, G.(1998). High-level dystrophin expression after adenovirus-mediated dystrophin minigene transfer to skeletal muscle of dystrophic dogs: prolongation of expression with immunosuppression. *Human Gene Therapy, v.* 9, pp. 629–34.

Huebner, KD; Jassal, DS; Halevy, O; Pines, M & Aanderson, JE. (2008). Functional resolution of fibrosis in *mdx* mouse dystrophic heart and skeletal muscle by halofuginone. *American journal of Physiology. Heart and Circulatory Physiology*, v. 294, pp. 1550-1561.

Jones, BR; Brennan, S; Mooney, CT; Callanan, JJ; Mcallister, H; Guo, LT; Martin, PT; Engvall, E & Shelton, GD. (2004). Muscular dystrophy with truncated dystrophin in a family of Japanese spitz dogs. *Journal of Neurological Science*, v. 217, pp. 143-149.

Kacsor, JJ; Hall, JE; Payne, E & Tarnopolsky, MA. (2007). Low intensity training decreases markers of oxidative stress in skeletal muscle of mdx mouse. *Free Radical Biology and Medicine*, v. 43, pp. 145-154.

Kerkis, I; Ambrosio, CE; Kerkis, A; Martins, DS; Zucconi, E; Fonseca, SAS; Cabral, RM; Maranduba, CMC; Gaiad, TP; Morini, AC; Vieira, NM; Brolio, MP; Sant'anna, OA; Miglino, MA & Zatz, M. (2008). Early transplantation of human immature dental pulp stem cells from baby teeth to golden retriever muscular dystrophy (GRMD) dogs: local or systemic? *Journal of Translational Medicine*, v. 6, p. 35, doi:10.1186/1479-5876-6-35.

Kimura, S; Ikesawa, M; Nomura, K; Ito, K; Ozasa, S; Ueno, H; Yoshioka, K; Yano, S; Yamashita, T; Matuskura, M & Miike, T (2006). Immobility reduces muscle fiber necrosis in dystrophin deficient muscular dystrophy. *Brain & Development*, v. 28, n. 7, pp. 473-6.

Koenig, M; Hoffman, EP; Bertelson, CJ; Monaco, AP; Feener, C & Kunkel, LM. (1987). Complete cloning of the Duchenne muscular dystrophy (DMD) cDNA and preliminary genomic organization of the DMD gene in normal and affected individuals. *Cell*, v.50, n. 3, pp.509–517.

Kornegay, JN; Li, J; Bogan, JR; Bogan, DJ; Chen, C; Zheng, H; Wang, B; Qiao, C; Howard Jr, JF & Xiao, X. (2010). Widespread Muscle Expression of an AAV9 Human Mini-dystrophin Vector After Intravenous Injection in Neonatal Dystrophin-deficient Dogs. *Molecular Therapy*, v. 18, n. 8, pp. 1501–1508.

Kornegay, JN; Sharp, NJH; Schueler, RO & Betts, CW. (1994). Tarsal joint contracture in dogs with golden retriever muscular dystrophy. *Laboratory Animal Science*, v. 44, pp. 331-333.

Kornegay, JN; Tuler, SM; Miller, DM & Levesaue, DC. (1988). Muscular dystrophy in a litter of golden retriever dogs. *Muscle nerve*, v. 11, pp. 1056-1064.

Landisch, RM; Kosir, AM; Nelson, SA; Baltgalvis & KA; Lowe, DA. (2008). Adaptative and nonadaptative responses to voluntary wheel running by mdx mice. *Muscle Nerve*, v. 38, pp. 1290-1303.

Liu, F; Nishikawa, M; Clemens, PR & Huang, L. (2001). Transfer of full-length Dmd to the diaphragm muscle of Dmd (mdx/mdx) mice through systemic administration of plasmid DNA. *Molecular Therapy*, v. 4, pp. 45–51.

Martin, PT; Shelton, GD; Dickinson, PJ; Sturges, BK; Xu, R; LeCouteur, RA; Guo, LT; Grahn, RA; Lo, HP; North, KN; Malik, R; Engvall, E & Lyons, LA. (2008). Muscular dystrophy associated with a-dystroglycan deficiency in Sphynx and Devon Rex cats. *Neuromuscular Disorders*, v. 18, pp. 942–952.

Mathur, S; Vohra, R; Germain, SA; Forbes, S; Bryant, ND; Vandenborne, K & Walter, G.A. (2011). Changes in muscle T2 and tissue damage after downhill running in mdx mice. *Muscle & Nerve*, v. 43, pp. 878-886.

McDonald, CM. (2002). Physical activity, health impairments, and disability in neuromuscular disease. *American Journal of Physical Medicine & Rehabilitation* , v. 81 Suppl 11, pp. 108-20.

Mercuri, E; Mayhew, A; Muntoni, F; Messina, S; Straub, V; Van Ommen, GJ; Voit, T; Bertini, E & Bushby, K. (2008). TREAT-NMD Neuromuscular Network: Towards harmonisation of outcome measures for DMD and SMA within TREAT-NMD. *Neuromuscular Disorders*, v. 18, n. 11, pp. 894-903.

Mokhtarian, A; Lefaucheur, JP; Even, PC & Sebille, A. (1999). Hindlimb immobilization applied to 21-day-old *mdx* mice prevents the occurrence of muscle degeneration. *Journal of Applied Physiology*, v. 86, n. 3, pp. 924-931.

Moxley, RT; Ashwal, S; Pandya, S; Connolly, A; Florence, J; Mathews, K; Baumbach, L; Mcdonald, C; Sussman, M & Wade, C. (2005). Practice Parameter: Corticosteroid treatment of Duchenne dystrophy. *Neurology*, v. 64, pp. 13-20.

Muntoni, F; Fisher, I; Morgan, JE & Abraham, D. (2002). Steroids in Duchenne muscular dystrophy: from clinical trials to genomic research. *Neuromuscular Disorders*, v. 12 (Suppl), pp. 162-165.

Nakamura, A &Takeda, S. (2011). Mammalian models of Duchenne Muscular Dystrophy: Pathological characteristics and therapeutic applications. *Journal of Biomedicine and Biotechnology*, v. 2011, 8p. doi:10.1155/2011/184393

Nguyen, F; Guigand, L; Goubault-Leroux, I; Wyers, M & Cherel, Y. (2005). Microvessel density in muscles of dogs with golden retriever muscular dystrophy. *Neuromuscular Disorders*, v. 15, pp. 154-163.

O'Brien, DP; Johnson, GC; Liu, LA; Guo, LT; Engvall, E; Powell, HC & Shelton, GD. (2001). Laminin alpha 2 (merosin)-deficient muscular dystrophy and demyelinating neuropathy in two cats. *Journal of Neurological Science*, v. 15, v. 189, pp. 37-43.

Ohlendieck, K & Campbell, KP. (1991). Dystrophin-associated proteins are greatly reduced in skeletal muscle from *mdx* mice. *Journal of Cell Biology*, v. 115, pp. 1685-1694.

Paola, JP; Podell, M & Shelton, GD. (1993). Muscular dystrophy in a miniature Schnauzer. *Progress in Veterinary Neurology*, v. 4, pp. 14-18.

Podhorska-Okow, M; Sandri, M; Zampieri, S; Brun, B; Rossini, K & Carraro, U. (1998). Apoptosis of myofibers and satellite cells: exercise-induced damage in skeletal muscle of the mouse. *Neuropathology and Applied Neurobiology*, v. 24, pp. 518-531.

Presthus, J & Nordstoga, K. (1993). Congenital myopathy in a litter of Samoyed dogs. *Progress in Veterinary Neurology*, v. 4, pp. 37-40.

Salvadori, C; Vattemi, G; Lombardo, R; Marini, M; Cantile, C & Shelton, GD. (2009). Muscular Dystrophy with Reduced b-Sarcoglycan. *Journal Compendium of Pathology*, v. 140, pp. 278-282.

Schatzberg, SJ; Olby, NJ; Breen, M; Anderson, LVB; Langford, CF; Dickens, HF; Wilton, SD; Zeiss, CJ; Binns, MM; Kornegay, JN; Morris, GE & Sharp, NJH. (1999). Molecular analysis of a spontaneous dystrophin 'knockout' dog. *Neuromuscular Disorders*, v. 9, pp. 289-295.

Sharp, N; Kornegay, J; Van Camp, SD; Herbstreith, MH; Secore, SL; Kettle, S; Hung, WY; Constantinou, CD; Dykstra, MJ & Roses, AD. (1992). An error in dystrophin mRNA processing in golden retriever muscular dystrophy, an animal homologue of Duchenne muscular dystrophy. *Genomics*, v. 13, pp. 115-121.

Shelton, GD & Engvall, E. (2005). Canine and feline models of human inherited muscle diseases. *Neuromuscular Disorders*, v. 15, n. 2, pp. 127-138.

Shelton, GD. & Engvall, (2002). E. Muscular dystrophies and other inherited myopathies. *Veterinary Clinics of North America - Small Animal Practice*, v. 32, n. 1, pp. 103-124.

Shelton, GD; Liu, LA; Guo, LT; Smith, GK; Christiansen, JS; Thomas, WB; Smith, MO; Kline, KL; March, PA; Flegel, T & Engvall, E. (2001). Muscular dystrophy in female dogs. *Journal Veterinary Internal Medicine*, v. 15, pp. 240-244.

Shelton, GD. (2010). Routine and specialized laboratory testing for the diagnosis of neuromuscular diseases in dogs and cats. *Veterinary Clinical pathology*, v. 39, pp. 278-295.

Shimatsu, Y; Yoshimura, M; Yuasa, K; Urasawa, N; Tomohiro, M; Nakura, M; Tanigawa, M; Nakamura, A; Takeda, S. (2005). Major clinical and histopathological characteristics of canine X-linked muscular dystrophy in Japan, CXMD. *ActaMyologica*, v. 24, n. 2, pp. 145-154.

Sicinski, P; Geng, Y; Ryder-Cook, A; Barnard, E; Darlison, M & Barnard, P. (1989). The molecular basis of muscular dystrophy in the *mdx* mouse: a point mutation. *Science*, v. 244, pp. 1578-1580.

Straub, V; Rafael, JA; Chamberlain, JS & Campbell, KP. (1997). Animal models for muscular dystrophy show different patterns of sarcolemmal disruption. *The Journal of Cell Biology*, v. 139, n. 2, pp. 375-385.

Strober, J.B. (2006). Therapeutics in duchenne muscular dystrophy. *NeuroRx*, v. 3, n. 2, pp. 225-34.

Tegeler, CJ; Grange, RW; Bogan, DJ; Markert, CD; Case, D; Kornegay, JN. & Childers, MK. (2010). Eccentric contractions induce rapid isometric torque drop in dystrophin-deficient dogs. *Muscle & Nerve*, v. 42, pp. 130-132.

Thibaud, JL; Monnet, A; Bertoldi, D; Barthelémy, I; Blot, S & Carlier, PG. (2007). Characterization of dystrophic muscle in golden retriever muscular dystrophy dogs by nuclear magnetic resonance imaging. *Neuromuscular disorders*, v. 17, pp. 575-584.

Uchikawa, K; Liu, M; Hanayama, K; Tsuji, T; Fujiwara, T &Chino, N. (2004). Functional status and muscle strength in people with Duchenne muscular dystrophy living in the community. *Journal of Rehabilitation Medicine*, v. 36, n. 3, pp.124-9.

Vainzof M. Ayub-Guerrieri, D; Onofre, PC; Martins, PC; Lopes, VF; Zilberztajn, D; Maia, LS; Sell, K & Yamamoto, L. (2008). Animal models for genetic neuromuscular disease. *Journal of Molecular Neuroscience*, v. 34, pp. 241-248.

Valentine, BA; Blue, JT; Shelley, SM & Cooper, BJ. (1990a) Increase Serum Alanine Aminotransferase Activity Associated with Muscle Necrosis in the Dog. *Journal of Veterinary Internal Medicine*, v. 4, pp. 140-143.

Valentine, BA; Cooper, BJ; Cummings, JF & Lahunta, AL. (1990b). Canine X-linked muscular dystrophy: morphologic lesions. *Journal of the Neurological Science*, v. 97,p p. 1-23.

Valentine, BA; Cooper, BJ; Delahunta, A; Oquinn, R & Blue, JT. (1988). Canine x-linked muscular-dystrophy - an animal-model of duchenne muscular-dystrophy - clinical-studies. *Journal of the Neurological Sciences*, v. 88, pp. 69-81.

Van ham, LM L; Roels, S . & Hoorens, JK. (1995). Congenital dystrophy like myopathy in a Brittany spaniel puppy. *Progress in Veterinary Neurology*, v. 6, pp. 135-138.

Van Putten, M; de Winter, C; van Roon-Mom, W; van Ommen, G; 't Hoen, PAC & Aartsma-Rus, A. (2010). A 3 months mild functional test regime does not affect disease parameters in young *mdx* mice. *Neuromuscular disorders*, v. 20, pp. 273-280.

Vignos, PJ; Wagner, MB; Karlinchak, B & Kairji, B. (1996). Evaluation of a program for long-term treatment of Duchenne muscular dystrophy. Experience at the University Hospitals of Cleveland. *Journal of Bone & Joint Surgery*, v. 78, n. 12, pp.1844-52.

Wentink, G; Linde-Sipman, JS & Van Der Meijer, AEFH. (1972). Myopathy with a possible recessive X-linked inheritance in a litter of Irish terriers. *Veterinary Pathology*, v. 9, pp. 328-349.

Wieczorek, LA; Garosi, LS & Shelton, GD. (2006). Dystrophin-deficient muscular dystrophy in an Old English sheepdog. *Veterinary Record*, v. 158, pp. 270-273.

Willmann, R; De Luca, A; Benatar, M; Grounds, M; Dubach, J; Raymackers, JM & Nagaraju, K.(2011). Enhancing translation: Guidelines for standard pre-clinical experiments in *mdx* mice. *Neuromuscular Disorders*. Article in Press

Willmann, R; Possekel, S; Dubach-Powell, J; Meier, T & Ruegg, M.A. (2009). Mammalian animal models for Duchenne muscular dystrophy. *Neuromuscular disorders*, v. 19, n. 4, 241-249.

Winand, N; Edwards, M; Pradhan, D; Berian, C & Cooper, B. (1994). Deletion of the dystrophin muscle promoter in feline muscular dystrophy. *Neuromuscular Disorders*, v. 4, pp. 433–445.

Yokota, T; Lu, QL; Partridge, T; Kobayashi, M; Nakamura, A; Takeda, S & Hoffman, E. (2009). Efficacy of systemic morpholino exon-skipping in duchenne dystrophy dogs, *Annals of Neurology*, v. 65, n. 6, pp. 667–676.

9

A Two Stage Model of Skeletal Muscle Necrosis in Muscular Dystrophy – The Role of Fiber Branching in the Terminal Stage

Stewart Head

Department of Physiology, School of Medical Sciences,
University of New South Wales, Sydney,
Australia

1. Introduction

Branched fibers are a well-documented phenomenon of regenerating dystrophic skeletal muscle. They are found in the muscles of boys with Duchenne muscular dystrophy (DMD) and in the muscles of *mdx* "aged" mice, an animal model of DMD. However, only a handful of studies have investigated how the contractile properties of these morphologically deformed fibers differ from those of normal fibers in aged muscle. These studies have found an association between the extent of fiber branching and susceptibility to damage from eccentric contractions. They have also found that branched muscle fibers cannot sustain maximal contractions and that branch points are sites of increased mechanical stress. New imaging techniques like second harmonic imaging have revealed that the sub-cellular myofibrillar structure is greatly disturbed at branch points. These findings have important implications for understanding the function of dystrophin. It is commonly thought that dystrophin's role is to mechanically stabilise the sarcolemma, as numerous studies have shown that eccentric contractions damage dystrophic muscle more than normal muscle. However, the finding that branched fibers are mechanically weakened raises the question: Is it the lack of dystrophin, or is it the fiber branching, that leads to the vulnerability of dystrophic muscle to contractile damage? The other question is how the presence of these branched fibers alters the contractile properties of "aged" dystrophic muscle. Throughout this chapter I will use the term branched to describe the malformed fibers. Most earlier studies use the terminology "split fiber", but because it conjures up images of a Y-shaped bifurcation, with one adult fiber giving rise to two daughter fibers it is somewhat misleading as we now know many fibers, if not most display a complex syncytia of interconnecting branches. Some branches do not originate from the main fiber but are results of incomplete regeneration with myotubes fusing to repair the damaged adult fiber. Branching, I feel, is a more accurate description of the malformed fiber morphology. With respect to the branching terminology I am following the lead of Ontell & Feng, 1981 where they state "the term branched has been preferred because it describes an existing condition while the term split implies a mode formation. Unfortunately there is no immediate apparent substitute the terms parent and daughter". Readers can make up their own mind on the split verse branched question by examining morphology of fibers in the following chapter.

2. Evolutionary aspects of fiber branching

2.1 Fiber branching in crustacean proprioceptors

Even though in mammalian skeletal muscle fiber branching occurs during the regenerative process, there are a group of muscles that normally show fiber branching. These are the intrafusal muscle fibers found in muscle proprioceptors, muscle fibers specialized for their role of proprioception. In crustaceans, using confocal laser scanning and conventional light microscopy, the morphology and organization of the muscle fibers in a proprioceptor, the thoracic coxal muscle receptor organ (TCMRO), and the associated 'extrafusal' promoter muscle were investigated in two species of decapod crustacean, the crayfish *Cherax destructor* and the mud crab *Scylla serrata*. The diameter of the TCMROs was shown to increase distally, with an increase up to 350% recorded for the crayfish. The tapered shape of the crayfish TCMRO was demonstrated to amplify movements mechanically at the transducer region where the afferent nerves attach. Serial sectioning of the TCMROs, showed that the fiber number increased in the proximal to distal direction from 14 to 30 fibers in the crayfish and from 7 to 20 in the crab. Optical sectioning with laser scanning confocal microscope revealed that the increase in fiber numbers was the result of muscle fibers branching in the distal third section of the TCMRO Fig. 1.

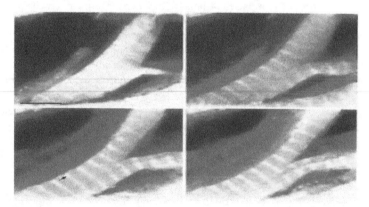

Fig. 1. Laser scanning confocal longitudinal sections of TCMROs from *Cherax destructor*. Fibers were stained with the F-actin binding dye phalloidin, conjugated with rhodamine, BODIPY, or fluorescein. — A. Preparation of a macerated crayfish TCMRO, showing a series of sections from the top of a single branched fiber stained with phalloidin/rhodamine through to the bottom section of the branch. Modified from Parkinson et al., 2001.

2.2 Fiber branching in mammalian proprioceptors

In the mammalian muscle spindle the intrafusal muscle fibers also exhibit branching, although it should be stressed that the evidence for this is not as strong as the case for crustacean propriorceptors. Vertebrate muscle spindle intrafusal fibers have been demonstrated to have the unique morphologies of the nuclear bag and nuclear chain fibers (Boyd, 1962). They are striated except for their central regions and branching has been reported in the central regions close to the area where the afferent nerve fibers originate (Barker & Gidumal, 1961). In the muscle spinal the branching of a small or intermediate fibers takes place over a distance of 60-90 micrometers. This largely occurs in the proximal pole or in the proximal part of the equatorial region of the muscle spindle. The two fibers produced may either taper off, or reunite in the distal pole or distal part of the equatorial region. The process of branching or reuniting is distinct from the condition where one fiber branches into two over a length of several hundred microns. Fig. 2 is a serial section from a mammalian muscle spindle and it clearly shows one fiber branching into two.

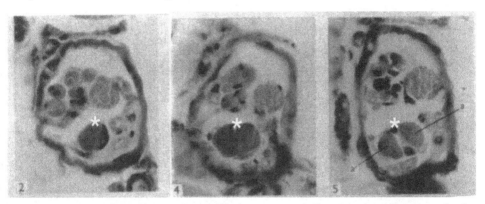

Fig. 2. Serial section through a single spindle from cat rectus femoris, the yellow * marks the position of a single intrafusal fiber as it branches into 2, in the first panel the diameter of the fiber is 11 micrometers. Serial transverse 12 micrometer paraffin sections stained with haematoxylin and eosin; numbers in the bottom left indicate the interval between segments. Modified from plate 2 in Barker & Gidumal, 1961.

2.2.1 What is the role of fiber branching in these systems?

In the crustacean receptor the tapered shape that results from fiber branching serves to amplify small movements, fine tuning the proprireceptor to respond to minor perturbations of its leg. However, overall it is tempting to speculate that fiber branching is protective and helps to protect the proprocepor intrafusal muscles from eccentric damages that occurs as a result of repeated eccentric length changes during locomotion.

3. What is a branched fiber?

A branched fiber is a skeletal muscle fiber composed of two or more cytoplasmically continuous strands. Some examples are shown in Fig.3 B–F and Fig.4. Branched fibers are demonstrable either by enzymatic muscle digestion (Head et al. 1990) or by reconstruction of serial cross-sections (Isaacs et al. 1973). Branching patterns vary greatly (Blaivas&Carlson, 1991;Tamaki et al. 1993), ranging from simple bifurcations (e.g. Fig. 3B) to complex, intertwining syncytia (e.g. Fig. 3E and Fig.4). Branched fibers have been found in muscular dystrophy (Swash & Schwartz, 1977; Ontell & Feng, 1981), in whole muscle transplants Fig.4 (Bourke & Ontell, 1984; Blaivas & Carlson, 1991), in muscles subjected to chemical or physical injury (Sadeh et al. 1985; Gutiérrez et al. 1991) and in overloaded muscles undergoing hypertrophy (Hall-Craggs, 1970; Eriksson et al. 2006).

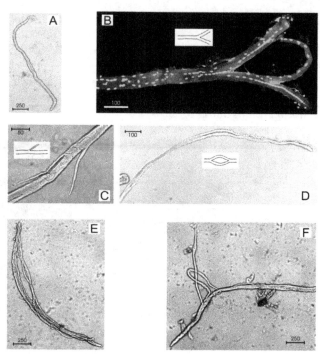

Fig. 3. **Examples of branched fibers.** Low power images of enzymatically dispersed single muscle fibers from EDL muscles of *mdx* mice. A, a morphologically normal, unbranched fiber. B, a branched fiber with bifurcations, imaged with confocal laser scanning microscopy and stained with ethidium bromide to highlight nuclei. Note the centrally located nuclei within the branches. C, a fiber with two small branches. D, a fiber that branches, then recombines. E, a fiber with highly complex branching patterns, forming an intertwining syncytium. F, another fiber with complex branching. Scale bar units are in microns. Modified from Chan *et al.*,2007.

3.1 How does branching occur?

Branching is most likely to result from the imperfect fusion of myogenic cells as they attempt to regenerate a fiber segment or complete fiber that has become necrotic (Schmalbruch, 1976; Ontell *et al.*1982). The association of branching with regeneration is evidenced by the frequent occurrence of centrally located nuclei in branched fibers (e.g. Fig. 3B; and see Schmalbruch, 1976; Ontell *et al.* 1982). Regenerating muscle has different functional characteristics from uninjured muscle. During regeneration, muscles display contractile differences such as reduced isometric force (Beitzel *et al.* 2004; Stupka *et al.* 2007; Iwata *et al.* 2010), longer twitch contraction and relaxation times (Beitzel *et al.* 2004; Stupka *et al.* 2007) and a dependence of contractility upon the extracellular Ca^{2+} concentration (Louboutin *et al.* 1996). Although branched fibers are a well-documented phenomenon of regenerating muscle, only a handful of studies have examined how their physiological properties may differ from those of morphologically normal fibers (Head *et al.* 1990, 1992, 2004; Chan *et al.* 2007; Lovering *et al.* 2009; Friedrich *et al.* 2010; Head, 2010).

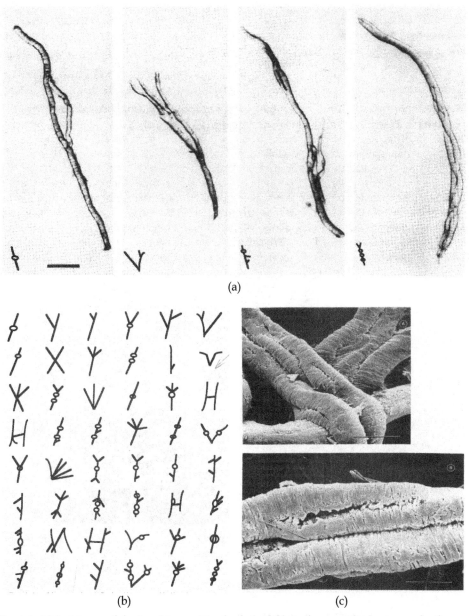

Fig. 4 A. LM pictures of dystrophin positive branched fibers form grafted rat muscle, the
stick drawing in the bottom left of each panel represents the branch pattern. scale bar 100
micrometers. B. Patterns of branching encountered in the dystrophin positive grafted
muscle. C. SEM of branched fibers, top panel arrows indicates branch points, * show a loop
scale bar 100 micrometers. Bottom panel high magnification of loop shown by * in both
panels Scale bar 50 micrometeres. Taken from Blaivas & Carlson, 1991.

3.1.1 Assessing intracellular continuity of branched fibers

It is essential to determine the actual boundaries of a single functional fiber to establish that these complex structures were not simply strong structural associations between more than one discrete cells. Intracellular continuity between the main body of the fibers and various appendages was assessed by a number of physiological techniques. The fluorescent dye, Lucifer Yellow, was ionophoresed into the intracellular environment of fibers (n = 9) of varying complexity at a single focal point. As is apparent in Fig. 5, Lucifer Yellow was able to diffuse from the point of injection to occupy the cytoplasm of all appendages of deformed fibers indicating that no barrier existed, at any junction within the fiber, to the internal diffusion of this dye. It was also possible to measure the resting membrane potential with an intracellular microelectrode at a number of locations in branches of deformed fibers. All values recorded from individual segments of a single, complex fiber were within a few millivolts, fiber depolarization, which was initiated with the impalement electrode, always lead to the contraction of all branches which constituted part of a single fiber. It was apparent, however, that the contraction of individual branches within a single fiber, as detected by video frame-by-frame analysis, was often unsynchronized, with some branches distal to the impalement electrode shortening before proximal branches (Head et al., 1990).

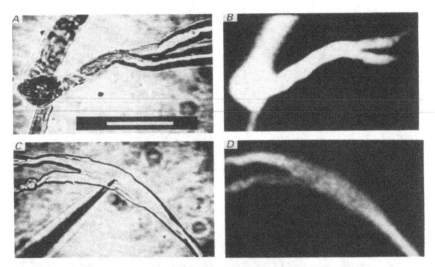

Fig. 5. Fluorescence images (B and D) of single intact dystrophic soleus muscle fibers (A and C). In each case in A & C an intracellular microelectrode was used to inject the dye just above the branch point, In C the tapering shadow of the electrode can be seen delivering dye. Scale bar 80 micrometers. From Head et al., 1990.

3.2 Do branched fibers exist in the intact muscle?

The early evidence for the presence of branched fibers within the skeletal muscle relied on reconstructing serial sections. In recent times collagenase has been used to digest the muscle so that entire isolated single fibers can be viewed, Head *et al.*, 1990 were among the first groups to apply this to mouse muscle, where it is now a key physiological tool worldwide. This has advanced our understanding of branched fiber physiology because it has allowed the

visualisation from tendon to tendon of the entire extent of branching in a fiber. It has also
enabled contractile physiology experiments to be carried out on branched fibers. It has been
suggested that fiber branching may be an artefact of the enzyme digestion technique, although
it is hard to explain why we do not see branching in normal muscle! Given the importance of
this point a study was undertaken in my laboratory using confocal laser scanning microscopy
to examine branched fibers *in situ*, as they lay within the muscle. This involves fixing the
muscle in formalin and then dehydrating the muscle in an alcohol series, before finally
clearing the tissue with methyl salicylate. Before fixation a micro electrode had been used to
fill 2 to 3 fibers within the muscle with the marker dye Lucifer yellow. The auto-fluorescence of
the fibers was such that it was possible to imaging all muscle fibers *in situ* in the muscle Fig 6.
Interestingly in fibers with simple Y-shaped bifurcating branches, both branches are aligned
along the longitudinal axis of the muscle Fig. 6 B&D. These *in situ* pictures of dystrophic
muscle fibers are also interesting because with they have caught branched fibers which have
been damaged and are undergoing necrosis Fig 6. E&F. (from Head et al., 1992)

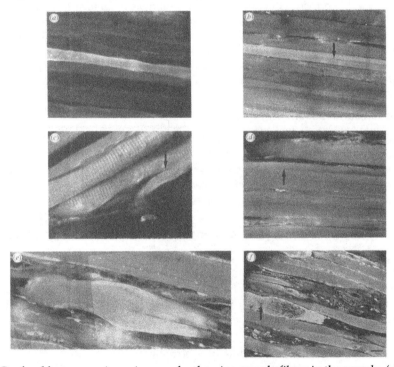

Fig. 6. Confocal laser scanning micrographs showing muscle fibers in the muscle. (a). A
single EDL fiber filled with Lucifer Yellow, note the surrounding fibers are visible because
they are auto-fluorescence. (b) Further along this same fiber a clear branch is evident (arrow).
(c) Auto-fluorescence image from an FDB muscle showing a fiber branching at the at the
attachment to the tendon(arrow). (d). A soleus fiber which branches into 2 asymmetrically
with a large and small daughter branch (arrow). (e) A deformed EDL muscle fiber which is
in the process of pathologically hyper-contracting and has detached from the tendons.(f) a
necrotic soleus muscle fiber. Scale bar (all are scaled in relation to the bar bottom right on
panel (f)) in micrometers: (a,b), 30; (c), 10; (d), 15; (e),15; (f), 30. From Head et al., 1992.

3.2.1 Myofibrillar micro branching within a muscle fiber

Friedrichs group has utilised a novel biological imaging technique which allows the microarchitecture of the myofibers in single muscle fibers to be visualised. Using their recently developed technique of second harmonic imaging they have elegantly demonstrated that in old *mdx* mice the myofibrils within muscle fibers are deformed, bifurcating into Y shaped branches which they term verniers Fig.7. Even in dystrophic fibers which appear to be macroscopically unbranched i.e. are straight fibers similar to those seen in control animals, the myofibrils branch into Y shaped verniers which are misaligned with the longitudinal axis of the fiber. The myofibril malformations in branched fibers are even more marked. Friedrich *et al.* 2010 have calculated that this alteration in the microarchitecture of the dystrophic fibers has a deleterious effect on the force output. From a biophysical standpoint because neighbouring sarcomere activation would be unsynchronized, myofibril misorientations in single mdx fibers can partly explain the decreased force in *mdx* muscle. Their image analysis provides the first quantitative estimate of an ultrastructure relate force deficit in *mdx* fibers. This deficit will vary among individual fibers, depending on the degree of myofibril twisting and local angle deviations. The force deficit is also inhomogeneous within fibers, depending on whether additional branches are present or not. They found normalized cosine angle deviations of up to 20% from the long axis that would not contribute to force output from the dystrophic muscle fiber (Friedrich et al., 2010).

3.2.2 Friedrich summarised

In the dystrophinopathies it is apparent that all the myofibrils are not pulling together and this worsens as the animal ages. As the force vectors are not aligned along the longitudinal axis the tendon doesn't get all the tension you would expect from the cross section of myofibrils. In effect the muscle is wasting energy because the cross bridges are working, burning up ATP, but the force is not being transmitted to the tendons.

4. Do branched fibers occur in human muscle disease especially DMD?

In recent years my laboratory and several others around the world, have used the *mdx* mouse model of DMD to demonstrate the importance of branched muscle fibers in the pathophysiology of dystrophic muscle function. One of the critiques of this work has been "YES, but does this phenomenon occur in boys with DMD, and also does it occur in other human myopathies?" The answer to these questions is a resounding "YES"!

4.1 Evidence for branched fibers in human dystrophy

In the 1970s and 1980s there was a large amount of detailed histological work carried out on human tissue. This work demonstrated unequivocally that branched fibers are present in DMD and other human myopathies. In fact the importance of fiber branching in human muscle diseases was the subject of an editorial in the Lancet in March 25, 1978 pp.646; *Muscle Fiber Splitting_ A Reappraisal.* Because of the importance of this question, i.e. does the *mdx* mouse model of fiber branching makes a good model for human DMD, in this section I am going to review the evidence that demonstrates that fiber branching is a major factor in DMD and also other human myopathies.

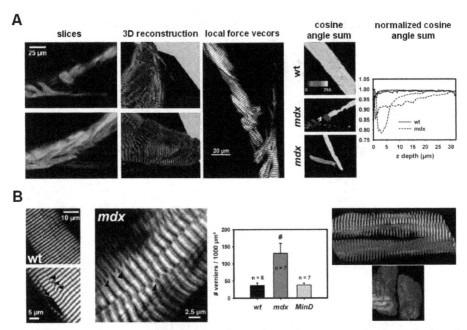

Fig. 7. SHG-microscopy reveals vastly altered sarcomere ultrastructure in intact single mdx fibers. **A,** example slices and 3D reconstruction of an *mdx* fiber (12 mo) show tilted myofibril geometry suggesting misorientated local force vectors. The degree of force drop from the geometry was quantified with gradient filter masks. The cosine angle sum is close to unity within wt single fibers (myofibrils run parallel) and reduced ~20 % in *mdx* fibers. **B,** magnified images show local disruptions of the sarcomere pattern ('verniers'). Their number is vastly increased in *mdx* but close to wt levels in minidystrophin (MinD) fibers. In *mdx* fibers, verniers run in streaks through the fiber centre (From Friedrich et al., 2010.).

4.1.1 The long history of branched fiber reports in human dystrophies

In humans fiber branching was first reported in boys with DMD by Erb in 1891, closely followed by Krosing in 1892. In the 20th century there have been reports by Greenfield *et al.* 1957; Adams *et al.* 1962; Pearce & Walton 1962; Bell and Conen 1968; Schwartz *et al.* 1976; Swash *et al.* 1977; Schmalbruch 1984 and Hamida *et al.* 1992.

4.2 Regenerated fibers in DMD: A serial section study by Schmalbruch (1984)

Fig. 8 shows a cross-section from two patients with Duchenne muscular dystrophy. Due to the importance of this result the 2 figures have been scanned and retain their orininal figure numbers and legend. They will be referred to as Figure1'and Figure 2'. In each case a sample cross-section from each patient is shown in the first panel while the second panel shows a reconstruction 6 mm long and from these cross-sections. In order to produce this very detailed reconstruction, 1200 sections were obtained from the 6 mm biopsy. Then every 10th section was photographed at X350. From these prints he reconstructed the fibers shown in the second panels. This rigorous approach allows the reconstruction of branched fibers and shows how they positioned *in situ* in the human muscle. This elegant study was one of the

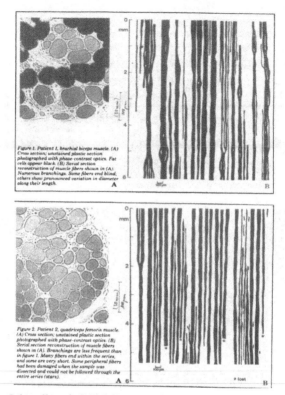

Fig. 8. Copied from Schmalbruch (1984) Figure 1 & 2.

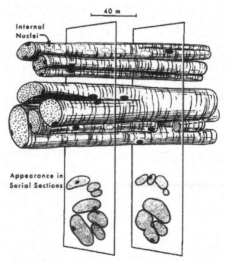

Fig. 8. A three-dimensional reconstruction from serial sections of branched fibers in DMD copied from Bell & Conen 1968.

first to link the degree of fiber branching to the severity of the disease. Patient one Figure 1'
was clinically more severely affected than patient two Figure 2', the creating kinase level
was higher and the biopsy specimen was heavily infiltrated with fat. As can clearly be seen
patient one Figure 1B'had a much higher degree of fiber branching.

4.2.1 Branched fibers in samples from 84 boys with Ducehenne muscular dystrophy

In another landmark study Bell & Conen 1968, obtained muscle biopsies from 84 DMD
patients and control samples from a further 72 children. All of the control fibers showed
predominantly normal histological features. All of the samples from the 84 DMD boys showed
branching. Fig.8. illustrates branched fibers serially reconstructed from cross-sections.

4.2.2 branched fibers occur in other human muscle diseases

It's not only in DMD that we see branched fibers, they are present in many other myopathies
(Swash & Schwartz 1977). demonstrates. Fig. 9 is taken from that paper to show some serial
sections taken from the quadriceps of a patient suffering from Kugelberg-Welander disease
of at least 10 years duration. This is a very nice illustration in humans of a large fiber
separating into three apparently separate fibers, but of course we know that the three
separate "daughter" fibers actually branch from a common trunk. Interestingly this panel
also illustrates a commonly observed phenomena associated with fiber branching that is the
presence of a "sentinel" nuclei near the membrane invagination at the stem of the branch

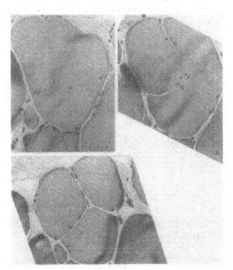

Fig. 9. Serial section of quadriceps. Arrows=branch formation, Kugelberg-Welander disease
H&E X 560.(a) One complete large fiber 250 micrometer in diameter.(b) 22 micrometers from
(a) two clefts associated with central nuclei (N); (C) 70 micrometers from (a) the fiber has
branched into three daughter fibers. From Swash & Schwartz 1977.

In this paper they also demonstrated fiber branching in Charcot-Marie-Tooth syndrome. In
humans fiber branching has also been reported in poliomyelitis, motor neuron disease and
limb girdle dystrophies.

4.2.3 Is fiber branching a compensatory respose to muscle loss?

Swash and Schwartz 1977 proposed that fiber branching represents a compensatory mechanism whereby the number of fibers and the overall mass of the diseased muscle is increased. This is a very teleological explanation and nowadays one I think that can be discounted in light of new information we have regarding the fact that fiber branching represents misguided skeletal muscle regeneration.

4.2.4 Some observations on branch formation in human myopahties

The paper by Schwartz et al., 1976, throws further light on the role of the nucleus in fiber branching. They used the electron microscope to look at early phase fiber branching and found that a zone of separation of myofibrils was often in close relation to a central nucleus. This zone consisted of granular cytoplasm containing glycogen granules and myofibrillar debris. Present, in nearly all cases, near the boundary of the dividing edge were large mitochondria and pinocytotic vesicles. In fact the membrane forming the dividing branch point seemed to be derived from the membrane formed during the extrusion of material by these pinocytotic vesicles. These observations require further investigation in order to understand the mechanisms involved.

4.2.5 Is there a fiber type bias for branching?

Several of these human studies have noted that the branching appears to affect type slow I fibers more commonly than their fast type II cousins. Studies on the *mdx* mouse also show that fiber branching is most prevalent in slow muscle (Head *et al.*,1992). This is an area which merits more investigation.

4.3 Microneurography studies on single human dystrophic muscle fibers

In humans branched fibers have complicated the interpretation of microneurography results obtained from patients with dystrophinopathies. Studies in Duchenne and Becker dystrophy by Stalberg 1977 and Hilton-Brown & Stalberg, 1983 have shown substantially increased fiber density. While typical multiple spike potentials have greatly increased duration there is also an increase in the duration of the mean interspike interval, these findings reflect an increased fiber size variation. Also there are occurrences of simultaneous blocking of two or more single muscle fiber action potentials in a multiple spike potential which is thought to be due to transmission failure at a neuromuscular junction of a muscle fiber branch. The increased fiber density reported in DMD and Becker dystrophy is at first site an apparent contradiction to the known loss of muscle fibers from the motor units in these conditions. However, the contradiction is resolved because the increased fiber density was interpreted to arise as a result of fiber branching. Each branch of a multiply branched fiber gives rise to a separate action potential, indistinguishable from true single muscle fiber action potentials; however, they are identified by a low jitter between action potentials. Thus the split fibers may account for a significant part of the increase fiber density in muscular dystrophy (Hilton-Brown et al., 1985).

5. Whole muscle and skinned fibers experiments show the susceptibility of branch points to damage

Enzymatically digesting soleus and EDL muscles from old *mdx* mice revealed that > 90% of fibers had some degree of branching, confirming numerous previous studies on dystrophic

muscle (Isaacs 1973; Ontell & Feng, 1981; Bourke & Ontell, 1984; Schmalbruch 1984; Head et
al 1990;1992; Tamaki et al. 1993; Pastoret & Sebille1995; Lefaucheur et al. 1995; Schafer et al.
2005; Bockhold et al. 1998; Chan et al. 2007; Lovering et al. 2009; Friedrich et al. 2010, Head,
2010). It seems clear that these branches occur as part of the regenerative process in *mdx*
muscles (Blaveri et al 1999). If the enzymatically isolated branched fibers are suspended in a
high relaxing solution (50mM EGTA) then they can be manipulated under a dissecting
microscope so that they can be attached to a force transducer in various configurations; i.e.
with or without a branch between the attachment points. It is also possible to liberate single
fibers from eccentrically damaged muscle and probe them with the membrane impermeable
dye, Evans blue, to see where the membrane integrity has been compromised. In skinned
fiber experiments the absence of the sarcolemma removes any contribution played by the
presence or absence of dystrophin to the stability of the surface sarcolemma. This is because
dystrophin, if present on the inner surface of the sarcolemma, is removed with the
membrane. When a fiber was activated (>50% of max) with a branch point between the
attachment points, in the majority of cases it broke: when the unbranched portion of the
same fiber was reattached to the transducer, the unbranched segment could generate a
normal force/pCa curve Fig. 10Ai/ii. (and see; Head et al.,1990; 2010)

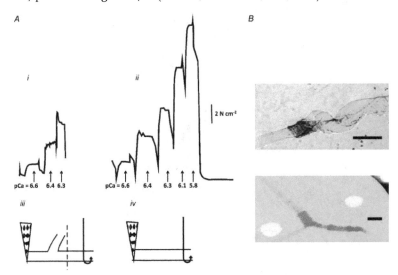

Fig. 10. *A*, generation of force–pCa curves in a branched EDL fiber from an *mdx* mouse. Top
traces are the force–pCa curves, with each peak representing the force developed by the fiber at
a certain value of pCa (i.e. −log10[Ca^{2+}]). The [Ca^{2+}] was progressively increased until maximal
force was reached or until the fiber broke. The schematic drawings below each force–pCa curve
indicate how the fiber was tied when generating that curve. When the fiber was tied as shown
in *Aiii*, with a branch point between the sites of attachment, the fiber broke before reaching
maximal activation (*Ai*). When the main trunk was retied as shown in *Aiv*, with no intervening
branches, a full force–pCa curve was obtained (*Aii*). *B*, two fibers from eccentrically contracted
EDL muscle from an *mdx* mouse, showing uptake of Evans Blue dye at branch points. Scale bar
represents 50 μm in upper picture, 30 μm in lower picture.(From Head, 2010).

When old *mdx* muscles were subjected to a moderate eccentric contraction (a contraction
which caused no damage in age matched controls or young mdx with less than 10% branched

fibers) the branched fibers were damaged at a branch point, fig. 10B shows examples of two branched enzymatically liberated fibers from the eccentrically contracted muscle. Evans blue will only penetrate damaged membrane and it is clear in this figure that the Evans blue uptake is in the vicinity of the branch points. These experiments support the hypothesis that it is the mechanical architecture of the fiber branches which weakens the fiber Fig. 10.

6. Reduced life span of mdx mice

Surprisingly there has been a misrepresentation in the literature to the effect that *mdx* mice have a normal lifespan. It's time to put this myth to rest, there have been several publications clearly demonstrating that *mdx* mice have a significantly reduced lifespan (Pastoret & Sebille 1995a,b; Lefaucheur, *et al.*, 1995). Most recently Chamberlain *et al.*, 2007 looking very old mice demonstrated a significantly reduced lifespan in both male and female *mdx* mice Fig. 11.

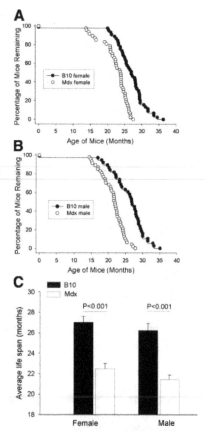

Fig. 11. Life span analysis for wild-type and mdx male and female mice. Graphs showing the age at death for the female (A) and male (B) mice. Circles denote the age at which each animal died. C) Histogram showing the average age at death of male and female wild-type (C57BL/10) and *mdx* mice. The average life span between wild-type and *mdx* males and between wild-type and *mdx* females was highly significant, as shown. From Chamberlain *et al.*, 2007.

They also noted as might be expected, that 24 month wild-type diaphragm muscles displayed no morphological abnormalities while aged matched *mdx* diaphragm showed a large degree of fibrotic infiltration and loss of muscle fibers. It is commonly accepted in the field that the diaphragm is the muscle with clinical features most similar to DMD. However, importantly and in direct contradiction to publications reporting that *mdx* muscle limb muscle do not display a DMD morphology, they noted they the *mdx* muscles displayed typical dystrophic features at each age examined. The dystrophic features included centrally located myofibers, necrotic fibers, small calibre regenerating fibers, moderate amounts of fibrosis, and some fatty infiltration. By 26 months of age fibrosis and fatty ill filtration were extreme. For example, they note increased necrosis fibrosis and adipocyte accumulation in the 26 months soleus compared with the same muscle group at 4 months. Interestingly they highlight the slow-twitch soleus as the most morphologically dystrophic limb muscle in the *mdx* mouse at any age. This correlates with early findings from my laboratory that the soleus muscle is the first to display extensive branching in the *mdx* mouse and reports (see section 4.2.5) that it is type I slow-twitch muscle fibers in humans which are most likely to be branched.

6.1 Aged mdx mice are an excellent model for Duchenne muscular dystrophy

Aged *mdx* mice represent the most advanced dystrophic condition that can be generated as a result of dystrophin deficiency in a small mammal model. The aged mouse phenotype resembles late stage DMD (Gregorevic et al., 2008). As detailed in this section the assumption that *mdx* skeletal muscle does not show dystrophic changes is because most of these studies were carried out on young animals of less than three months of age, when the dystrophic phenotype has not fully developed.

6.2 The main age related dystrophic change in the *mdx* mouse is the formation of branched fibers

The major skeletal muscle changes that you see with age in the *mdx* mouse is an increase in the number of branched fibers, both in the number of branched fibers present within the muscle and the number of branches on an individual muscle fiber (Head *et al.*, 1992; Tamaki *et al.*, 1993; Bockhold *et al.*, 1998; Chan *et al.*, 2007; Lovering *et al.*, 2009; Friedrich *et al.*, 2010; Head 2010). Since branched mature myofibers are not present at the time of onset of clinical symptoms, they must be formed as a secondary consequence of the absence of dystrophin Fig. 12.

6.2.1 Contractile abnormalities of aged muscles with branched fibers

Numerous studies have shown that old *mdx* dystrophin deficient skeletal muscles resembles the DMD phenotype, due to space constraints only a selection is given here, (Pastoret & Sebille,1995; Lefaucheur *et al.*, 1995; Lynch *et al.*, 2001; Chan *et al.*, 2007; Claflin & Brooks, 2008; Lovering *et al.*, 2009; Friedrich *et al.*, 2010; Head,2010; Mouisel *et al.*, 2010; Wooddell *et al.*, 2010; Hakim *et al.*, 2011). Old *mdx* muscles generate less specific force and are more easily damaged by mild eccentric contractions when compared with young *mdx* dystrophin deficient muscles.

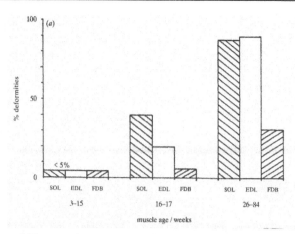

Fig. 12. Percentage of fibers with branched in different age groups of mdx mice, From Head et al., 1992.

6.2.2 Both young and old mdx muscle lack dystrophin so why should old mdx be more susceptible to damage? We know its not aging per se

So the primary question is; given dystrophin is absent from both young and old muscles, why is absence of dystrophin linked to major membrane damage only in old muscles? My laboratory has carried out a key study in this field (Chan *et al.*, 2007). We developed a mild eccentric contraction protocol which had no significant effect on normal muscle. When this contraction protocol was carried out on young *mdx*, there was no difference compared to young age matched controls. When the same contraction protocol was given to aged *mdx* where over 80% of the muscle fibers were extensively branched then there was a massive 60% drop in force. My thesis and the theme of this chapter is: The drop of force is not due to an absence of dystrophin, but is due to the presence of branched fibers. Wooddell *et al.*, 2010 exercised young and old *mdx* mice and compare the degree of muscle damage by the use of the membrane impermeable dye Evans blue. Evans blue is only taken up by damaged cells. There was significant threefold increase of dye uptake only in old *mdx* mice 12 to 19 month of age. Young *mdx* mice were not affected and there was little dye uptake. They also confirm this finding by measuring the creating kinase levels (a marker of muscle damage) which was only significantly elevated in old *mdx* mice. Once again it has been shown branched fibers are mechanically weak and more easily damaged when they contract (Chan *et al.*, 2007; Friedrich *et al.*, 2010; Head *et al.*, 1990,1992; Head 2010; Lovering *et al.*, 2009;). So it is reasonable to conclude that Wooddell *et al.*, 2010 results are explained by the presence of branched fibers in the old *mdx*. It must be emphasised that other factors such as age and absence of dystriophin have been taken into account and do not play a major role.

6.2.3 Even when not damaged old mdx muscles generate less force and power

Lynch *et al.*, 2001 showed differences in the effect of age on structure-function relationships of limb muscles of *mdx* mice compared to control mice. They demonstrated that limb muscles from 24- to 28-month-old *mdx* mice are smaller and weaker with lower normalised force and power; once again age matched studies showed that this was not an ageing phenomenon but was due to the disease process. These findings were supported and extended by Mouisel et al., 2010. Given that both young and old mdx lack dystrophin I propose that the force and power deficits are due to the presence of branched fibers. It has been shown that the architecture of the branched fiber compromises the coordinated activation of the fiber in the longitudinal axis of the muscle fiber (Friedrich et al., 2010; Head, 2010)

7. Branched fibers in other systems are also susceptible to damage: Lamininopathies and regeneration in normal tissue

The129/ReJ dy/dy mouse lacks laminin-alpha-2 and has a severe muscular dystrophy phenotype. It shares three fundamental characteristics with Duchenne muscular dystrophy; progressive and severe muscle weakness, progressive degeneration and disappearance of skeletal muscle with a massive degree of fibrosis and increased serum activity of sarcoplasmic enzymes (Rowland, 1985). In some respects it is a superior functional mouse model for DMD. By three months of age animals are unable to use their hind legs. Enzyme digests have demonstrated the presence of extensive complexed fiber branching in limb muscles in the laminopathies (Head et al., 1990, 2004).

7.1 Skinned fiber studies in the dy/dy mouse show branched fiber weakness

In an early study we utilised the skin fiber technique to tie up single branched fibers on the force transducer, such that a branch was between the connection points, the large majority of cases the these fibers broke at a branch point. Importantly the muscle fiber was not itself intrinsically weak in itself because when the same broken fiber was retied with no branch between the points of attachment fibers could sustain maximal force development (Head et al., 1990).

7.1.1 Intact dy/dy muscles cannot sustain isometric stimulation and the subsequent force drop is directly connected to the number of branched fibers lost

When these branched fibers were present in the intact muscle and the isolated muscle stimulated repeatedly with maximal isometric contractions then the muscle force loss was around 35% (after allowing for the effects of fatigue and in comparison to age matched controls). Because of large amounts of connective tissue present in the dy/dy mouse enzyme digests were particularly successful and it proved possible to view almost the entire population of fibers after digestion. This facilitated the very important discovery that after repeated isometric stimulation there was a 35% drop of force and this force loss was correlated with a 40% loss of branched fibers (Head et al., 1990)!

8. Passive properties of mdx mice, if you stretch an old mdx muscle it pulls apart

In the most recent publication on the effect of age on the mdx mouse Hakim et al., 2011 looked at the passive properties of fast-twitch edl muscle in two month old mice compared with 20 months old mdx mice. What they did to the EDL was to passively stretch it, i.e. the muscle was not contracting actively, and look at the effect on muscle integrity. Surprisingly when they gave the muscle a very large stretch from 110% Lo to 160% Lo; in 2 month old mdx mice a partial tear was observed only at the proximal end of the muscle, at 6 months of age there was some separation across the entire muscle belly, although there were still substantial attachment and finally in 14 and 20 month old *mdx* mice the muscle simply pulled apart. The important point here is that the damage in age matched control was minimal! It is instructive to compare this finding with results from my laboratory which show a strong correlation in the degree of eccentric contraction damage and the age related increase in branched fibers and the increased complexity of the branching (Chan *et al.* 2007). Once again it is important to bear in mind that both the young and old *mdx* mouse lack dystrophin, and the age matched control animals demonstrated age in itself is not a significant factor. So logically it is reasonable to infer that some other disease process, which increases with age, is causing the muscle weakness in the aged dystrophin deficient *mdx* mouse. The branched fibers are the obvious, and I would suggest, the only candidate to account for the age related increase in susceptibility to damage in dystrophinopathies.

9. Young muscles are not unaffected by the absence of dystrophin

This chapter focuses on old *mdx* muscle and branched fibers, however, I do not wish to imply that young dystrophin deficient non-branched muscle fibers are normal. As I detail in the final section of this chapter the hypothesis is that muscular dystrophy is a two-stage process. In the first stage in the dystrophinopathies, around the time when the animal starts to use their skeletal muscles, there is a rise in cytosolic calcium which acts as a trigger for fiber necrosis. This starts the cycle of degeneration and regeneration which produces the branched fiber phenotype. Initially it was thought absence of dystrophin weakened the sarcolemma and when the muscle was activated micro-tears appeared allowing a pathological influx of calcium. Most current research shows that this explanation was too simplistic and not supported by experimental data. It now seems clear that dystrophin plays a role in organizing and aggregating ion channels in the membrane.

9.1 The role of free radicals, stretched activated ion channels and calcium in dystrophic damage

Eccentric contraction studies on non-branched dystrophic fibers showed that there was a long time delay between the contraction and subsequent increase in intracellular calcium (see Allen & Whitehead, 2010 for a review). If the muscle membrane simply ripped then the calcium would go up immediately, as is the case in branched fibers, where the contraction induced damage leads to an almost instantaneous explosive rise in intracellular calcium (Head, 2010). A similar argument applies to the proposal that the dystrophic membrane contains population of abnormal stretch activated channels, in this case you would predict that the calcium would rise as soon as the muscle is stretched, the significant delay allows this mechanism to be discounted. However, blocking the stretch activated channel does prevent he delayed rise in intracellular calcium, so clearly they do have a role to play (see Allen *et al.*, 2010 for a review). So what's happening? It seems stretching the dystrophic muscle causes a higher than normal free radical oxygen production and it is these free ROS molecules that activated the stretch activated channels allowing the delayed influx of calcium to occur (Whitehead *et al.*, 2006). This calcium triggers fiber necrosis, followed by regeneration producing branched fibers. The branched fibers are mechanically weak and as mentioned before strong activation will directly allow calcium to rush in through membrane ruptures.

10. Dystrophinopatheis a 2 stage pathology: The importance of branched fibers in the aetiology of muscular dystrophy

I propose that the skeletal muscle pathophysiology of the dystrophinopathies is a twofold process see Fig. 13. Initially, before the animal becomes mobile the muscle fibers are normal in appearance, although the plasma creating kinase is elevated. There are several studies on the *mdx* mouse which show that if muscles are immobilised either by denervation or mechanically using rods or a cast, dystrophic changes do not occur in the muscle (see for example; Mokhtarian et al., 1999). So the absence of dystrophin is thought to either weaken the membrane and/or alter the activity of membrane ion channels. The alteration of stretch activated ion channels is mediated by abnormal free radical formation that occurs during dystrophic muscle contraction. This first stage leads to muscle fiber degeneration and initiates a cycle of degeneration and regeneration which results in the accumulation branched fibers. Branched fibers are mechanically compromised and cannot sustain the normal stresses and strains of everyday contraction. It is the presence of these branched fibers which terminally weaken the muscle.

10.1 Implications for the pathogenesis of Duchenne muscular dystrophy

The fact that fiber branching in itself can increase muscle damage during eccentric contractions challenges our current understanding of dystrophin's function as a mechanical and ion channel stabiliser of the sarcolemma. It has important implications for our understanding of the progression of dystrophin-deficient muscular dystrophy.

10.2 The branch initiating dystrophic event in straight fibers

The initiating event that triggers fiber necrosis in *mdx* mice must occur while the fibers are still unbranched, as branching results from regeneration following necrosis. Hence, to ascertain the function of dystrophin, it is necessary to study fibers before they become branched. The studies mentioned in this chapter which found greater force deficits for *mdx* mice compared with wild-types all used mice which were older than 6-8 weeks, at which age it is known that 17% of fibers are already branched (Chan *et al.*, 2007). Thus not clear whether they are examining the primary pathological event, or the downstream consequences, resulting from a loss of dystrophin. Any supposed mechanical weakness resulting from an absence of dystrophin is confounded by the mechanical weakness resulting from fiber branching. It is just as likely that the initiating event is an influx of Ca^{2+} through malfunctioning ion channels (Carlson, 1998), rather than contraction-induced damage to a mechanically compromised sarcolemma. Several classes of ion channels, reviewed in Allard, 2006, have been observed to function abnormally in mdx muscle fibers. It has been proposed that Ca^{2+} entering through these channels activates enzyme mediated cell damage pathways, leading to fiber necrosis. Another class of ion channel that may allow excessive Ca^{2+} influx is stretch-activated channels, which may be abnormally activated in *mdx* fibers through mechanisms involving reactive oxygen species (ROS) (Allen *et al.*, 2010; Allen & Whitehead, 2010).

My argument may be summarised in the flowchart in Fig. 13. We envisage dystrophinopathy in the *mdx* mouse as a two-stage process. The immediate consequences of losing dystrophin's normal functions might be referred to for simplicity as a "primary stage" in which the loss of dystrophin initiates muscle damage, in the absence of any pre-existing fiber deformity. The regenerated fibers formed during the primary stage are branched. It is the progressive increase of branching which initiates the secondary stage. In the secondary stage the branched fibers are mechanically weak and damage in this terminal phase enters into a positive feedback loop.

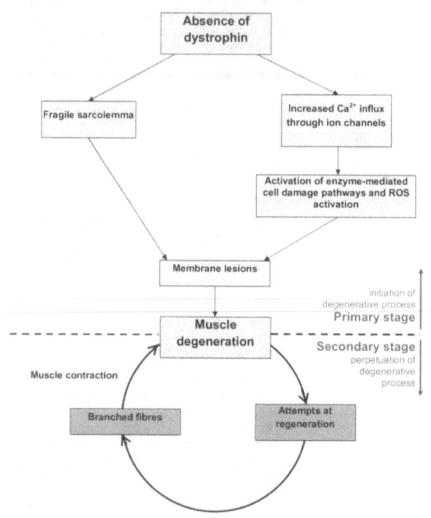

Fig. 13. **Proposed pathogensis of dystrophinopathy in _mdx_ mice.** The primary effects of dystrophin's absence could be either a mechanical weakening of the sarcolemma (_left_) or an influx of Ca^{2+} through malfunctioning ion channels (_right_). Whatever the mechanism, muscle degeneration ensues. The secondary stage is a cycle in which attempted regeneration produces branched fibers, which are structurally compromised and easily damaged by contractile activity, resulting in further degeneration. In this scheme, research into dystrophin's function would be best directed at the primary stage, before fiber branching contributes to any observed susceptibility to contraction-induced damage in dystrophin-deficient muscle.

11. Conclusion and clinical implications of the two stage model

The two stage dystrophic process explains why there is a loss of muscle function over time, i.e. why the muscles are not simply destroyed on first use. Clinically this is potentially a very important point because it means if the initial pathological increase in calcium is prevented the disease process will be halted before it enters the 2nd stage degeneration/ regeneration cycle and the mechanically compromised branched fibers will not form. Research suggests the unbranched dystrophin-negative fibers are relatively normal in regard to their contractile properties (Williams *et al.*, 1993; Lynch *et al.*, 2001; Chan *et al.*, 2007). Thus if the initial calcium influx is prevented the dystrophin-negative muscle fibers will serve for day to day activities possibly for a normal life span.

12. References

Allen, D.G.; Gervasio, O.L., Yeung, E.W. & Whitehead, N.P. (2010). Calcium and the damage pathways in muscular dystrophy. *Can J Physiol Pharmacol* Vol., 88, pp. 83-91.

Allen, D.G. & Whitehead, N.P. (2010). Duchenne muscular dystrophy – What causes the increased membrane permeability in skeletal muscle? *Int J Biochem Cell Biol*, doi: 10.1016/ j.biocel .2010.11.005.

Barker, D. and Gidumal, J. L. (1961). The morphology of intrafusal muscle fibres in the cat. *Journal of Physiology*, Vol., 157: pp.513–528.

Beitzel, F; Gregorevic, P., Ryall, J.G., Plant, D.R., Sillence, M.N. & Lynch, G.S. (2004). β2-Adrenoceptor agonist fenoterol enhances functional repair of regenerating rat skeletal muscle after injury. *J Appl Physiol*, Vol., 96, pp. 1385–1392.

Bell, C.D. & Conen, P.E. (1968). Histopathological changes in Duchenne muscular dystrophy. *Journal of the Neurological Sciences*, Vol., 7, pp. 529-544.

Blaivas, M. & Carlson, B.M. (1991). Muscle fiber branching -- difference between grafts in old and young rats. *Mechanisms of Ageing and Development*, Vol.,60 pp. 43-53.

Blaveri, K.; Heslop, L., Yu, D.S., Rosenblatt, J.D., Gross, J.G., Partridge, T.A. & Morgan, J.E. (1999). Patterns of repair of dystrophic mouse muscle: studies on isolated fibers. *Dev Dyn.*, Vol., 216, pp. 244-56.

Bockhold, K.J.; Rosenblatt, J.D. & Partridge, T.A. (1998). Aging normal and dystrophic mouse muscle: analysis of myogenicity in cultures of living single fibers. *Muscle Nerve*, Vol., 21, pp. 173-83.

Bourke, D.L. & Ontell, M. (1984). Branched myofibers inlong-term whole muscle transplants: a quantitative study. *Anat Rec*, Vol., 209, pp. 281–288.

Boyd, I. A. (1962). The structure and innervation of the nuclear bag muscle fibre system and the nuclear chain muscle fibre system in mammalian muscle spindles. *Proc. R. Soc.*, B Vol., 245, pp. 81-136.

Chamberlain, J. S.; Metzger, J., Reyes, M., Townsend, D. &. Faulkner, J.A. (2007). Dystrophin-deficient mdx mice display a reduced life span and are susceptible to spontaneous rhabdomyosarcoma. *FASEB J.*, Vol.,21, pp. 2195–2204.

Chan, S. & Head, S. I., (2010). The role of branched fibres in the pathogenesis of Duchenne muscular dystrophy. *Exp Physiol* Vol., 96.6 pp. 564–571.

Chan, S.; Head S. I. & Morley, J. W. (2007). Branched fibers in dystrophic mdx muscle are associated with a loss of force following lengthening contractions. *Am J Physiol Cell Physiol*, Vol., 293, pp. C985–C992.

Claflin, D.R. & Brooks, S.V. (2008). Direct observation of failing fibers in muscles of dystrophic mice provides mechanistic insight into muscular dystrophy. *Am J Physiol Cell Physiol*, Vol., 294, pp. C651-658.

Eriksson, A.; Lindström, M., Carlsson, L. & Thornell, L.E. (2006). Hypertrophic muscle fibers with fissures in power-lifters; fiber splitting or defect regeneration? *Histochem Cell Biol.*, Vol.,126, pp. 409-417.

Friedrich, O.; Both, M., Weber, C., Schurmann, S., Teichmann, M.D.H., von Wegner, F., Fink, R.H.A., Vogel, M., Chamberlain, J.S. & Garbe, C. (2010). Microarchitecture is severely compromised but motor protein function is preserved in dystrophic mdx skeletal muscle. *Biophys J* Vol., 98, pp. 606-616.

Gregorevic, P.; Blankinship, M.J., Allen, J.M. & Chamberlain JS. (2008). Systemic microdystrophin gene delivery improves skeletal muscle structure and function in old dystrophic mdx mice. *Mol Ther.*, Vol., 16, pp. 657-64.

Gutiérrez, J.M.; Núñez, J., Díaz, C., Cintra, A.C., Homsi-Brandeburgo, M.I. & Giglio, J.R. (1991). Skeletal muscle degeneration and regeneration after injection of bothropstoxin-II, a phospholipase A2 isolated from the venom of the snake Bothrops jararacussu. *Exp Mol Pathol* Vol., 55, pp. 217-229.

Hakim, C.H.; Grange, R.W. & Duan, D. (2011). The passive mechanical properties of the extensor digitorum longus muscle are compromised in 2- to 20-mo-old mdx mice. *J Appl Physiol.*, Vol., 110, pp. 1656-63.

Hall-Craggs, E.C. (1970). The longitudinal division of fibres in overloaded rat skeletal muscle. *J Anat* Vol., 107, pp. 459-470.

Head, S.I. (2010). Branched fibres in old dystrophic mdx muscle are associated with mechanical weakening of the sarcolemma, abnormal Ca2+ transients and a breakdown of Ca2+ homeostasis during fatigue. *Exp Physiol* Vol., 95, pp. 641-656.

Head, S.I.; Bakker, A.J. & Liangas, G. (2004). EDL and soleus muscles of the C57BL6J/dy2j laminin-a2-deficient dystrophic mouse are not vulnerable to eccentric contractions. *Exp Physiol* Vol., 89, pp. 531-539.

Head, S.I.; Stephenson, D.G. & Williams, D.A. (1990). Properties of enzymatically isolated skeletal fibres from mice with muscular dystrophy. *J Physiol* Vol., 422, pp. 351-367.

Head, S.I.; Williams, D.A. & Stephenson, D.G. (1992). Abnormalities in structure and function of limb skeletal muscle fibres of dystrophic mdx mice. *Proceedings of the Royal Society of London - Series B: Biological Sciences* Vol., 248, pp. 163-169.

Hilton-Brown, P. & Stålberg, E. (1983). *Electroencephalography and Clinical Neurophysiology* , Vol., 56, pp.S99-S99.

Hilton-Brown, P.; Stålberg, E., Trontelj, J. & Mihelin, M. (1985). Causes of the increased fiber density in muscular dystrophies studied with single fiber EMG during electrical stimulation. *Muscle Nerve.* Vol., 8, pp. 383-388.

Isaacs, E.R.; Bradley, W.G. & Henderson, G. (1973). Longitudinal fibre splitting in muscular dystrophy: a serial cinematographic study. *J Neurol Neurosurg Psychiatry* Vol., 36 pp. 813-819.

Iwata, A.; Fuchioka, S., Hiraoka, K., Masuhara, M. & Kami, K. (2010). Characteristics of locomotion, muscle strength, and muscle tissue in regenerating rat skeletal muscles. *Muscle Nerve* Vol., 41, pp. 694–701.

Lefaucheur, J.P.; Pastoret, C. & Sebille, A. (1995). Phenotype of dystrophinopathy in old mdx mice. *Anat Rec,* Vol., 242, pp.70–76.

Louboutin, J.P.; Fichter-Gagnepain, V. & Noireaud, J. (1996). External calcium dependence of extensor digitorum longusmuscle contractility during bupivacaine-inducedregeneration. *Muscle Nerve* Vol., 19, pp. 994–1002.

Lovering, R.M.; Michaelson, L. & Ward, C.W. (2009). Malformed mdx myofibers have normal cytoskeletal architecture yet altered EC coupling and stress-induced Ca2+ signaling. *Am J Physiol Cell Physiol* Vol., 297, pp. C571-580.

Lynch, G.S.; Hinkle, R.T., Chamberlain, J.S, Brooks, S.V., & Faulkner, J.A. (2001). Force and power output of fast and slow skeletal muscles from mdx mice 6-28 months old. *J Physiol*, Vol., 535, pp. 591-600.

Mokhtarian, A.; Lefaucheur, J. P., Even, P. C. & Sebille, A. (1999). Hindlimb immobilization applied to 21-day-oldmdx mice prevents the occurrence of muscle degeneration. *Journal of Applied Physiology*, Vol. 86, pp. 924-931.

Mouisel, E.; Vignaud, A., Hourdé, C., Butler-Browne G. & Ferry, A. (2010). Muscle weakness and atrophy are associated with decreased regenerative capacity and changes in mTOR signaling in skeletal muscles of venerable (18-24-month-old) dystrophic mdx mice. *Muscle Nerve.*, Vol., 41, pp. 809-18.

Ontell, M. & Feng, K.C. (1981). The three-dimensional cytoarchitecture and pattern of motor innervation of branched striated myotubes. *Anat Rec.*, Vol., 200 No.1, pp. 11-31.

Ontell ,M.; Hughes, D. & Bourke, D. (1982). Secondary myogenesis of normal muscle produces abnormal myotubes. *Anat Rec* Vol., 204, pp. 199-207.

Parkinson, A.L.; Bakker, A.J. & Head, S.I. (2001). Morphology and organization of muscle fibres in the thoracic coxal muscle receptor organ and the associated promoter muscle, in a crayfish, Cherax destructor , and mud crab, Scylla serrata. *Acta Zoologica* (Stockholm) Vol., 82, pp. 251–260.

Pastoret, C. & Sebille, A. (1995a). Age-related differences in regeneration of dystrophic (mdx) and normal muscle in the mouse. *Muscle Nerve*, Vol., 18, pp. 1147-54.

Pastoret, C. & Sebille, A. (1995b). mdx mice show progressive weakness and muscle deterioration with age. *J Neurol Sci*, Vol., 129, pp. 97-105.

Sadeh, M.; Czyewski, K. & Stern, L.Z. (1985). Chronic myopathy induced by repeated bupivacaine injections. *J Neurol Sci* Vol., 67, pp. 229-238.

Stalberg, E. (1977) A course in Single Fibre Electromyography, Uppsala, Sweden.

Schäfer, R.; Zweyer, M., Knauf, U., Mundegar, R.R. & Wernig A. (2005). The ontogeny of soleus muscles in mdx and wild type mice. *Neuromuscul Disord*, Vol.,15, pp. 57-64.

Schmalbruch, H. (1976). The morphology of regeneration of skeletal muscles in the rat. *Tissue Cell* Vol., 8, pp. 673-692.

Schmalbruch, H. (1984). Regenerated muscle fibers in Duchenne muscular dystrophy: a serial section study. *Neurology*, Vol., 34, pp. 60-65.

Schwartz M. S.; Sargeant, M. & Swash, M. (1976). Longitudinal fibre splitting in neurogenic muscular disorders—its relation to the pathogenesis of 'myopathic' change. *Brain* vol., 99, pp. 617-636.

Stupka, N.; Schertzer, J.D., Bassel-Duby, R., Olson, E.N. & Lynch, G.S. (2007). Calcineurin-Aα activation enhances the structure and function of regenerating muscles after myotoxic injury. *Am J Physiol Regul Integr Comp Physiol* Vol., 293, pp. R686–R694.

Swash, M. & Schwartz, M.S. (1977). Implications of longitudinal muscle fibre splitting in neurogenic and myopathic disorders. *J Neurol Neurosurg Psychiatry* Vol., 40, pp. 1152-1159.

Tamaki, T.; Sekine, T., Akatsuka, A., Uchiyama, S. & Nakano, S. (1993). Three-dimensional cytoarchitecture of complex branched fibers in soleus muscle from *mdx* mutant mice. *Anat Rec.*, Vol.,237, pp. 338-344.

Whitehead, N.P.; Streamer, M., Lusambili, L.I., Sachs, F. & Allen, D.G. (2006). Streptomycin reduces stretch-induced membrane permeability in muscles from mdx mice. *Neuromuscul Disord*, Vol., 16, pp. 845-54.

Williams, D.A.; Head, S.I., Lynch, G. & Stephenson, D.G. (1993). Contractile properties skinned muscle fibres from young and adult normal and dystrophic mdx mice. *Journal of Physiology*, Vol., 460, pp, 51-67.

Wooddell, .CI.; Zhang, G., Griffin, J.B., Hegge, J.O., Huss, T. & Wolff, J.A. (2010). Use of Evans blue dye to compare limb muscles in exercised young and old mdx mice. *Muscle Nerve.*, Vol., 41, pp. 487-99.

Permissions

The contributors of this book come from diverse backgrounds, making this book a truly international effort. This book will bring forth new frontiers with its revolutionizing research information and detailed analysis of the nascent developments around the world.

We would like to thank Dr Arunkanth Ankala and Dr Madhuri Hegde, for lending their expertise to make the book truly unique. They have played a crucial role in the development of this book. Without their invaluable contribution this book wouldn't have been possible. They have made vital efforts to compile up to date information on the varied aspects of this subject to make this book a valuable addition to the collection of many professionals and students.

This book was conceptualized with the vision of imparting up-to-date information and advanced data in this field. To ensure the same, a matchless editorial board was set up. Every individual on the board went through rigorous rounds of assessment to prove their worth. After which they invested a large part of their time researching and compiling the most relevant data for our readers. Conferences and sessions were held from time to time between the editorial board and the contributing authors to present the data in the most comprehensible form. The editorial team has worked tirelessly to provide valuable and valid information to help people across the globe.

Every chapter published in this book has been scrutinized by our experts. Their significance has been extensively debated. The topics covered herein carry significant findings which will fuel the growth of the discipline. They may even be implemented as practical applications or may be referred to as a beginning point for another development. Chapters in this book were first published by InTech; hereby published with permission under the Creative Commons Attribution License or equivalent.

The editorial board has been involved in producing this book since its inception. They have spent rigorous hours researching and exploring the diverse topics which have resulted in the successful publishing of this book. They have passed on their knowledge of decades through this book. To expedite this challenging task, the publisher supported the team at every step. A small team of assistant editors was also appointed to further simplify the editing procedure and attain best results for the readers.

Our editorial team has been hand-picked from every corner of the world. Their multi-ethnicity adds dynamic inputs to the discussions which result in innovative outcomes. These outcomes are then further discussed with the researchers and contributors who give their valuable feedback and opinion regarding the same. The feedback is then collaborated with the researches and they are edited in a comprehensive manner to aid the understanding of the subject.

Apart from the editorial board, the designing team has also invested a significant amount of their time in understanding the subject and creating the most relevant covers. They scrutinized every image to scout for the most suitable representation of the subject and create an appropriate cover for the book.

The publishing team has been involved in this book since its early stages. They were actively engaged in every process, be it collecting the data, connecting with the contributors or procuring relevant information. The team has been an ardent support to the editorial, designing and production team. Their endless efforts to recruit the best for this project, has resulted in the accomplishment of this book. They are a veteran in the field of academics and their pool of knowledge is as vast as their experience in printing. Their expertise and guidance has proved useful at every step. Their uncompromising quality standards have made this book an exceptional effort. Their encouragement from time to time has been an inspiration for everyone.

The publisher and the editorial board hope that this book will prove to be a valuable piece of knowledge for researchers, students, practitioners and scholars across the globe.

List of Contributors

Yuko Miyagoe-Suzuki and Shin'ichi Takeda
Department of Molecular Therapy, National Institute of Neuroscience, National Center of Neurology and Psychiatry, Osaka University, Japan

So-ichiro Fukada
Department of Immunology, Graduate School of Pharmaceutical Sciences, Osaka University, Japan

Pietro Spitali and Annemieke Aartsma-Rus
Leiden University Medical Center, The Netherlands

T. Iannitti
Department of Physiology, School of Medicine, University of Kentucky Medical Center, Lexington, USA

D. Lodi
Department of Nephrology, Dialysis and Transplantation, University of Modena and Reggio Emilia Medical School, Modena, Italy

V. Sblendorio and B. Palmieri
Department of General Surgery and Surgical Specialties, University of Modena and Reggio Emilia Medical School, Surgical Clinic, Modena, Italy
Present address: Unit of Pharmacology, Department of Pharmacobiology, Faculty of Pharmacy, University of Bari, Italy

V. Rottigni
Department of General Surgery and Surgical Specialties, University of Modena and Reggio Emilia Medical School, Surgical Clinic, Modena, Italy

Jennifer Morgan
The Dubowitz Neuromuscular Centre, UCL Institute of Child Health, London, UK

Hala Alameddine
UMRS 974, UMR7215, Institut de Myologie, Paris, France

Taeyoung Koo, Linda Popplewell, Alberto Malerba and George Dickson
The Biomedical Sciences, Royal Holloway, University of London, Egham, Surrey, UK

Sasha Bogdanovich
University of Pennsylvania School of Medicine and Pennsylvania Muscle Institute, Department of Physiology, Philadelphia, Pennsylvania, USA
Current address: University of Kentucky College of Medicine, Department of Ophthalmology and Visual Sciences, Lexington, Kentucky, USA

Emidio E. Pistilli
West Virginia University School of Medicine, Division of Exercise Physiology, Morgantown, West Virginia, USA

Nikolaos P. Mastroyiannopoulos, Andrie Koutsoulidou and Leonidas A. Phylactou
Department of Molecular Genetics, Function & Therapy, The Cyprus Institute of Neurology & Genetics, Cyprus

Thais Gaiad
Department of Physical Therapy, University of Jequitinhonha and Mucuri Valley – UFVJM, Brazil

Karla Araujo
Department of Surgery, Sector of Anatomy, University of São Paulo – USP, Brazil

Fátima Caromano
Department of Physical Therapy, University of São Paulo – USP, Brazil

Carlos Eduardo Ambrosio
Department of Basic Science, University of São Paulo – USP, Brazil

Stewart Head
Department of Physiology, School of Medical Sciences, University of New South Wales, Sydney, Australia